THE COMPLETE GUIDE TO

FamilyTree**DNA**

Y-DNA, Mitochondrial,
Autosomal and X-DNA

THE COMPLETE GUIDE TO

FamilyTree**DNA**

Y-DNA, Mitochondrial,
Autosomal and X-DNA

ROBERTA ESTES

Genealogical Publishing Company

Published by Genealogical Publishing Company
Baltimore, Maryland
2024

ISBN 9780806321400

Cover design by Kate Boyer

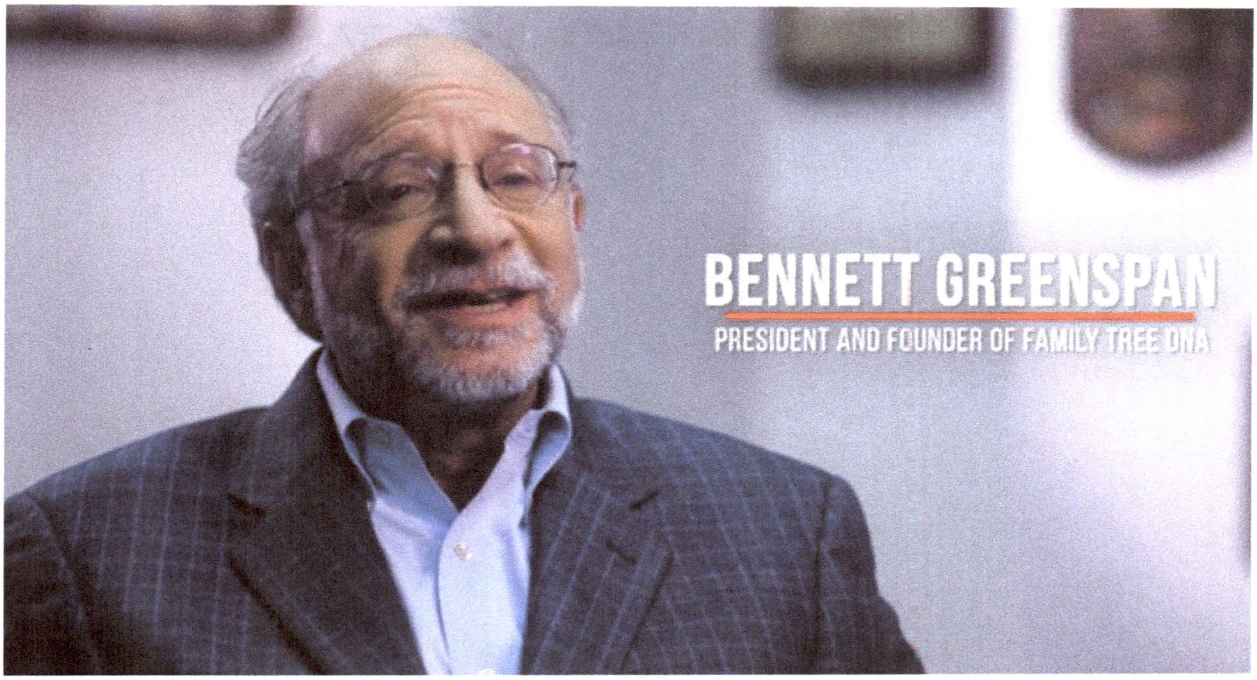

This book is dedicated to
BENNETT GREENSPAN,
Founder and now President Emeritus of FamilyTreeDNA,
without whose curiosity, tenacity, vision, and dedication,
direct-to-consumer genetic genealogy might never have existed.

Bennett founded a business that grew
into an industry that launched a revolution in genealogy
and changed the world by changing the way we see ourselves
and our connection to others.

People told Bennett his idea would never work,
that no one would ever "buy that."
Thankfully, he didn't listen and proceeded to pursue his dream,
driven by one burning desire - to find his family,
both close and distant – around the world.

In Bennett's words,
Our history is written into our cells,
and we are all related.

CONTENTS

Chapter 3

Chapter 5

Chapter 6

Chapter 7

Chapter 8

Chapter 9

Chapter 10

Chapter 11

ACKNOWLEDGMENTS

Thank you to the millions of people who have tested their DNA. Their investment helps them find their ancestors, but it also helps us find ours through intersections and interaction with others. We are all interconnected.

Thank you, Bennett Greenspan and Max Blankfeld, for being visionary pioneers who founded FamilyTreeDNA in 2000, and for more than two decades of investment in science, genealogy, and genealogists.

Thank you to Dr. Lior Rauchberger, CEO of Gene by Gene, the parent company of FamilyTreeDNA, for continuing their rich legacy.

Thank you to my colleagues Dr. Paul Maier, Population Geneticist at FamilyTreeDNA; Goran Runfeldt, Head of Research and Development at FamilyTreeDNA; Dr. Miguel Vilar, Genographic Project Lead Scientist; Michael Sager, Y-DNA phylogeneticist, and John Detsikas, Discover™ Front End Developer, for the research initiatives, innovation, and advancements that keep this field interesting and new. Advances in the Y-DNA tree and the Million Mito Project are rewriting the history of humanity, while the Discover™ Reports are making those discoveries personal, interesting, and relevant to everyone.

Thank you, Janine Cloud, FamilyTreeDNA Group Projects Manager, who, in addition to overseeing groups, administrators, and countless conferences and events, was kind enough to edit this book.

Thank you to the thousands of project administrators who founded and administer projects. Their passion and dedication facilitate collaboration by encouraging testers to join projects of interest and relevance to their family research. I think of them as genetic shepherds assisting their project members.

Thank you to my mother, who was an early DNA tester. One of her final words of encouragement to me was to "use genetics to find people's ancestors and tell their stories."

Genetic genealogy didn't yet exist when my stepfather assured me that I could do anything. He was a visionary beyond his time, and I'm so grateful for his words of encouragement.

Thank you to my husband, Jim, who has faithfully supported my genealogy addiction and joins me as I chase those elusive ancestors from place to place around the world.

Thank you for reading this book. I hope these tools help you find your ancestors too.

INTRODUCTION

FamilyTreeDNA, originally written as Family Tree DNA, was founded by Bennett Greenspan in Houston, Texas, more than two decades ago to solve puzzles for genealogists.[1]

In 1999, Bennett, a genealogy enthusiast, wanted to determine whether two men with the same surname were, in fact, descended from the same family.

The families had originated in the same ancestral village in the Crimea, one immigrating to Argentina and one to the United States. The only clues Bennett had were the same surname and the common ancestral village.

Bennett had previously read articles about the use of the Y chromosome to reveal information about both the paternal line of the Jewish priestly tribe, the Cohanim, and Thomas Jefferson's family. The Y chromosome is passed directly from father to son, remaining essentially unchanged over generations, except for occasional small, genealogically relevant mutations.

If testing the Y chromosome could solve those mysteries, Bennett thought maybe it could solve his, too. However, Bennett needed to find someone to test those two same-surname men.

Bennett reached out to Dr. Michael Hammer at the University of Arizona, who explained that he did not run tests like that for the public, nor did he know anyone who did.

As Bennett relates, he didn't know what to say, and during a long, pregnant pause in the conversation, Hammer uttered the words that would ricochet through the genealogy community, **"Someone should start a company like this; I get phone calls from crazy genealogists like you all the time."** A short time later, Bennett had a proof of concept and preliminary business plan.

Bennett eventually joined with business partner Max Blankfeld, building FamilyTreeDNA, the first genetic genealogy company, whose mission was to provide genetic tools for those "crazy genealogists." Not only did his perseverance and vision launch a company, but also founded the entire genetic genealogy industry.

Initially, FamilyTreeDNA launched by offering 12 marker Y-DNA tests for genealogists, followed shortly by a basic mitochondrial DNA test.

Two men with a similar surname could both take a Y-DNA test to see if their 12 markers matched. If so, then their paternal line was likely related. If not, then their line was probably from a different paternal lineage.

---

1 https://dna-explained.com/2016/12/15/lifetime-achievement-awards-for-bennett-greenspan-and-max-blankfeld/

You might notice that today, I'm using the words "likely" and "probably." We know a lot more about DNA matching and relationships today than we did more than two decades ago.

In August of 2000, the first surname project, Mumma, was created for genealogist Doug Mumma.[2]

From the beginning, surname projects would be the launching pad for genetic genealogy, providing an avenue to answer questions left unanswered when paper trail documents were not available or were inconclusive.

For the first time in history, two men could test and, based on how closely they matched or didn't match, determine whether they descended from a common ancestor.

By the end of 2001, Y-DNA testing had expanded to 25 markers, and by 2003, to 37 markers. In 2006, the 67-marker test was added, and in 2011, 111 markers.

Today, utilizing two different types of Y-DNA tests, combined, we can reliably tell men whether they are related on their paternal line in a genealogical timeframe, and we can tell them approximately when.

The Big Y test was added in 2013 and has been continually refined since that time. The current iteration, Big Y-700, introduced in 2019,[3] provides genealogists with the most information in terms of matching and the greatest refinement in terms of understanding how long ago two men shared a common ancestor on their direct paternal line.

---

2 https://www.familytreedna.com/groups/mumma/about/background

3 https://dna-explained.com/2019/01/30/the-big-y-test-increases-again-to-big-y-700/

HOW TO USE THIS BOOK

If you're experienced with genetic genealogy, you may simply want to read this book.

However, if not, you may want to open your results at FamilyTreeDNA and follow along so you can use this book as a guide.

Or, if you're like me, you may want to read this book once to understand the big picture and concepts, then go back and use it as a reference manual and step-by-step guide.

My web page and blog at **www.dnaexplain.com** provide more than 1700 articles and several resource pages. DNAexplain is fully keyword searchable, so if you wonder about a term or want to read more about something, just enter the word or phrase in the search box in the upper right-hand corner.

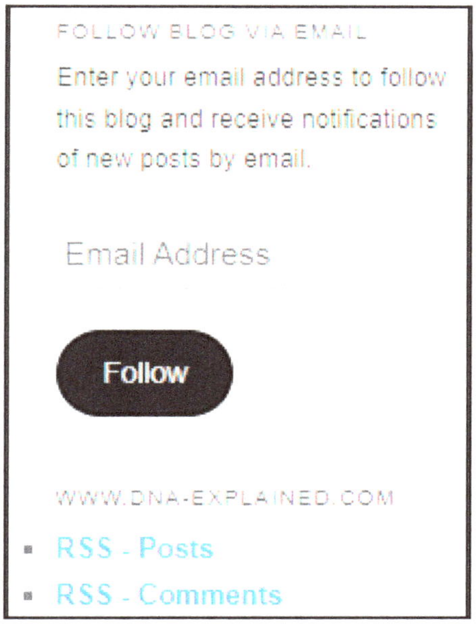

TIP: You can subscribe to receive an email every time I publish an article. It's free, and the articles come directly to you. I publish about two articles each week and have since 2012. Just enter your email address and click on "Follow." I never share your email address or any other information with anyone, ever.

Education and Instruction

All vendors change their websites, bringing their customers new features and other improvements. I've written this book with that in mind. This book was authored at a specific point in time, understanding that the best way for you to utilize any vendor's tools is to understand the foundational genetic concepts.

Therefore, I've explained how DNA works, how to navigate the FamilyTreeDNA website and products, and how to interpret your discoveries for your genealogy. As the website is updated, you will have a firm educational foundation, and the changes should not be disconcerting.

Evolution

While we discuss the individual tests and terminology later in the book, this section provides an overview of how testing has evolved over time. All three types of genealogy DNA tests,[4] Y-DNA, mitochondrial DNA, and autosomal DNA, have improved as more people have tested and new features have been added. Of course, every improvement is reflected in the number and quality of matches and useful information provided to testers.

Mitochondrial DNA

Mitochondrial DNA testing began more than two decades ago with a basic test and provided testers with matching information and a high-level haplogroup. Today, the entire mitochondrial genome is tested, and every customer receives a detailed haplogroup – both of which improve the usefulness of the test with more refined matches for genealogy.

Y-DNA

Y-DNA testing has progressed from 12 Short Tandem Repeat (STR) markers to 700 STR markers, plus a lot more.

More advanced Single Nucleotide Polymorphism (SNP) testing has now surpassed what STR testing[5] could provide to genealogists by testing an exponentially larger number of markers that are vastly more stable. What was often inferred years ago can now be confirmed, and many red herrings have been eliminated.

4 https://dna-explained.com/2012/10/01/4-kinds-of-dna-for-genetic-genealogy/

5 https://dna-explained.com/2014/02/10/strs-vs-snps-multiple-dna-personalities/

Autosomal Testing

Autosomal DNA testing began with providing an individual's percentages of basic ancestral origin locations, popularly referred to as "ethnicity," and a list of genetic matches from the pool of other testers. Today, results have been refined to include:

- Shared matches
- Chromosome Browser to compare DNA segments
- Family Matching, also called bucketing. By connecting your known matches to their corresponding profiles on your uploaded or created family tree, the proprietary algorithm identifies those matches as maternal, paternal, or both.
- Family Finder Matrix to view groups of matches to determine whether your matches also match each other
- myOrigins® population-based ethnicity
- Shared Origins which compares your population-based origins with those of your matches
- myOrigins® Chromosome Painter
- ancientOrigins which provides comparisons to the autosomal DNA of ancient European groups

Better yet, many of these products and features can be combined in various ways to provide information not available anyplace else to genealogists.

The genealogist's quiver is, indeed, full.

It's an exciting time to be a genealogist!

Chapter 1

TYPES OF TESTING – Y-DNA, MITOCHONDRIAL DNA, AUTOSOMAL, AND X-DNA

At FamilyTreeDNA, you can order three different types of tests, and within those test types, you can order different flavors. Think of this as dessert. You can select cake, pie, or ice cream, then select, add, or refine flavors and toppings within that category.

We will talk in general about each one, then take a deep dive into how you can benefit from using each type of test. After all, it's not really about the test – it's about the results and how they enhance your genealogy. In order to reap the greatest benefit, it's important to understand how these tests work, how to use them, and what the results are and are not telling you.

Each type of DNA has specific characteristics and is used in different situations. Some types of DNA are inherited differently by the son and daughter in our example, below.

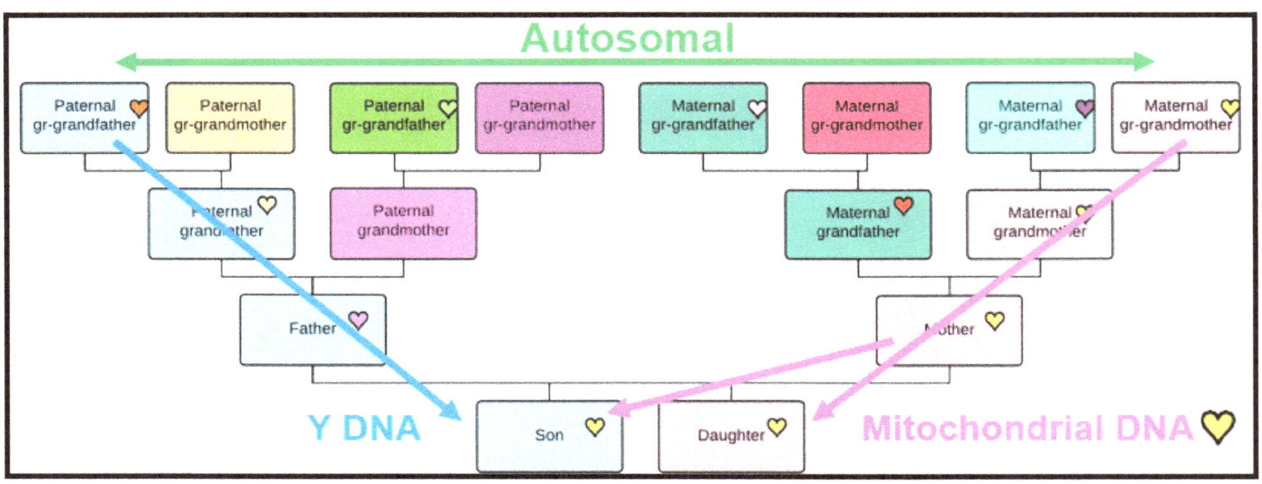

In these examples, everything is from the perspective of the son or daughter as testers.

Y-DNA testing is only available for males because only males have a Y chromosome, which is inherited directly from their father, as shown by the blue arrow. In other words, the son has the father's Y chromosome (and generally his surname,) but the daughter does not have a Y chromosome.

Previously, Y-DNA 12, 25, 37, 67, and 111-marker STR panel tests were sold, but today, those options have been consolidated into 37 and 111-marker tests, which are now considered entry-level. Prices have dropped accordingly, too.

In addition to STR marker testing, which includes the 37- and 111-marker tests mentioned above, the Big Y-700 test[6] uses NGS scan technology to add at least another 589 STR markers, PLUS scans more than 50 million SNP locations on the Y chromosome to provide very specific, personal, leaf-level tip-of-the-branch haplogroup assignments.

The two types of Y-DNA tests examine different types of markers and are compatible, additive, comprehensive, and necessary to wring as much as possible out of Y-DNA testing.

Y chromosome testing can often provide paternal surnames and matches that are closely related and recent in time, those that are more distantly related and reach far back in time, or both. It can also be combined with Family Finder autosomal testing to provide additional relationship information.

Mitochondrial DNA**,** often abbreviated as mtDNA, can be tested by everyone since both males and females inherit it from their mothers. Mitochondrial DNA is inherited from the direct matrilineal line, as shown by the pink arrows and the yellow hearts. Both the son and daughter can test for their mother's mitochondrial DNA.

The colored hearts in our example show the inheritance path of mitochondrial DNA for each individual in our tree. For example, the father inherits his mitochondrial DNA from his mother, who inherited it from her mother.

Originally, three versions of the mitochondrial DNA test were offered. The HVR1 (Hypervariable Region 1) and HVR2 (Hypervariable Region 2) tests each tested about 500 locations, respectively. The FMS or Full Mitochondrial Sequence (mtFull) test was introduced later, tests the entire 16,569 locations of the mitochondrial sequence, and is the only test available today.

Laser Focus

Both Y-DNA and mitochondrial DNA can reach far back in time, but are also very informative of recent connections. Neither Y-DNA nor mitochondrial DNA are ever mixed with the DNA of the other parent, so the DNA is not diluted or divided over the generations.

Think of Y-DNA and mitochondrial DNA as having the ability to provide recent genealogy information and connections, plus a deep dive on just one particular line without having to try to sort out and filter the results from your other ancestral lines.

Both Y-DNA and mitochondrial DNA tests are deep, not broad. They test one line each, focusing like a laser beam.

Y-DNA and mitochondrial DNA will both be able to tell you whether **that specific** ancestral line is European, African, Native American, Asian, Jewish, and so forth. Additionally, both tests offer matching at FamilyTreeDNA, information about where other testers' ancestors are found in the world, and more.

6 https://blog.familytreedna.com/wp-content/uploads/2019/03/big-y-700-white-paper_compressed.pdf

Both Y-DNA and mitochondrial DNA can be used in conjunction with autosomal testing results to identify relationships.

On my blog at **www.dnaexplain.com**, I provide both Y-DNA[7] and Mitochondrial DNA[8] comprehensive Resource pages.

Autosomal DNA

Autosomal DNA is the DNA contributed to you on Chromosomes 1-22 by your ancestors from across all of your ancestral lines in your tree.[9]

Everyone receives half of their autosomal DNA from each parent, with the exception of Chromosome 23, which has a different inheritance pattern for males and females. The 23rd chromosomes are the sex chromosomes, X and Y, which we discuss separately.

Because each parent's autosomal DNA divides in half with each generation, the contributions of more distant ancestors' DNA are reduced over time with each successive generational division.

Eventually, those distant ancestors' DNA is in pieces so small that it's no longer discernible and attributable to a particular ancestor. Over the generations, many ancestors' DNA eventually disappears altogether.

Autosomal DNA is broad across many lines, as the Autosomal green arrow at the top of the pedigree chart shows, but cannot reach back deeply into distant generations.

Ancestral autosomal DNA divides randomly and unevenly during inheritance from parent to child in each generation. While you DO inherit half your DNA from each parent, you do NOT necessarily inherit exactly half of the DNA they received from each ancestor which was mixed together randomly in a process called *recombination*. You could receive all of the DNA that your parents inherited from a specific ancestor, none of it, or some portion.[10] For example, you might not inherit any Native American autosomal DNA from your Native ancestor, depending on how far back they are located in your tree, combined with the randomness of inheritance. You also can't inherit what your parents didn't inherit. There is no "skipping a generation."

I wrote extensively about methodologies for identifying your Native American ancestry in my book, *DNA for Native American Genealogy*.[11] [12]

TIP: Your genealogical tree and your genetic tree will differ.

Your genealogical tree, shown in red below, includes all of your ancestors, and the blue portion shows the DNA you inherited from specific ancestors, which constitutes your genetic tree.

---

7 https://dna-explained.com/y-dna-resources/

8 https://dna-explained.com/mitochondrial-dna/

9 https://dna-explained.com/2022/11/30/chromosomes-and-genealogy/

10 https://dna-explained.com/2017/06/27/ancestral-dna-percentages-how-much-of-them-is-in-you/

11 https://dna-explained.com/2021/11/12/dna-for-native-american-genealogy-hot-off-the-press/

12 https://genealogical.com/store/dna-for-native-american-genealogy/

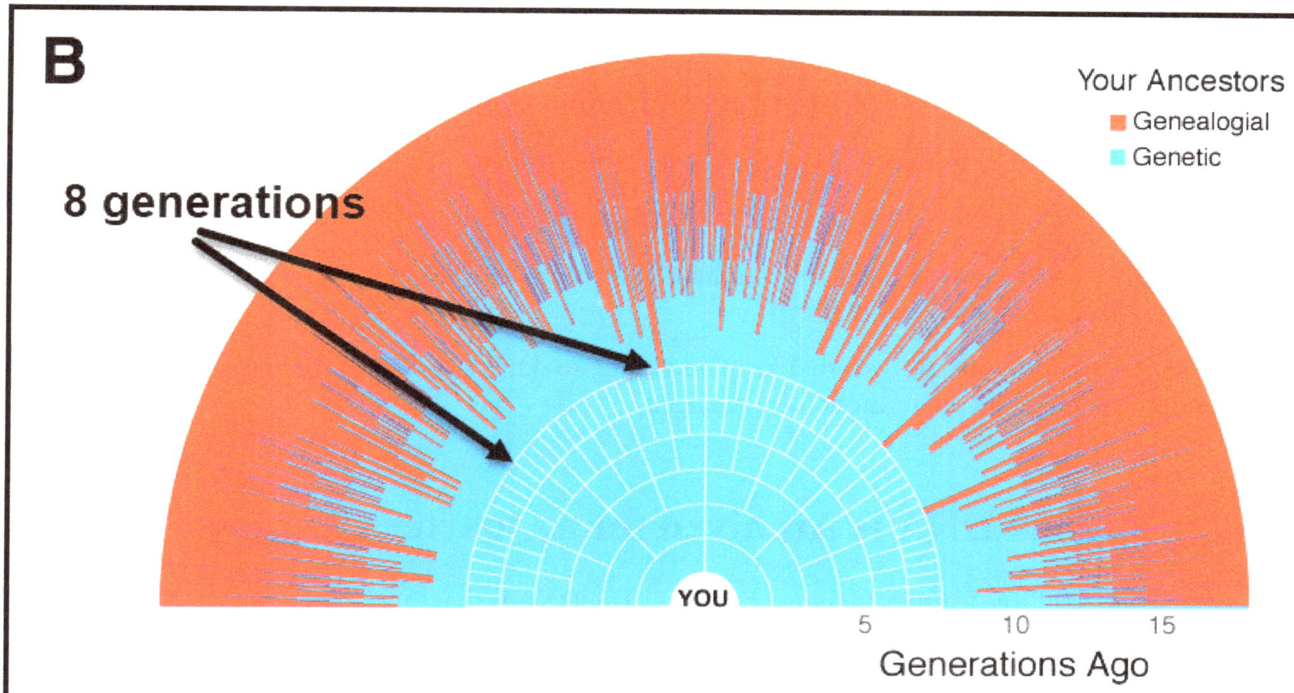

Figure 5. (A) You have an exponentially increasing number of genealogical ancestors, but a much smaller number of genetic ones. Your genealogical ancestors outnumber the world population less than 1,000 years ago. This is because most of your ancestors are duplicated in your family tree. (B) Most of your ancestors from 15 generations ago contributed no DNA to you, due to random genetic recombination, and finite space in the genome.

This figure created by Dr. Paul Maier at FamilyTreeDNA, from the *MyOrigins 3.0 White Paper*[13], illustrates that around seven or eight generations back in time, the amount of blue genetic contribution of a lineage starts to vary, then disappears entirely in some lines. Larger blocks or higher percentages of blue DNA indicate relationships closer in time, and smaller amounts of blue DNA indicate more distant ancestors. In other words, the DNA of the ancestors represented by red has disappeared in you, but they are still your ancestors. You just don't carry an individually discernible amount of the red ancestors' DNA today.

It's unlikely that you are completely missing DNA from one of your ancestors within the past six generations or so[14], but beyond that, it becomes increasingly likely that you inherited either no DNA from some ancestors or fragments too small to detect and be reported by DNA testing vendors as matches.

Translated, this means that autosomal DNA matching is most reliable in the closer and closest generations.

There is no documented occurrence of second cousins who don't match each other. 90% of third cousins match, and about 50% of fourth cousins. I wrote about that in the article, *Why Don't I Match My Cousin?*[15]

13 https://blog.familytreedna.com/wp-content/uploads/2021/08/myOrigins_3_WhitePaper.pdf

14 Assuming that they are in fact your ancestor.

15 https://dna-explained.com/2013/09/29/why-dont-i-match-my-cousin/

The Gift That Keeps on Giving

Remember, all of these tests at FamilyTreeDNA are evergreen, meaning three things:

- FamilyTreeDNA continues to improve the tools and content
- People continue to test, so you'll have new matches over time
- You pay once, when you make the purchase, but results are updated as new features are added and more people test

These DNA tests literally are the tests that keep on giving, so don't forget to check back regularly to see if you have new matches and what might have changed.

Your DNA is Archived for a Quarter Century

One of the wonderful free features included by FamilyTreeDNA is that they archive your DNA for at least 25 years. This is also known as biobanking and means that family members of many original testers, who are now deceased, were - and are - able to order new tests or upgrade the existing tests of their departed family members. I was able to use my mother's stored DNA for the autosomal Family Finder test in 2011, five years after she passed away. This means two things:

- FamilyTreeDNA often has a full generation of testers who never tested elsewhere. Many were no longer able to provide a DNA sample by the time the other testing companies began offering autosomal tests. You will never find them at Ancestry or 23andMe because those companies don't accept uploads, and you may never find them in any other database, either.
- Because FamilyTreeDNA offers multiple products, and because the DNA is archived, you can upgrade and add products over time, often without submitting a new DNA sample.

Chapter 2

SETTING YOURSELF UP FOR SUCCESS

Luck favors the prepared. Genealogy and DNA testing are much like anything else. The better you understand your tools and the more you prepare, the "luckier" you get.

Before we review each tool, let's look at what you need to do to make yourself successful. Your work helps others, too. A rising tide lifts all ships.

Let's review some basic setup information to make sure you have all your bases covered.

At the upper right-hand side of your personal page, you'll see your name and kit number.

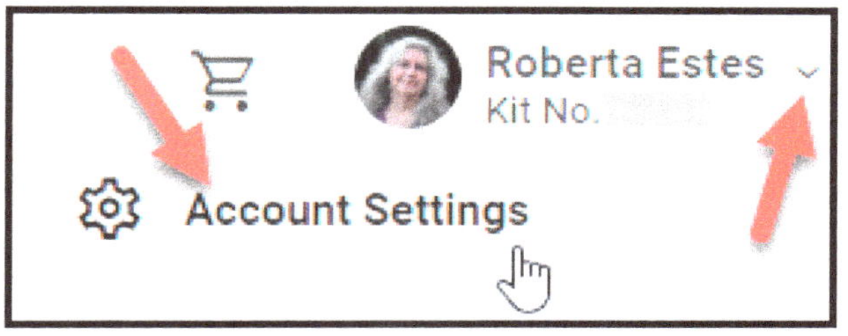

Account Settings

Click on the little down arrow to reveal "**Account Settings**."

Please note that on all Account Settings pages, there is a little *Help* button with a question mark in the far upper right-hand corner that explains each option. You'll also see a little "i" in a circle which means more information is available if you mouse over that location.

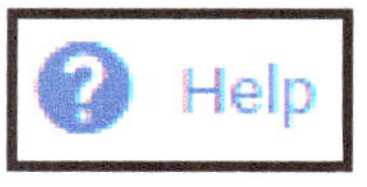

▶ I encourage everyone to take a few minutes to review **Account Settings** to ensure that your account is set up the way you wish and that all fields that will assist your genealogy are complete.

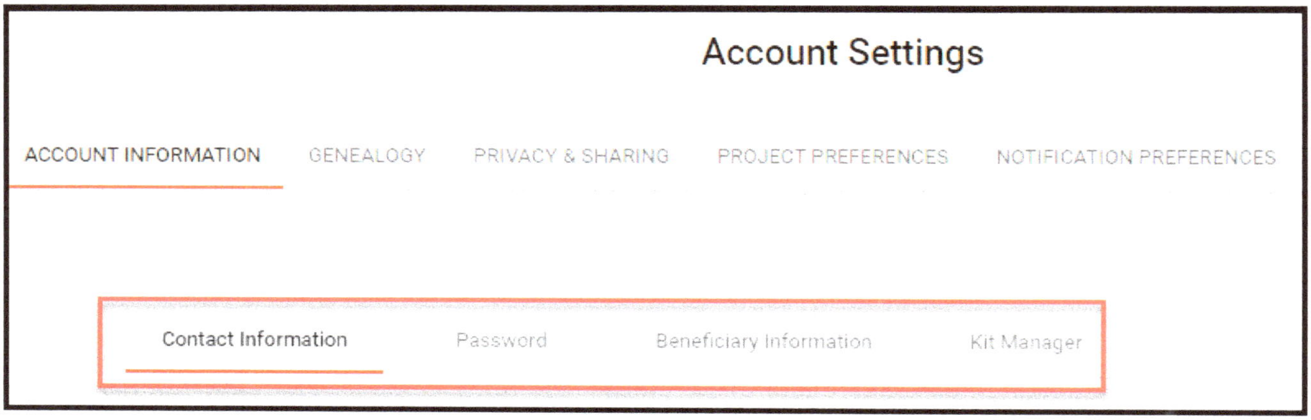

On your Account Settings page, you'll see five categories across the top. The lower options change when you click on the tabs on the top row.

In particular, please pay particular attention to:

- Account Information - Current email, phone number, and mailing address, all of which are important for password recovery.
    - Note that neither your matches nor Group Project Administrators (unless you've granted them advanced access) can see your full address. Only you and FamilyTreeDNA Customer Service can. Group Project Administrators can only see your city, state, and country. Password change is also found here.
    - Please complete your Beneficiary Information to provide access to someone else after you've gone to meet your ancestors. You can designate a project administrator, which means they could order (and pay for) upgrades to your kit when new technology becomes available in the future. What a great way to keep your DNA giving.
    - If the test-taker is not managing the kit, complete the Kit Manager information so that customer service knows they can communicate with that person on your behalf and about your DNA results.
- Genealogy – Surnames List (with locations) and Earliest Known Ancestors (with locations) are both utilized throughout the various products to enhance your experience and that of your matches as well. These two fields DO NOT cross-populate.
- Privacy and Sharing - You select and adjust your matching preferences on this tab.
    - To view your matches, you MUST opt in to matching.[16]
    - To share your population (ethnicity) origins with matches, you must opt in.

16 https://www.familytreedna.com/legal/consent/matching

- If you are opted-in to matching, you can also opt in to or opt out of Investigate Genetic Genealogy matching[17], which is entirely separate from standard matching.
- Project Preferences – Each project, and administrator is authorized separately for various access levels.[18]

- Notification Preferences – Email notification preferences for various match levels.

TIP: If you disable matching for lower-level tests, such as the 12-111 marker Y-DNA tests, you may miss a notification about a match with someone whose genealogy you share, but who either did not take a higher-level test or doesn't match you at a higher level. They may have information that you need, and vice versa. Maybe all they need is some encouragement to upgrade.

Account Information

You'll want to review each category. Be sure to complete your contact information. Your email is only displayed to matches, but if FamilyTreeDNA needs to contact you, they will use this information. You also change your password here.

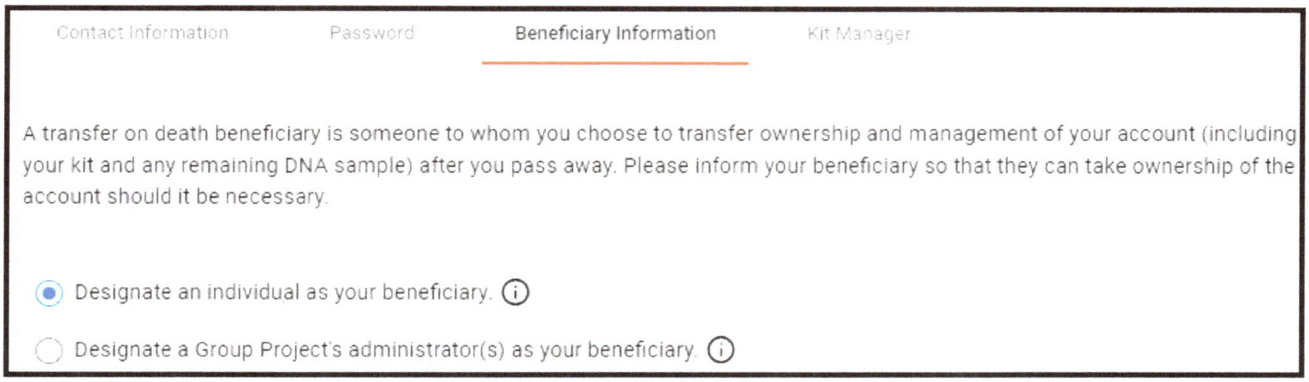

Make sure to complete the Beneficiary Information to ensure that someone has access to your DNA results once you've joined your ancestors. This is critical if an upgrade would be beneficial or for a myriad of other functions.

If your beneficiary contacts FamilyTreeDNA, this information will be essential to that process.

Genealogy

Next, click on the "Genealogy" tab.

You'll see the "Surnames" link first.

17 https://help.familytreedna.com/hc/en-us/articles/4413980253967-Investigative-Genetic-Genealogy-Matching-IGGM-Introduction

18 https://learn.familytreedna.com/project-administration/group-administrator-access-levels-and-permissions/

Upload Surnames

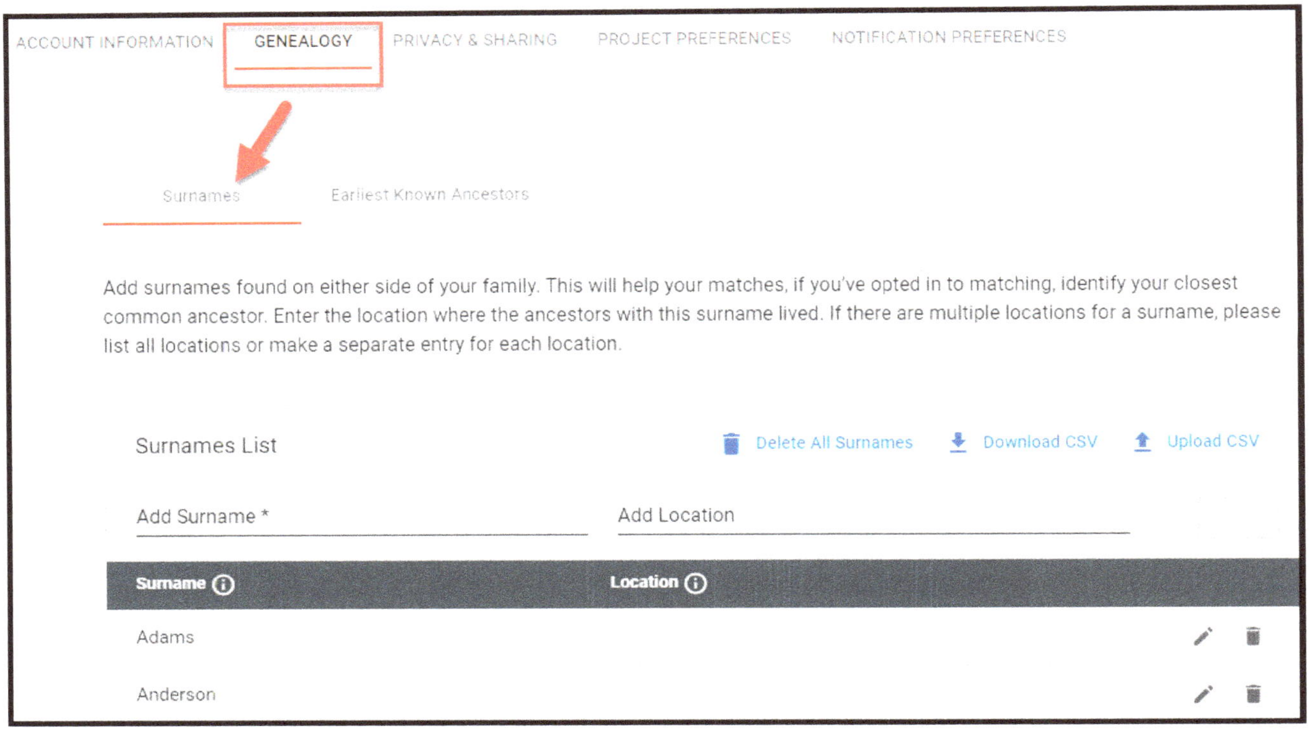

It's important to either manually enter or upload your ancestral surnames from a .csv (comma-separated values) file so that FamilyTreeDNA can inform you of common surnames with your matches. I created a spreadsheet by making a list of all my ancestral surnames AND locations, 12 generations back in time. Create as extensive a list as you can, although there's not much need to go beyond a dozen generations. Do not include people whose surname is unknown.

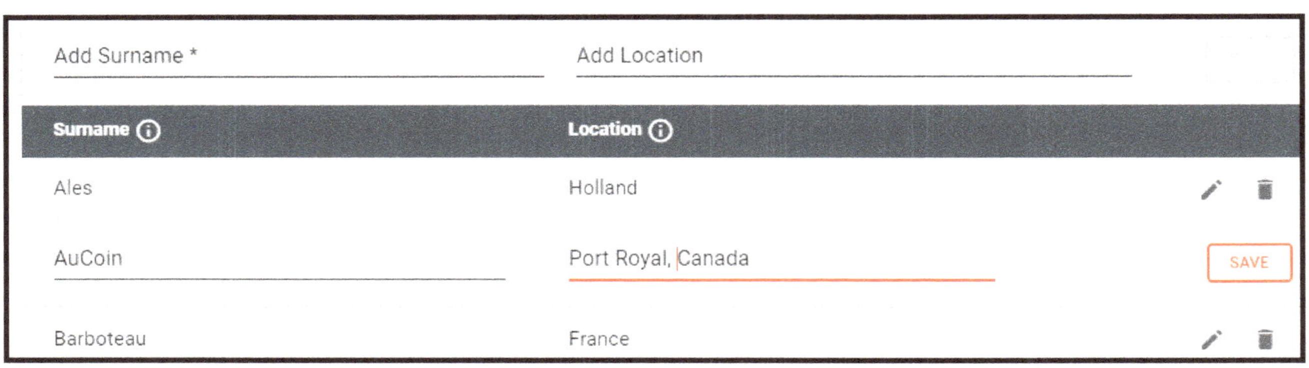

TIP: Make sure you save your spreadsheet as a comma-separated values file (CSV) that includes two columns with the headers formatted as "Surname,Location" with no space after the comma. This exact formatting is critical to a successful upload.

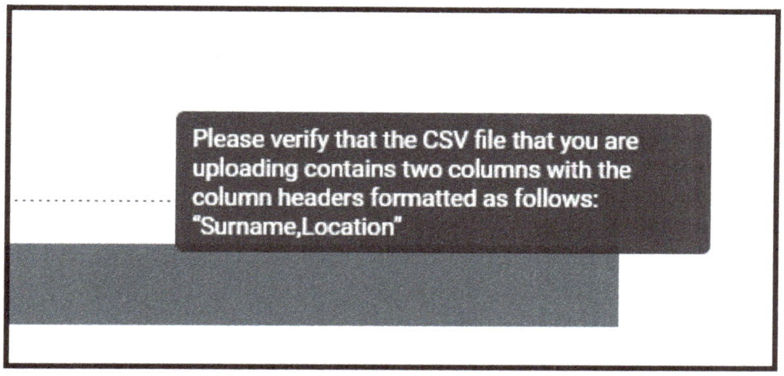

If you've already entered your information, but have since discovered a location, for example, click on the pencil to edit.

TIP: If you uploaded a GEDCOM file at some point in the past, your surnames might not have been auto-populated, so you will need to add them. However, if you upload a tree today, the surnames of only your direct line ancestors will automatically populate the surname field. You might think that the best way to populate the surname field would be to delete your current tree and upload a new one - but you'll need to connect all of your matches to their profile cards again if you upload a new tree.

Uploading surnames is important because FamilyTreeDNA provides a list of Matched Surnames to each of your Family Finder matches. If you and your match don't both provide your ancestral surnames, you won't be able to view your common surnames.

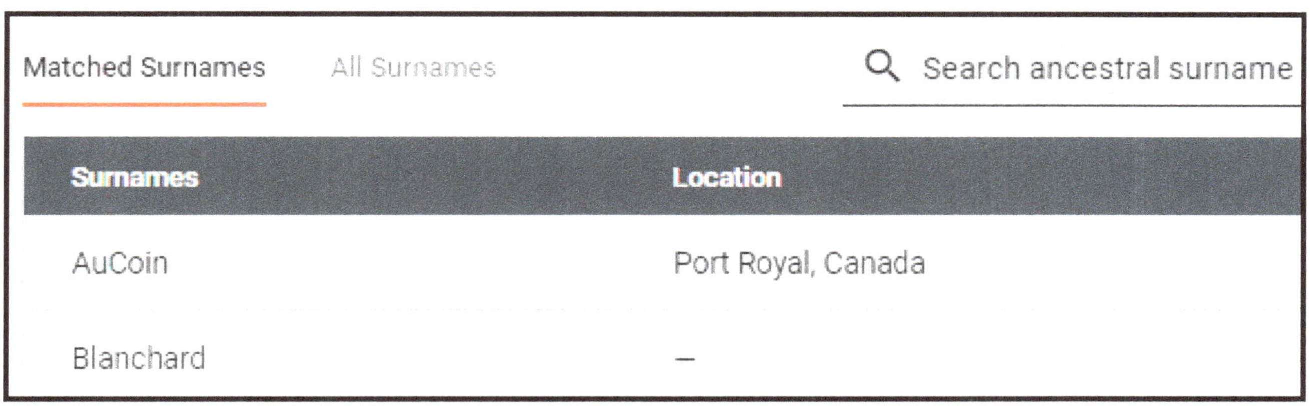

Next, click on the "Earliest Known Ancestor."

Earliest Known Ancestor

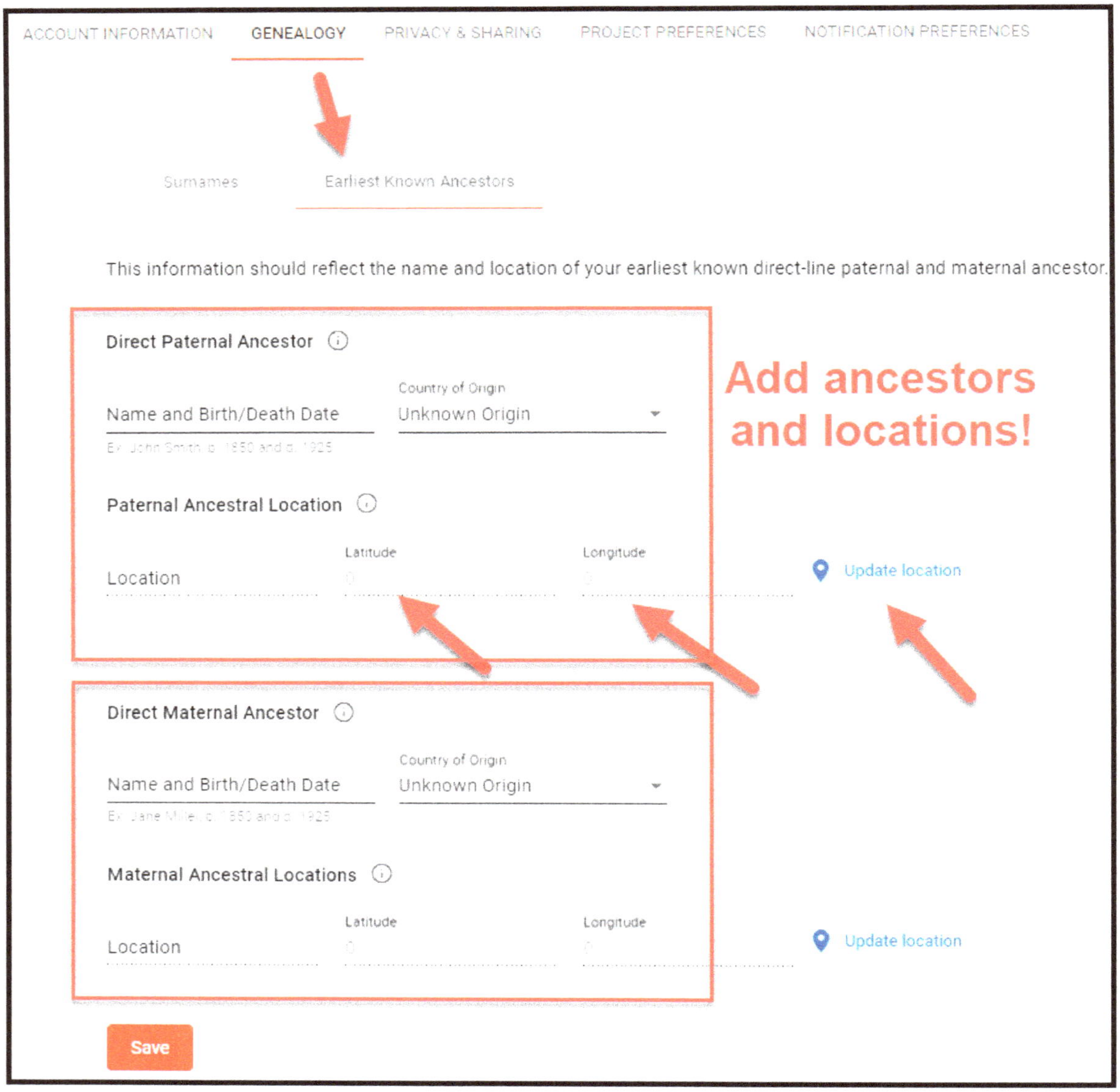

The top half of this page is asking ONLY for your direct paternal, meaning patrilineal, ancestor. This is your father's father's father's line, which in men correlates to the Y-DNA line. Please complete this information, **even if you are a female**, because the Origins Sharing map displays both your direct paternal and direct maternal ancestors.

The next section is asking ONLY for your direct maternal, meaning matrilineal, ancestor. This is your mother's mother's mother's line, which correlates to your mitochondrial ancestor.

Complete these fields even if you're NOT taking those tests.

TIP: Be sure to click "Save" when you're finished.

You can see that the "Location: Latitude and Longitude" are empty, so click on "Update Location" after filling in the name and country location of your ancestor.

That link takes you to a map titled "Plot Ancestral Locations."

Plot Ancestral Locations

You can either enter a search location or drop a pin on the map. When finished, be sure to **"Save"** your information.

When you return to your **Earliest Known Ancestors** page, you'll notice the updated location information there.

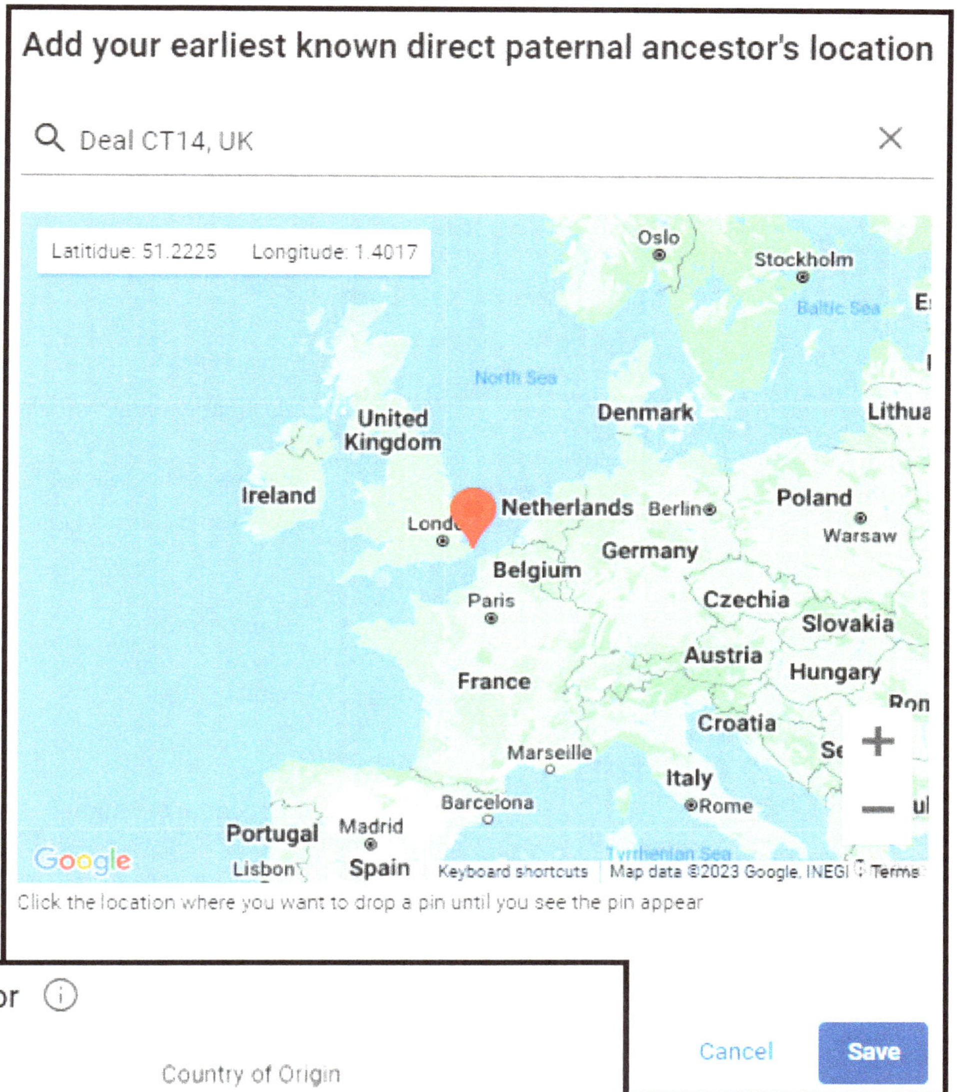

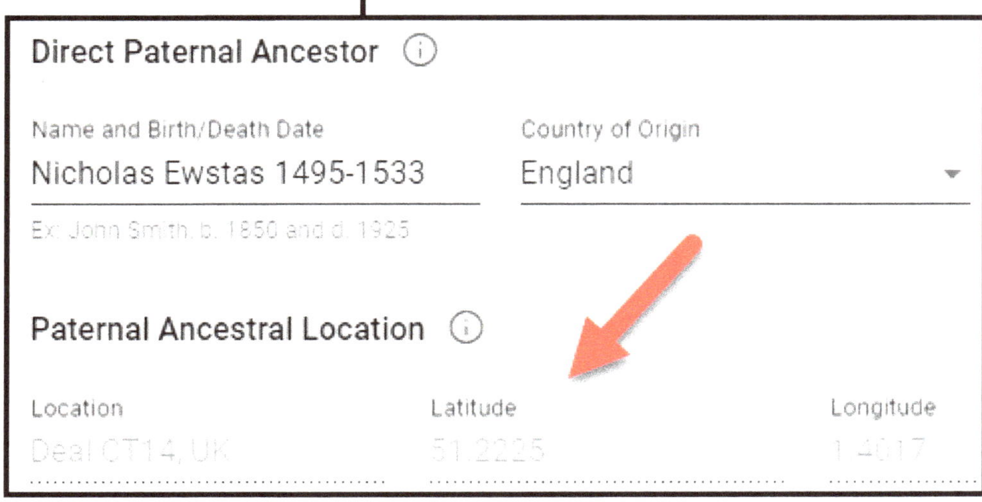

Completing This Information is Essential

Why is completing this information essential? Let's look at an example.

I've signed in to my mother's kit so you can see her match to me.

Without clicking on my name, you can easily see that I've taken the mtFull test, and I've listed several surnames. By clicking on my name as the match, you can view additional information, at right.

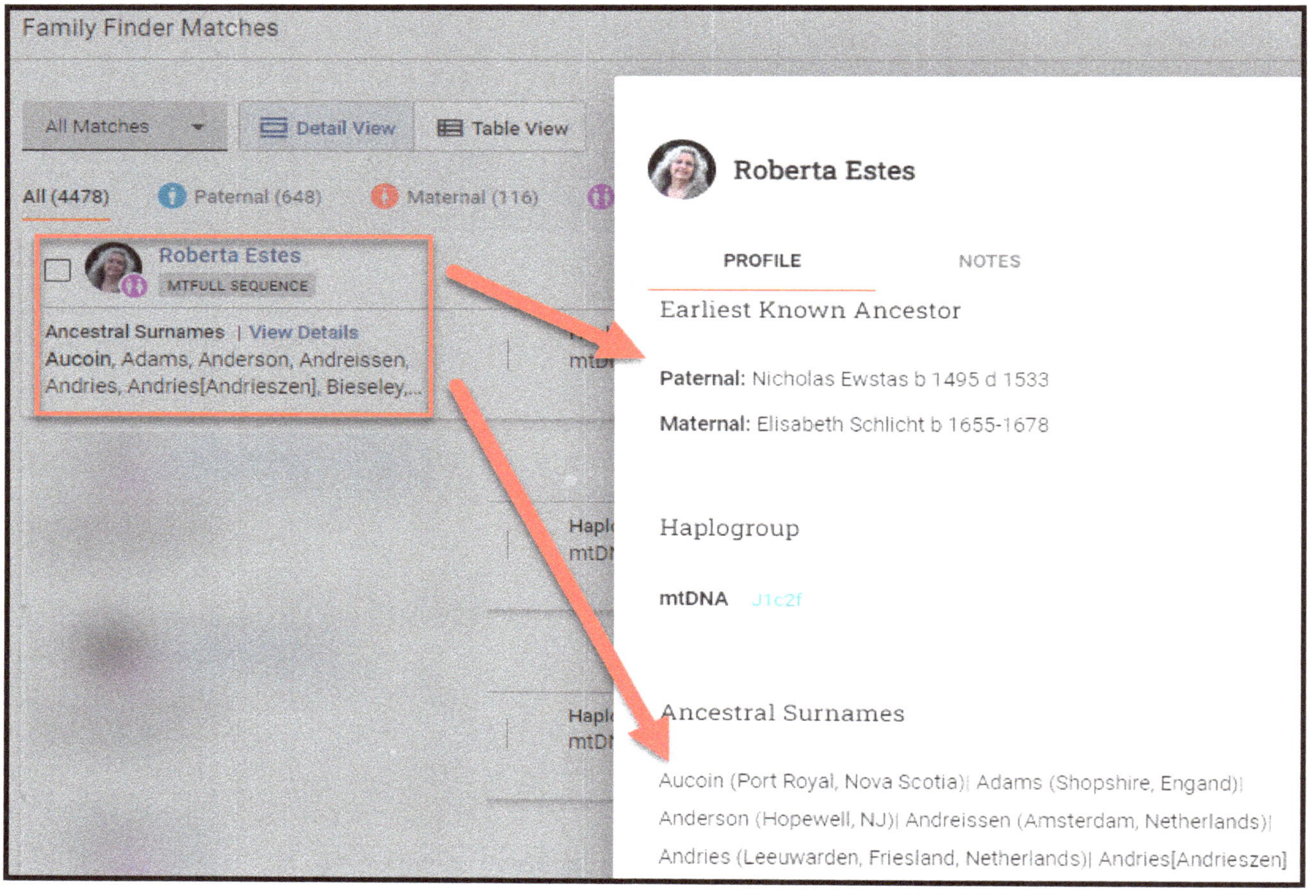

You can view my direct paternal and maternal ancestors, my haplogroup, and a list of my ancestral surnames plus associated locations. How cool is this? Have you ever wondered which of your matches share your ancestors' surnames? Even if your surnames don't match, perhaps a common location will provide the clue you need.

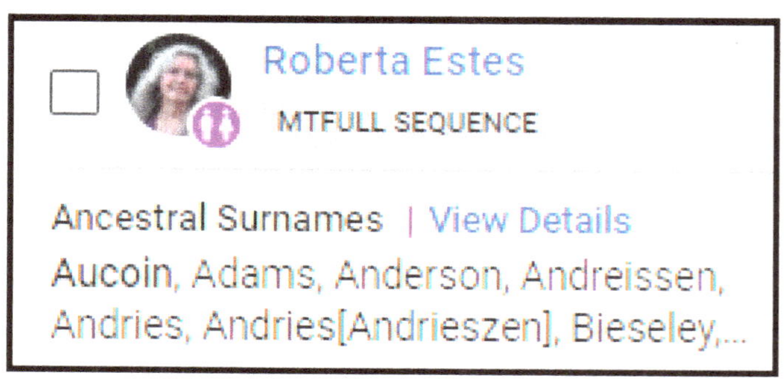

The bolded surnames are found in your surname list and that of your match, too. By clicking on "View Details," you can select to view all surnames for your match, or just your matching surnames in common.

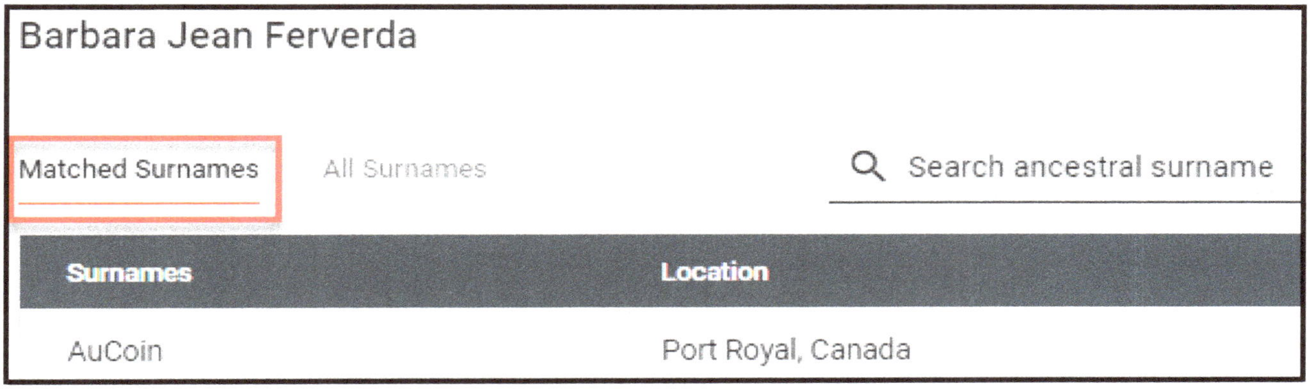

You can search for a specific surname for this match, such as AuCoin.

You can also return to your match page and search for matches with any of your surnames. A list of matches who have that surname themselves, or who have that surname in their list of Ancestral Surnames will be shown.

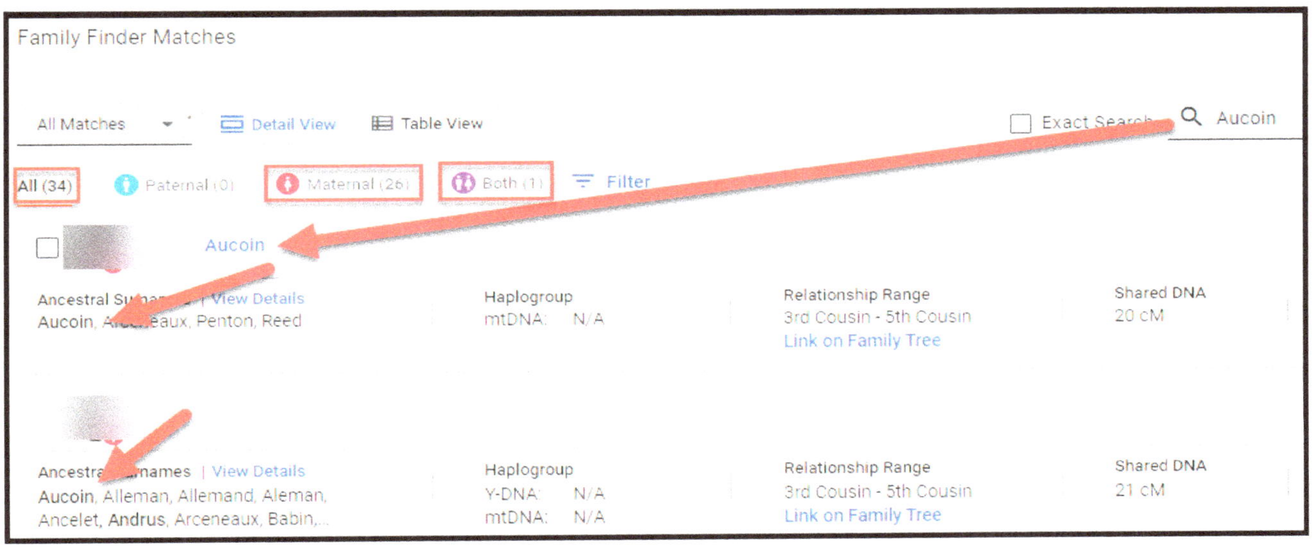

You can see on my mother's match list that there are 34 people with the surname Aucoin listed, 26 of whom are bucketed or assigned to her maternal side through Family Matching, and one of which (me) matches my mom on both her maternal and paternal sides.

IMPORTANT TIP – Searching for a surname does NOT access your matches' trees, just the surnames listed under Ancestral Surnames, or their own surname. You can do tree-matching by utilizing Genetic Affairs[19] on top of your Family Finder test. We'll discuss that option in the Genetic Affairs section.

Now you understand why entering or uploading a list of Ancestral Surnames and completing your Earliest Known Ancestors are such important steps.

19 https://dna-explained.com/2020/08/13/genetic-affairs-instructions-and-resources/

Privacy and Sharing

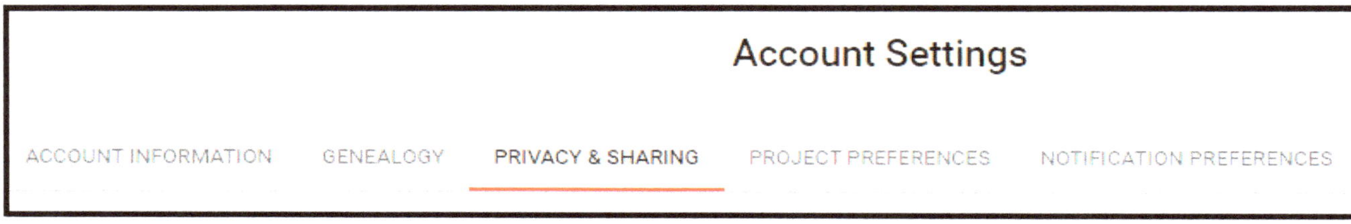

The defaults for Privacy & Sharing work well for most people, except for two fields to which I'd like to draw your attention. However, everyone should review each option.

TIP: Be aware that if you disable any of the matching options, you won't match people you would otherwise match, which may cause a significant amount of confusion and perhaps lead to unwarranted conclusions about WHY people aren't matching you, or why you aren't matching other people. There is no way for your matches to know you've disabled matching.

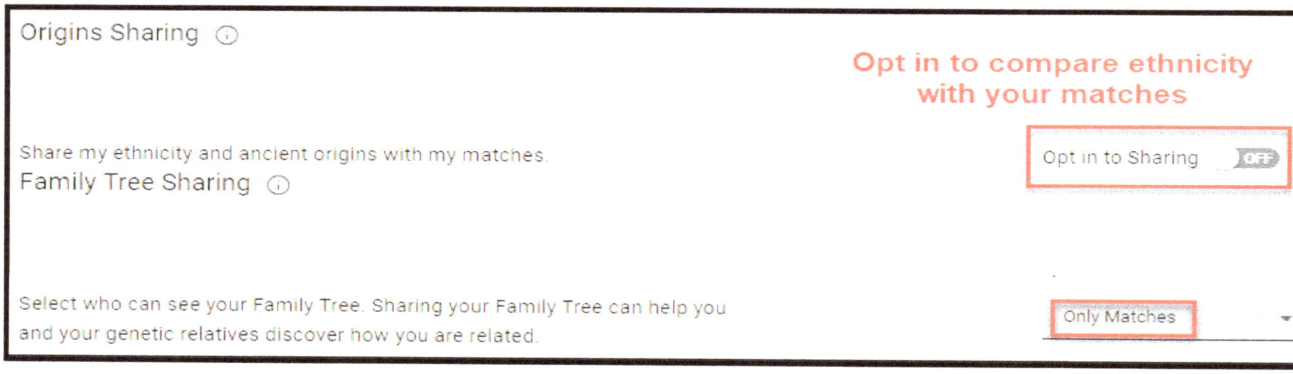

The two default matches you may want to change are Origins Sharing and Family Tree Sharing.

If you opt-in to Origins Sharing, you will be able to use the Compare Origins tool to compare your myOrigins ethnicities with your Family Finder matches. If you do NOT opt in, your matches will not be able to see your percentages, and you won't be able to see theirs.

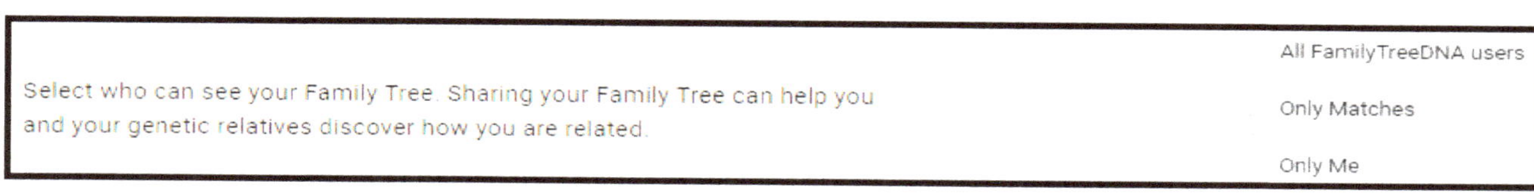

If you change your Share Family Tree selection to "Only Me," your matches will NOT be able to view your tree. Many people have created "accidentally private" trees by making this selection.

"Only Matches" means that your matches can view your tree.

If you select "All FamilyTreeDNA users," it means that if you are linked to one of your match's trees, and that match shares their tree, or one of their matches views their tree, your information can be displayed.

Trees and Why They Are Important

Genealogy is about ancestors and family trees. FamilyTreeDNA has incorporated tools into its product that leverage trees, locations, ancestors, and matches.

This is very important, because you may have ancestors who are found in the trees of other testers. Furthermore, confirming segment matches is one form of proof[20] that you do, in fact, descend from that specific ancestor or ancestral couple.

You'll want to do one of three things:

- Upload your tree to FamilyTreeDNA via a GEDCOM file from your genealogy software
- Download a tree you've created at either Ancestry, MyHeritage, or elsewhere in a GEDCOM file format, and upload to FamilyTreeDNA[21]
- Create a tree at FamilyTreeDNA

My preferred option is to upload a GEDCOM file to FamilyTreeDNA.[22]

TIP: Huge files aren't necessary. You will want your direct ancestors and their descendants in order to link your matches.

I maintain my "life's work tree" on my computer, but there's no need to upload a massive file. The goal is to be able to connect relatives who have tested that you can identify. I uploaded a file with 12 generations of direct line ancestors, making sure to include (or extend) to cover all of my Y-DNA and mitochondrial DNA lines. I include at least the grandchild generations of those ancestors, and, when I identify a match, extend the line to the present.

20 https://dna-explained.com/2020/12/16/triangulation-resources-in-one-place/

21 https://dna-explained.com/2020/06/30/download-your-ancestry-tree-and-upload-it-elsewhere-for-added-benefit/

22 FamilyTreeDNA has announced the intention of utilizing the MyHeritage trees, beginning sometime in 2024.

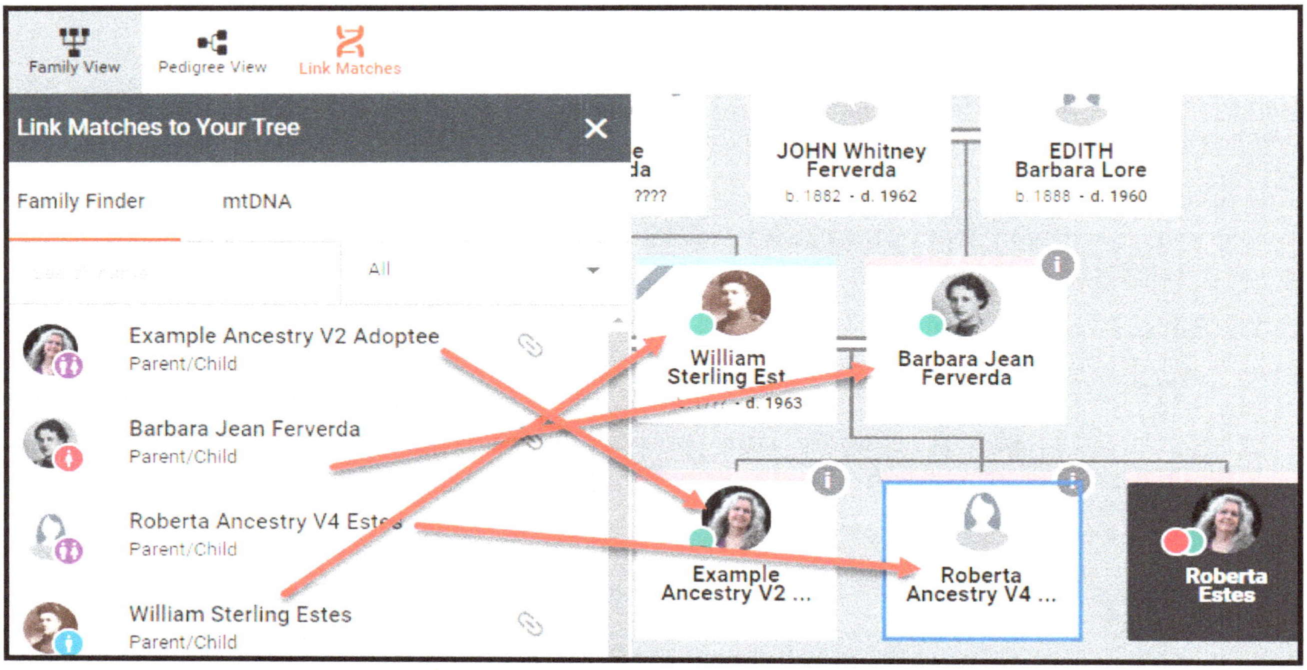

When I figure out how a match at FamilyTreeDNA is related, if that line is not extended sufficiently to connect that person to their proper place in my tree, I extend their branch and connect them at that time, as illustrated above.

Once you've linked matches to their profiles in your tree, you probably won't want to upload a different or replacement tree because you'll have to relink everyone again.[23] If you do upload a modified tree, remember that you may need to add those lines and relink your matches. Be sure to check your tree or download your match list first, so you have a record of which matches were previously linked.

Connecting relatives on your tree allows FamilyTreeDNA's system to triangulate between you and known cousins and assign matches maternally or paternally.[24]

TIP: Many people offer to test all upstream close relatives – parents, grandparents, aunts and uncles, and so forth if their grandparents haven't tested. I figure a DNA test is about the price of a book, and I'd order a book in a heartbeat if I thought the key to my ancestor even MIGHT be in there.

The goal is to capture as much of the DNA of my ancestors as possible so that when someone else matches me on that same segment, FamilyTreeDNA knows that match is on my paternal side, for example. Because I linked my paternal family member to my tree in the appropriate place, FamilyTreeDNA can assign that new match paternally.

23 https://dna-explained.com/2020/11/10/genealogy-tree-replacement-should-i-or-shouldnt-i/

24 https://dna-explained.com/2019/11/06/triangulation-in-action-at-family-tree-dna/

Furthermore, by definition, those matches are automatically phased, meaning assigned maternally or paternally (or both) and triangulated,[25 26] too.

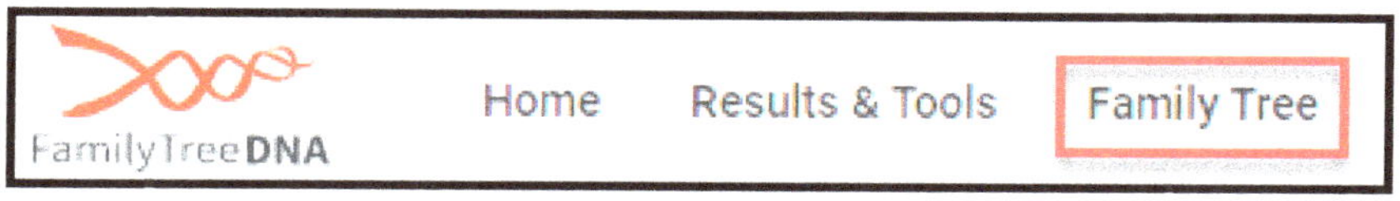

You'll be prompted at numerous places during account setup to upload a tree, but you can upload a tree anytime by clicking at the top of your personal page on "Family Tree."

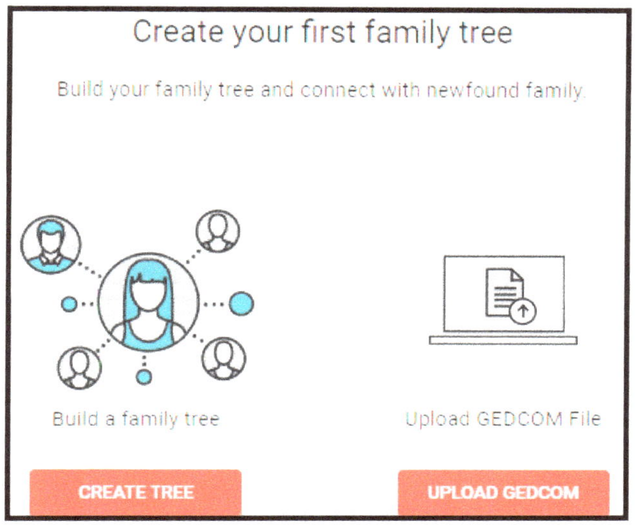

You'll be asked to create a tree or upload a GEDCOM file.

You can also click on "Family Tree" in the "Other Tools" section.

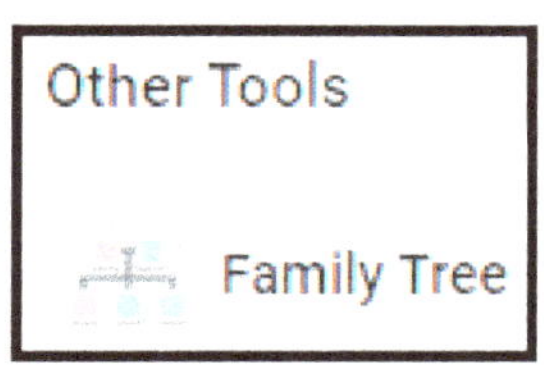

DNA, trees, and genealogical records work in tandem, so you want to do everything possible to leverage your results.

TIP: The matches surname search at FamilyTreeDNA does not search the trees, only the surnames that you upload. Today, when you upload a tree, FamilyTreeDNA adds your ancestral surnames to the Surname list, but if you uploaded a tree earlier, or created a tree at FamilyTreeDNA, you'll need to add those surnames manually.

25 https://dna-explained.com/2017/05/16/concepts-why-genetic-genealogy-and-triangulation/

26 https://dna-explained.com/2019/11/06/triangulation-in-action-at-family-tree-dna/

Chapter 3

Y-DNA – YOUR FATHER'S STORY

The Y chromosome is magical for genealogy because it is passed from father to son, generation after generation, with the DNA changing just enough over time to be genealogically useful. Those changes are called mutations and, in this context, do not have any negative health implications.

Y-DNA never mixes with any of the mother's DNA, so unlike autosomal DNA, Y-DNA doesn't lose potency over time, nor do you have to figure out which ancestor it came from. Females don't have a Y chromosome. So, if you're a female, you can't test directly, but you can, hopefully, recruit a male from the surname line you want to learn more about. In the case of your father, he can test, or your full brother or paternal half-brother can test, or your paternal uncle can test to represent your father's line. You may need to go back up your tree a few generations to find a male descendant who carries the surname and, of course, by implication, the Y-DNA of that line.

TIP: You can find Y-DNA candidates in other lines using the same methodology.

One of the challenges is, of course, that DNA testing as a whole can expose closely held family secrets. You might discover a non-paternal event, NPE, also called a non-parental event, not- (the) parent-expected, or misattributed parentage. In other words, it's possible that you'll discover that your Y-DNA does not match the surnames of the lineage you expect, meaning there is a genetic break or genetic difference someplace in the line. That disconnect could be in a recent generation, many generations back in time, or someplace in between.

Making unexpected discoveries[27] is always a possibility with DNA testing.

Y-DNA Goals

Your Y-DNA testing goals may include:

- Determining or discovering the direct paternal line. This is clearly a very important test for male adoptees or males in search of their paternal (patrilineal)[28] connection.
- Confirming a patrilineal line of descent from a particular ancestor or ancestral family.
- Discovering who you do or don't match. Y-DNA testing can be used for excluding relationships as well as confirming them.

---

27 https://dna-explained.com/2018/02/18/unexpected-discoveries-through-dna-testing/

28 https://dna-explained.com/2018/11/28/concepts-paternal-vs-patrilineal-and-maternal-vs-matrilineal/

- Sorting testers into genetic lineages to determine which branch of a particular family you descend from.
- Learning more about the history of the paternal line. Think clans here, or historical figures like Somerled[29] or Brian Boru[30] - both before and after the adoption of surnames.
- Delving into the patrilineal history before the advent of surnames, such as Celts or Yamnaya, for example.
- To determine the origin of the lineage, meaning Native American, European, African, Asian, Jewish, Pacific Islander, etc.
- Understanding your ancestor's migration path.
- Determining when you share the most recent common ancestor (MRCA) with other men who have taken a Y-DNA test.
- Learning about ancient DNA connections, where they are found, and how long ago you shared a common paternal ancestor.
- Have fun by discovering notable connections.
- Joining Y-DNA projects to collaborate with other researchers.

FamilyTreeDNA provides customers with more than 20 tools to understand your Y-DNA results and what they mean to you.

Two Types of Y-DNA Markers

Y-DNA testing utilizes two types of mutations, Short Tandem Repeats, known as STRs, and Single Nucleotide Polymorphisms, known as SNPs.[31] [32]

These two types of mutations are different and serve different functions, but work together[33] for the highest resolution, most detailed genealogy information available for Y-DNA testing.

STR panels, such as the Y-12, 25, 37, 67, and 111, are used for matching against other testers in the database. While only Y-37 and Y-111 are now available for purchase, you may still receive matches at the legacy levels, which are no longer being sold individually since those levels are included in the available panels. For example, the Y-37 panel includes Y-12 and Y-25, while the Y-111 includes those plus the Y-37 and Y-67 panels. Big Y-700 also includes all 111 markers plus an additional 589 or more STRs that come from Big Y data.

So, what are STR markers? Let's take a step back to explain the underpinnings of DNA so it's easier to understand the message of markers and matching.

---

29 https://en.wikipedia.org/wiki/Somerled

30 https://en.wikipedia.org/wiki/Brian_Boru

31 https://dna-explained.com/2014/02/10/strs-vs-snps-multiple-dna-personalities/

32 https://dna-explained.com/2023/08/10/haplogroups-dna-snps-are-breadcrumbs-follow-their-path/

33 https://dna-explained.com/2021/12/03/strs-and-snps-are-str-markers-still-useful-for-y-dna/

Building Blocks of DNA

The smallest units of DNA are made up of 4 base nucleotides, DNA words, if you will, that are represented by the following letters:

A = Adenine
C = Cytosine
G = Guanine
T = Thymine

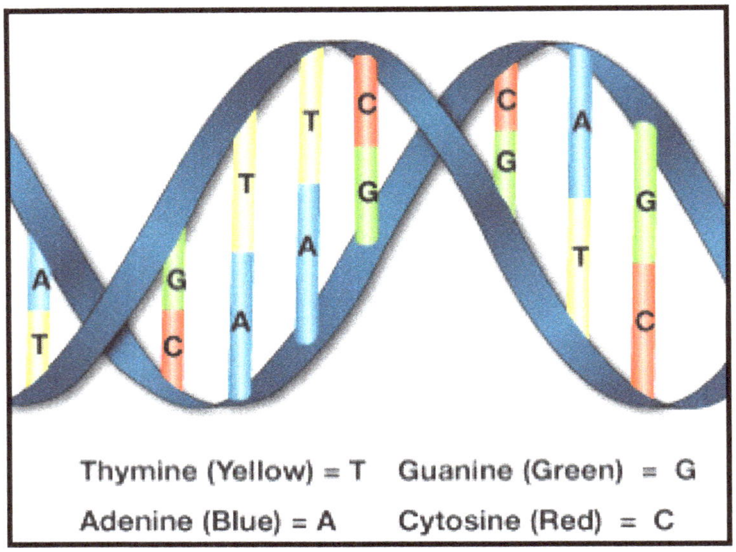

The order in which these are found is called your DNA sequence, also known as your haplotype. You don't need to remember the base names or even the letters, just remember that in analyzing DNA results, we are looking for pattern matches of contiguous nucleotides of DNA.

Your DNA, when transcribed on paper, looks like a string of beads. There are 4 kinds of beads, each representing one of the nucleotides above. One segment of your DNA might look like this:

ATTCTAATTT

A mutation would be defined as any type of change from the standard, or reference, sequence in your haplotype, meaning your personal DNA results. These cumulative differences not only provide matching within families, but more broadly, they define your family Y-DNA or mitochondrial DNA haplogroup (ancestral clan).

STRs – Short Tandem Repeats

An STR or Short Tandem Repeat is analogous to a genetic stutter, a replication error. Think of the copy machine getting stuck. In the transcription we mentioned, we see a group of nucleotides that form a pattern. That pattern repeats at a specific, named location on the chromosome and is then counted and displayed as a numeral. The values at those named locations can then be compared against the database to look for other testers who have the same number value.

ATTCTCTCTCTCTAATTT

For example, in the sequence above, you have the bases CT, then followed by CT repeated four times in that specific order, for a value of 5, meaning 5 total repeats of CT at that specific location on the Y chromosome.

Because STR markers mutate fairly often, and documenting lineages depends on a mutation occurring that is identifiable with a specific lineage, STR marker mutations were perfect for genealogy. At least in the beginning.

TIP: DYS locations are the names of STR markers, such as DYS393. D stands for DNA, Y stands for the Y chromosome, and S is a unique segment.

Initially, genealogists were excited to have 12 markers to compare with other men.

Y-DNA - Standard Y-STR Values | Help

PANEL 1 (1-12)											
Marker	DYS393	DYS390	DYS19 **	DYS391	DYS385	DYS426	DYS388	DYS439	DYS389I	DYS392	DYS389II ***
Value	13	25	14	12	11-14	12	12	12	13	13	29

Today, these first 12 markers form Panel 1. Every tester has values associated with each individual marker.

PANEL 1 (1-12)		
Marker	DYS393	DYS390
Value	13	25

For example, marker DYS393, above, has a value of 13 for this tester, meaning the Y-DNA shows 13 repeats at this location. DYS390 has 25 repeats, and so forth.

FamilyTreeDNA compares testers against each other, reporting matches as they are found. Testers don't have to match exactly. FamilyTreeDNA allows for some number of mutation differences[34] at each panel level. We will look at examples in the STR Results and Matching section.

However, since STRs mutate more rapidly, they are also somewhat unreliable because they may randomly change between any generation.

Furthermore, back mutations happen from time to time, making it appear as if a mutation never occurred. Forward mutations happen, too, adding a repeat to the sequence from one generation to the next.

Clearly, these situations can really throw a monkey wrench into the works, given that we need to be able to depend on the results to identify, set forth, and track lineages to determine relationships.

34 https://help.familytreedna.com/hc/en-us/articles/4408063356303-Y-STR-Results-Guide

This brings us to SNPs, a second type of mutation.

SNPs, or Single Nucleotide Polymorphisms

A Single Nucleotide Polymorphism, generally called a SNP, pronounced "snip," is a change at a single location on the chromosome. It may be a change from one base to another, the addition of a base, or even the subtraction of one.

Going back to our bead sequence:

ATTCTAATTT

An example of a SNP mutation would be if the first A above were to change to T, G, or C as in the sequence below:

TTTCTAATTT

A subtraction, called a deletion, would occur if the leading A were simply gone.

TTCTAATTT

An addition, called an insertion, would occur if a new bead were inserted in the sequence at that location.

AGTTCTAATTT

SNPs are a single nucleotide change at one location, or position, not a stutter insertion of multiple bases.

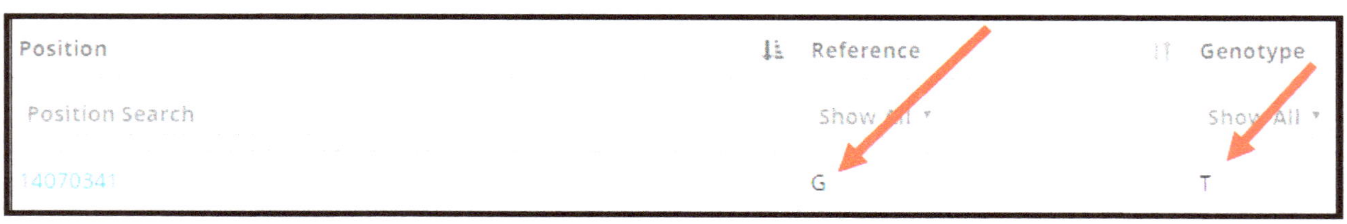

In this example from a Big Y Private Variant test result, the typical or reference nucleotide is a G in the human reference genome[35], but this tester has a T at that position.

SNP mutations are used to define haplogroups, which are branches of the Y-DNA haplotree, the tree of mankind. For example, R-M269 is a very common high-level haplogroup present in about half of European men. R indicates haplogroup R, and M269 is the location where a specific mutation is found. All men who are assigned to haplogroup R-M269, or subgroups beneath R-M269, descend from the first man in which that mutation occurred.

35 https://www.genome.gov/genetics-glossary/Human-Genome-Reference-Sequence

Name	Position (GRCh38)	Ancestral	Derived
M269	20577481	T	C

R-M269 is identified when C, Cytosine, replaces T, Thymine, at position 20577481. You don't have to care about the underlying specifics, but you will very much care about the genealogical message that haplogroups and other mutations provide for genealogy.

High-level haplogroups, such as R-M269, are predicted from STR-only tests, such as the 37 and 111-marker test panels. However, much more specific and refined haplogroups with greater granularity are assigned when testers purchase the Big Y-700[36] test, which includes:

- At least 700 STR values.
- A scan that targets approximately 23.6 million of the 59 million base pairs on the Y chromosome to detect relevant STR and SNP mutations.

While STR tests focus only on a small number of specific locations, the Big Y-700 test scans the majority of that portion of the Y chromosome that provides the most relevant information for genealogy, searching for all mutations. Not only will the Big Y-700 test find mutations inherited from earlier generations, but much more recent mutations, too. These novel mutations are known as private variants. When found in more than one man and determined to be of sufficient quality, private variants are assigned a name, becoming a haplogroup. New haplogroups form new branches of the Y-DNA haplotree, which now has more than 60,000 branches.[37]

For example, my Estes line now falls 26 branches below R-M269, which is about 7,650 years old[38], into haplogroup R-ZS3700[39] that dates to Moses Estes, who was born in 1711. That's a HUGE difference in Time to Most Recent Common Ancestor (TMRCA), 7,650 years ago to 300 years ago - thanks to the Big Y test. Better yet, any other man who falls into haplogroup R-ZS3700 knows that he, too, descends from Moses Estes.

Big Y matching occurs separately from STR matching and uses SNPs, meaning that Big Y testers receive STR matches plus Big Y SNP matches, along with several unique tools available only with SNP or Big Y testing.[40]

36 https://blog.familytreedna.com/wp-content/uploads/2019/03/big-y-700-white-paper_compressed.pdf

37 https://dna-explained.com/2022/10/04/familytreedna-to-surpass-60000-y-dna-haplogroups-and-introduces-new-time-tree/

38 https://discover.familytreedna.com/y-dna/R-M269/story

39 https://discover.familytreedna.com/y-dna/R-ZS3700/story

40 https://dna-explained.com/2023/10/11/new-discover-tool-compare-haplogroups-more-at-familytreedna/

Haplogroup Names

This is a good place to mention that you may see Y-DNA haplogroup names mentioned in two ways.

At one point in time, haplogroups followed a number-letter-number naming pattern, such as R1b1c. As new branches were discovered, more letters and numbers were added. Eventually, as many new haplogroups were discovered, that name became unwieldy and too long to remember or work with, so that naming format was replaced by the letter of the base haplogroup, such as R, plus the SNP, or mutation, that defines that particular haplogroup branch, such as R-M269. Therefore, R1b1c from 2005-2008 became R1b1a2, which in turn became R-M269 in 2014. Since R-M269 is a SNP name, it will never change.[41]

TIP: A haplogroup branch and a downstream haplogroup are the same thing. The word "branch" simply means the new haplogroup branches from or occurs beneath a branch, as a descendant of the older or parent haplogroup.

If you see a Y-DNA letter-number-letter format haplogroup today, you're probably dealing with significantly outdated information.

TIP: The ISOGG Haplogroup Tree tracked the evolution of haplogroups names for 15 years, but stopped in 2020.[42] Today, FamilyTreeDNA updates their tree daily with customer, academic and ancient sequences, and is the standard scientific and genealogical haplotree resource, passing 75,000 branches in 2023 based on more than 285,000 tests.[43]

Mitochondrial DNA haplogroups are still named in the letter-number-letter pattern today. Mitochondrial haplogroup names aren't as long, but the Million Mito Project[44] may change that format.[45]

Haplogroup Age Terminology

Conversationally, sometimes people refer to older or younger haplogroups or use terms like high-level or mid-level. We mention that high-level haplogroups have lots of matches, and more recent ones don't. Not only is this confusing, it may lead to assumptions about what is "good" and "bad," which aren't necessarily accurate.

---

41 https://dna-explained.com/2014/05/09/2014-y-tree-released-by-family-tree-dna/

42 https://isogg.org/tree/

43 https://www.familytreedna.com/public/y-dna-haplotree/A

44 https://dna-explained.com/2020/03/17/the-million-mito-project/

45 https://dna-explained.com/2022/04/13/million-mito-project-team-introduction-and-progress-update/

Haplogroup Terminology	Meaning & Source	Relative Age	What's Better – Next Step
Base haplogroup, such as haplogroup R which is the prefix for R-M207	The "top" or root of a particular branch of the haplotree where this haplogroup was first named. The oldest haplogroup, which is highest in this branch of the haplotree.	Depends on the haplogroup, but thousands of years. R-M207 is the base of haplogroup R and was formed about 28,000 years ago.	Any descendant haplogroup that can be obtained by STR testing, a Family Finder haplogroup, or the Big Y-700 test.
High-level haplogroup	A haplogroup still relatively high in the tree, but can be reliably predicted by STR markers without SNP testing, such as R-M269.	Closer in time than a base haplogroup. R-M269 was formed about 4,350 BCE or 6,350 years ago.	An intermediate-level haplogroup, provided by the Family Finder test, or by the most refined haplogroup possible from the Big Y-700 test.
Intermediate-level haplogroup – high-level haplogroups from STR tests are updated to intermediate-level if they have taken a Family Finder test	Generally, a haplogroup closer in time than a high-level haplogroup and is SNP-confirmed. May be produced by a Family Finder test.	Estes men are receiving R-DF49 from the Family Finder test, which was formed about 4,350 years ago.	Most refined SNP haplogroup obtained by Big Y-700 test.
Most refined haplogroup – the youngest, most recent, or best haplogroup	The most genealogically relevant haplogroup that places men who've taken the Big Y test into family lineages.	In the Estes lineage, R-BY154784 originated about 190 years ago, or 1830.	When other men in the same line test, sometimes new haplogroups are formed, providing additional refinement.

While genealogists are always focused on older generations, in this case, the most relevant haplogroup information is the most refined, youngest, most recently formed haplogroup because only men in that branch of the tree will share that mutation. In other words, Y-DNA mutations resemble our traditional pedigree chart.

Unlike autosomal DNA, where lots of matches are a good thing, the various types of Y-DNA testing refine your matches to the most relevant and most recently related, so there probably won't be as many of them, certainly not as many as in autosomal tests.

For example, the highest or oldest haplogroups will have the most matches, but that only tells you, in the case of R-M207, the base of haplogroup R, how many men descend from a common ancestor 28,000 years ago. You match all of them at that level. While that's interesting, and so is the path of haplogroup R out of Africa, it's not helpful to more recent genealogy.

Haplogroup	Haplogroup Type	Haplogroup Formation	Downstream Haplogroup Branches	SNP-Confirmed Testers	Countries
R-M207	Base	26,000 BCE 28,000 years ago	35,511	134,142	213
R-M269	Predicted High Level	4,350 BCE 6,350 years ago	29,575	107,126	184
R-DF49	Intermediate from Family Finder	2,350 BCE 4,350 years ago	7	8,296	35
R-BY482	Big Y – Estes haplogroup	1500 CE	3 + 2 unnamed lineages	18	2 US & UK
R-BY490	Big Y	1650 CE	2 + 11 unnamed lineages	15	2
R-ZS3700	Big Y	1700 CE	1 + 2 unnamed lineages	4	2
R-BY154784	Big Y	1850 CE	0 today	2	1

In this example, R-BY482 is shared by all Estes men who descend from the Estes lineage in Kent, near Ringwould, England. R-BY482 has three branches that can further define your genealogical lineage, with two more lineages waiting for additional testers in order to be named. R-BY490, a descendant haplogroup of R-BY482, is found only in the American lines, and R-ZS3700 is found only in Moses, the son of Abraham, the Virginia immigrant. Today, if a man takes the Big Y-700 test and discovers that he falls in haplogroup R-ZS3700, or a subgroup, we know immediately that he descends from Moses Estes's sons. If he falls into R-BY154784, he knows he descends from Moses's son, John.

The Y-DNA portion of the surname projects I administer benefits immensely from Big Y testing, which allows comparisons of multiple men from a specific lineage.

When my McNeill cousin's Big Y test completed, I wrote the article "*Y-DNA: Step-by-Step Big Y Analysis*"[46] to help people understand what to expect when they receive their results. There have been new features added since that time, but it's still a good genealogical discussion about the benefits of Big Y testing and how to use the results.

The case study, "*The Ancestors are SPEAKing: An 18-Year Y-DNA Study That Led Us Home,*" utilizes STR markers, select Big Y testers, and autosomal results combined with genealogy, and, of course, a dash of luck.[47]

From a genealogical perspective, the best test for Y-DNA is clearly the Big Y-700 test, but other tests are available and useful. What you order depends on your goals.

Which Test Should I Order? STR 37/111 or Big Y-700 SNP-Based Test?

The evolution of the Y-DNA testing field did not happen overnight. For a long time, STR markers were used for "recent" genealogical matching, and SNPs were for deep lineage only. That hasn't been the case in several years, meaning that the timeframes overlap and SNPs are generally substantially more useful for genealogy, but old "advice" sometimes dies hard.

Today, every male needs to take a Big Y[48] test if they are interested in genealogical placement at the most refined location on the tree, which translates to the most accurate comparisons to other men. Only two circumstances come to mind in which someone might NOT order the Big Y test today:

- When a Y-DNA test is being done solely as an exclusionary test. In other words, to see if John Doe is from a specific male Doe line. If so, then an upgrade can later be purchased to the Big Y-700. If not, the original tester did not spend the additional funds only to discover that the tester was not from the hoped-for Doe line. I often sponsor or grant scholarships for tests, but only for descendants of my specific line. The least expensive way to confirm a common lineage is a 37-marker Y-DNA test. However, keep in mind that occasionally men who match on the Big Y-700 do not match on STR tests alone.

46 https://dna-explained.com/2020/05/30/y-dna-step-by-step-big-y-analysis/

47 https://dna-explained.com/2022/11/05/the-ancestors-are-speaking-an-18-year-y-dna-study-that-led-us-home-52-ancestors-381/

48 https://blog.familytreedna.com/wp-content/uploads/2018/06/big_y_700_white_paper_compressed.pdf

- When purchase price is a constraining factor. It's always better to have something than nothing, and a Y-37 or Y-111 test plus a Family Finder test may, in some circumstances, prove more useful for a specific genealogical goal.

Big Y testers receive everything STR testers receive, plus additional features and MUCH more specificity and granularity.

To begin with, the Big Y testers receive both STR and SNP values, which provide them with two kinds of testing and matching. Big Y testers obtain their genealogically closest matches, and the results place each tester at the tip or end of their branch of the tree, often with a family-level haplogroup, especially if multiple family members have tested.

Feature	STR 37 & 111-Marker Tests	Big Y-700 Test
Number of STR markers	37 or 111 (111 includes 37)	111 + 589, possibly more
Haplogroup	High level, predicted[49]	Most refined possible, SNP confirmed, end-of-branch
Number of SNPs	None included, some available for purchase	Targets more than 23.6 million scanned locations, finds previously known plus unknown SNPs
Matching	At the level you tested	At all STR levels plus SNPs through Big Y
Migration Map	Yes	Yes, more detailed map + Globetrekker
Y STR Results	Yes	Yes
Matches Map	Yes	Yes
Ancestral Origins	Yes	Yes
Haplogroup Origins	Yes	Yes
Haplogroup & SNP Tree	Yes	Yes
Projects	Yes	Yes
Previously Discovered Haplogroup SNP Mutations	Predicted high level haplogroup	Yes - complete scan of all SNPs
Ability to Discover New Haplogroup Mutations	No	Yes
Block Tree	No	Yes

49 A high-level predicted haplogroup essentially means that FamilyTreeDNA provides STR testers with the best branch possible based on a haplogroup prediction utilizing STR markers. Generally, this is a branch midway up the tree, or the top of an existing branch that was formed several thousand years ago. The Big Y test confirms haplogroups in the current era.

Discover™ Haplogroup Story	Discover™ Haplogroup Reports Tool, for predicted haplogroup provided	Discover™ Haplogroup Reports Tool, at advanced level
Discover™ Time Tree	Discover™ Haplogroup Reports Tool, for predicted haplogroup provided	Discover™ Haplogroup Reports Tool, at advanced level
Discover™ Ancestral Path	Discover™ Haplogroup Reports Tool, for predicted haplogroup provided	Discover™ Haplogroup Reports Tool, at advanced level
Discover™ Ancient Connections with time to most recent common ancestor (TMRCA)	Discover™ Haplogroup Reports Tool, for predicted haplogroup provided	Discover™ Haplogroup Reports Tool, at advanced level
Discover™ Notable Connections with time to most recent common ancestor (TMRCA)	Discover™ Haplogroup Reports Tool, for predicted haplogroup provided	Discover™ Haplogroup Reports Tool, at advanced level
Discover™ Country Frequency	Discover™ Haplogroup Reports Tool, for predicted haplogroup provided	Discover™ Haplogroup Reports Tool, at advanced level
Discover™ Suggested Projects	Discover™ Haplogroup Reports Tool, for predicted haplogroup provided	Discover™ Haplogroup Reports Tool, at advanced level
Discover™ Scientific Details – Age Estimate	Discover™ Haplogroup Reports Tool, for predicted haplogroup provided	Discover™ Haplogroup Reports Tool, at advanced level
Discover™ Scientific Details - Variants	Discover™ Haplogroup Reports Tool, for predicted haplogroup provided	Discover™ Haplogroup Reports Tool, at advanced level
Discover™ Ancestral Path	Discover™ Haplogroup Reports Tool, for predicted haplogroup provided	Discover™ Haplogroup Reports Tool, at advanced level
Discover™ Globetrekker	No	Available only for Big Y testers from their account page
Discover™ Compare Haplogroups	Yes	
Upgradable	Yes	No, this is presently the highest level but is updated with new discoveries
Perpetual updates providing lifetime analysis	Yes, receive new STR matches	Yes, new STR and Big Y matches PLUS new haplogroup branches on the tree as they are discovered

Let's start with the Y-DNA Dashboard where you'll find your results.

Y-DNA Dashboard

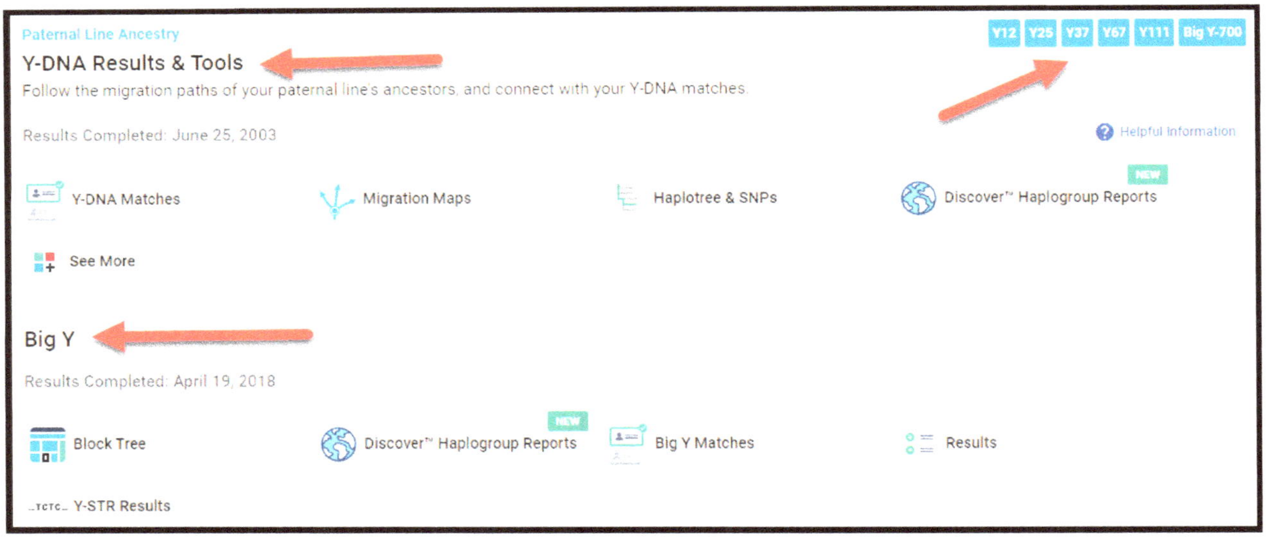

Testers can easily see their testing level at the upper right corner of their personal page.

If a man has taken the Big Y-700 test, the Big Y-700 button will be blue, and the Big Y section will be displayed with several tabs.

If someone has not taken the Big Y test, that button will be grey. It's easy to upgrade by clicking on the Big Y-700 button.

The Big Y-500 is an earlier version of the Big Y-700, and can be upgraded to the Big Y-700, which includes:

- A much broader scan using updated lab processes and newer technology, reaching portions of the Y chromosome not previously possible
- Significantly better coverage, going from 11.5-12.5 million base pairs to 16-22 million base pairs, with fewer no-calls
- Potentially, new haplogroups for men who previously tested with the Big Y-500 and thought they were at the end of the line
- More than the 200 additional STR markers

In the Estes DNA project, four new haplogroups were discovered in one lineage when Big Y-500 men upgraded to the Big Y-700. The upgrade was genealogically very useful, breaking the line down into several descendant branches. The Discover™ Time Tree told us when the various lineages had split from their parent haplogroups and was accurate within 50 years of the proven genealogy.

STR Testing Tools

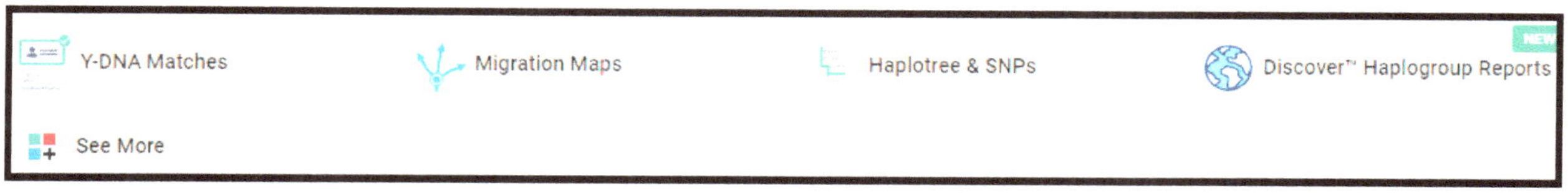

When ordering a 37 or 111-marker Y-DNA test or working with STR test results, you receive the following tools on your personal page:

- Y-DNA Matches
- Migration Maps
- Haplotree & SNPs
- Discover™ Haplogroup Reports – the new Discover™ Haplogroups Reports pages which include several tools

Under the "See More" tab:

- Ancestral Origins
- Matches Maps
- Haplogroup Origins
- Y STR Results

Let's begin by looking at STR results and Y-DNA tools.

STR Results and Matching

Your Y-STR Results are your actual marker values.

In the Y-DNA Results & Tools section, click on See More, then Y-STR Results.

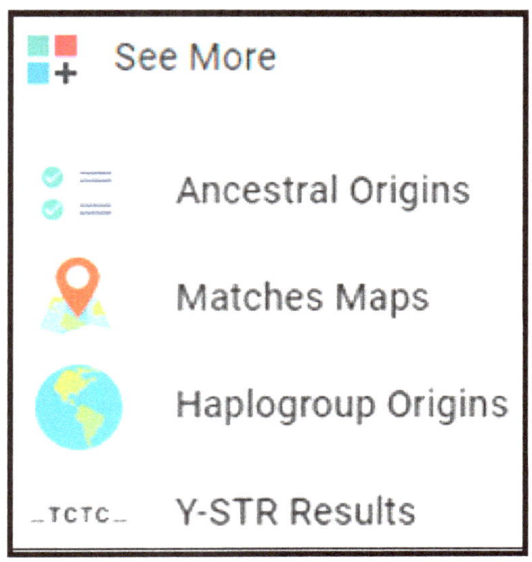

Your marker values appear by panel, under the marker name, but these values are only useful and relevant when compared to other testers.

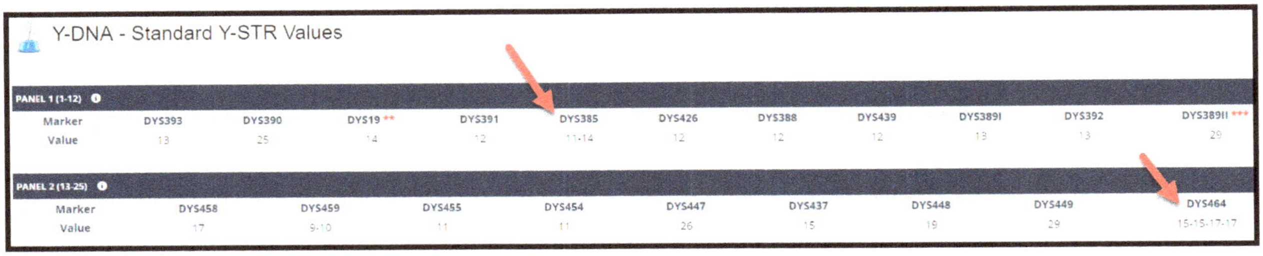

There is no hidden or inherent meaning in the numbers themselves. Some markers have two (or more) values, like DYS385, which shows a result of 11-14. Treat these as normal marker values. The only difference is in how they are counted if you don't match,[50] but you don't need to worry about those details because FamilyTreeDNA calculates matches using the same criteria for everyone.

The gold is in your matches.

Y-DNA Matches

Y-DNA Matches is the button you are looking for.

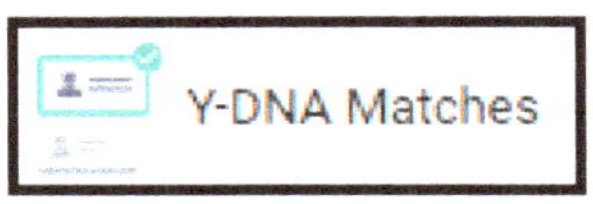
Y-DNA Matches

Your matches will be shown at several different testing levels that can be selected across the top. In this case, my Estes cousin has 32 STR matches at 111 markers, displayed in closest to most distant match order.

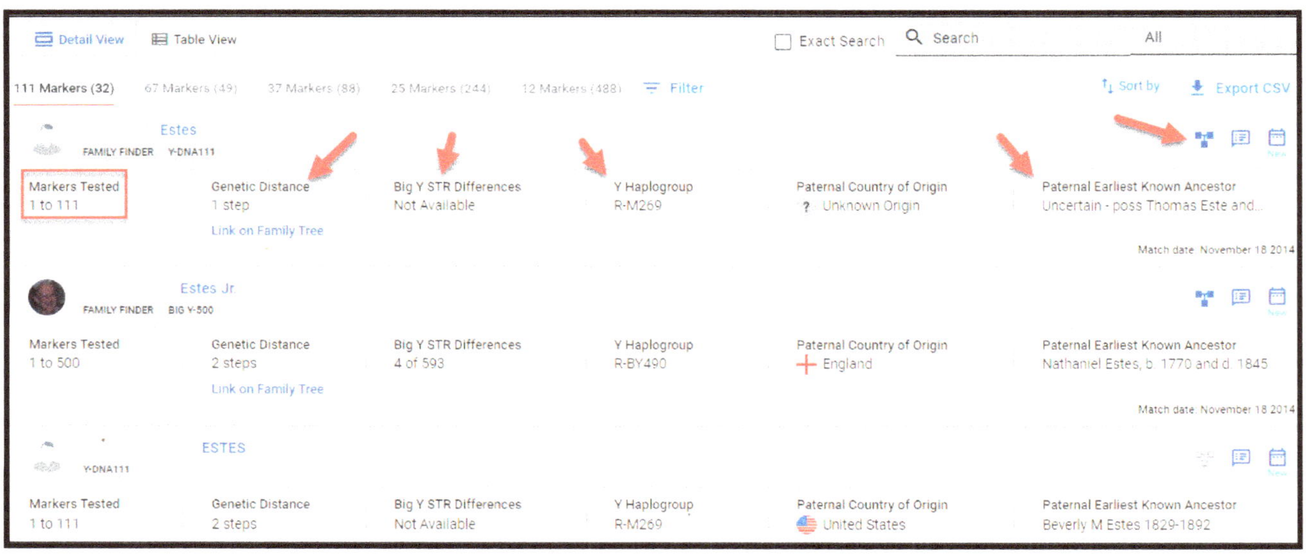
Detail View
Table View
Exact Search
Search
All
111 Markers (32)
67 Markers (49)
37 Markers (88)
25 Markers (244)
12 Markers (488)
Filter
Sort by
Export CSV
Estes
FAMILY FINDER Y-DNA111
Markers Tested 1 to 111
Genetic Distance 1 step
Link on Family Tree
Big Y STR Differences Not Available
Y Haplogroup R-M269
Paternal Country of Origin ? Unknown Origin
Paternal Earliest Known Ancestor Uncertain - poss Thomas Este and...
Match date November 18 2014
Estes Jr.
FAMILY FINDER BIG Y-500
Markers Tested 1 to 500
Genetic Distance 2 steps
Link on Family Tree
Big Y STR Differences 4 of 593
Y Haplogroup R-BY490
Paternal Country of Origin England
Paternal Earliest Known Ancestor Nathaniel Estes, b. 1770 and d. 1845
Match date November 18 2014
ESTES
Y-DNA111
Markers Tested 1 to 111
Genetic Distance 2 steps
Big Y STR Differences Not Available
Y Haplogroup R-M269
Paternal Country of Origin United States
Paternal Earliest Known Ancestor Beverly M Estes 1829-1892

50 https://dna-explained.com/2016/07/27/y-dna-match-changes-at-family-tree-dna-affect-genetic-distance/

Whether two men match or not is determined by markers 1-111. If they do not match at one of these levels, they won't show on the STR match list. Two men may match at one testing level and not match at another depending on where and how many differences are measured between their DNA.

For someone to be listed as your match, they need to have no more than the following total number of mutations different from your results.

Markers in Panel Tested	Maximum Number of Mutations Allowed for a Match
12	0 unless in a common project, then 1
25	2
37	4
67	7
111	10

For example, if you have three mutations in the first 12 markers, as compared to someone else, you won't be listed as a match at that level or at 25 markers. However, if those are still your only three mutations at 37 markers, then you will be listed as a match at the 37-marker level.

Each testing level has its own match threshold,[51] and the number of mismatches is known as Genetic Distance.[52] A Genetic Distance of "2 steps" means you have two mismatches with that person at the level you're viewing.

The haplogroup of your match is shown, as is their Country of Origin and that all-important Paternal Earliest Known Ancestor. That's why it's important to enter the names and locations of your ancestors.

Don't neglect that little pedigree icon, shown below on the bottom left. If it's darkened, that means your match has a tree. Everyone loves matches with testers who have either created or uploaded their trees.

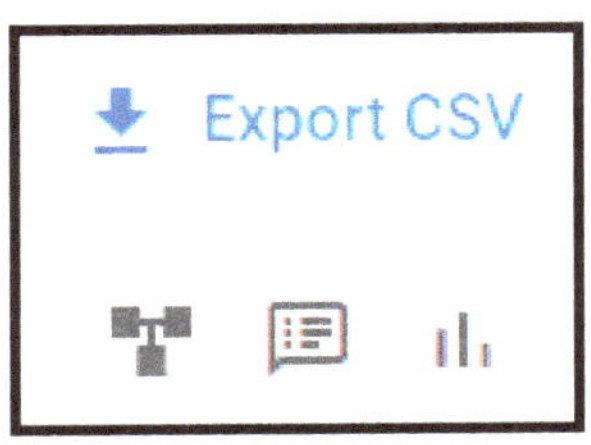

You can download your list of matches by clicking on the "Export CSV," at upper right.

51 https://help.familytreedna.com/hc/en-us/articles/4408063356303-Y-STR-Results-Guide-

52 https://dna-explained.com/2016/06/29/concepts-genetic-distance/

You can also switch to Table View for a more compact display, as shown below.

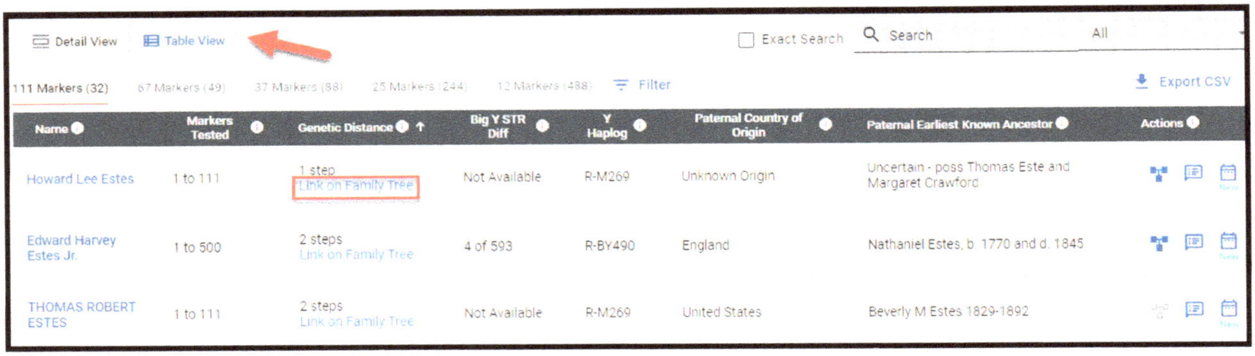
Detail View
Table View
Exact Search
Search
All
111 Markers (32)
67 Markers (49)
37 Markers (88)
25 Markers (244)
12 Markers (488)
Filter
Export CSV
Name
Markers Tested
Genetic Distance
Big Y STR Diff
Y Haplog
Paternal Country of Origin
Paternal Earliest Known Ancestor
Actions
Howard Lee Estes
1 to 111
1 step
Link on Family Tree
Not Available
R-M269
Unknown Origin
Uncertain - poss Thomas Este and Margaret Crawford
Edward Harvey Estes Jr.
1 to 500
2 steps
Link on Family Tree
4 of 593
R-BY490
England
Nathaniel Estes, b. 1770 and d. 1845
THOMAS ROBERT ESTES
1 to 111
2 steps
Link on Family Tree
Not Available
R-M269
United States
Beverly M Estes 1829-1892

TIP: To view additional information, including the email address for your match, click on their name to display their profile card.

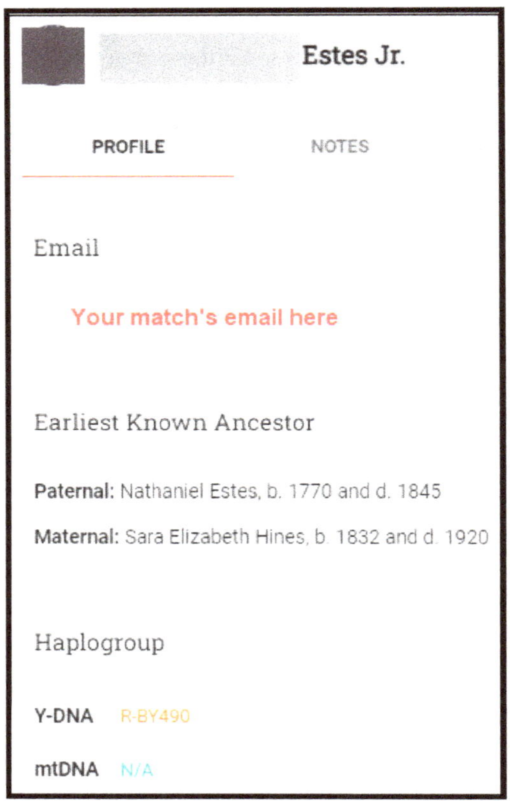

Genetic Distance

Genetic Distance[53] simply means the number of mutations difference between you and another tester at a specific level of testing. It does NOT mean generations, a common misconception.

A smaller number of genetic distance steps = better, and generally means a closer, more meaningful match.

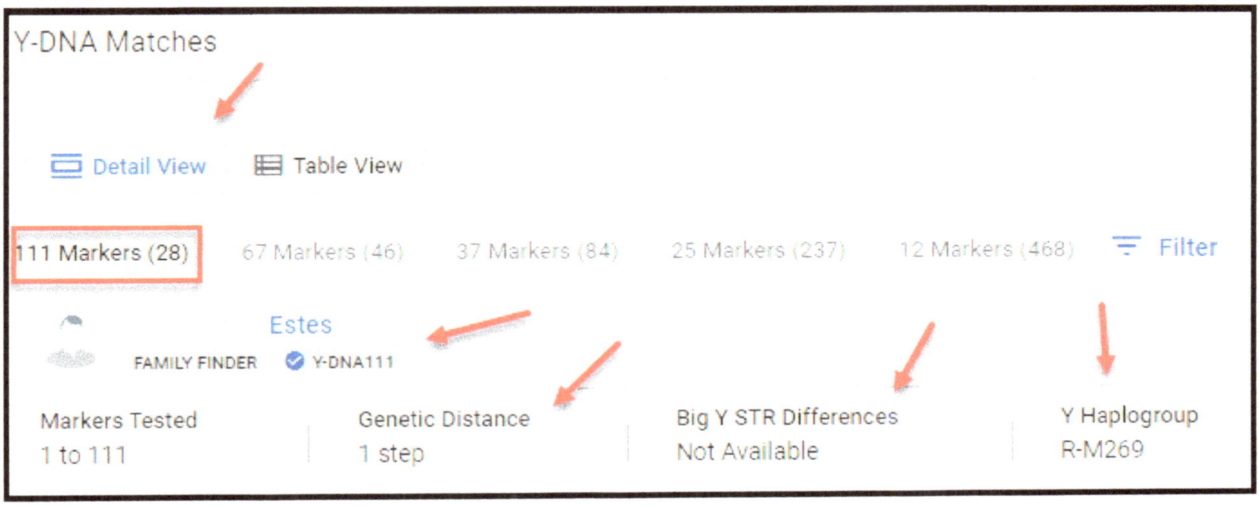

A genetic distance of "1 step" means these men mismatch by a value of one at one marker location. Genetic Distance for "Big Y STR Differences" is calculated separately for the markers above 111 that are tested only in the Big Y. Men who have not taken the Big Y test won't have any value available, of course.

Generally, each mutation is counted as 1 step, meaning a genetic distance of 1.

However, there are some exceptions in how steps are calculated.

For example, in some cases, multi-copy markers that have more than one value are scored differently.[54]

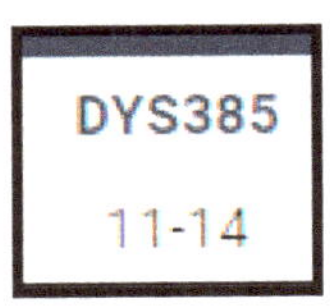

TIP: Marker scoring can be very technical. My advice is to simply utilize the information provided by FamilyTreeDNA, understanding that they are using the same criteria for everyone. If you want to get down in the weeds, I've written several articles,[55] found in the footnotes.[56] You can also read the articles on the Y-DNA Resource page.[57]

---

53 https://dna-explained.com/2016/06/29/concepts-genetic-distance/

54 https://dna-explained.com/2016/07/27/y-dna-match-changes-at-family-tree-dna-affect-genetic-distance/

55 https://dna-explained.com/2018/12/13/big-y-500-str-matching/

56 https://dna-explained.com/2019/01/30/the-big-y-test-increases-again-to-big-y-700/

57 https://dna-explained.com/y-dna-resources/

How Can I View My Matches' Marker Values?

Genetic Distance tells you how closely you match, but it doesn't tell you the values of your markers when compared to each other.

For example, three men can match each other at a Genetic Distance of 1, and all 3 men mismatch each other on a different marker. On the other hand, you can mismatch two men at a distance of 1, and they match each other on the marker where they both mismatch you. They both are a GD of 1 to you, but they match each other exactly.

In order to sort men into family lines using STR markers, you need to know both how closely people match, and the values on mismatching markers.

You can't see other people's marker values on your match page, but you can if your matches have joined DNA projects.

Viewing the public Estes DNA Project[58], I can see all of the STR values of the men in the project from markers 1-111 on the Y-DNA Classic or Y-DNA Colorized Reports page. I'm only displaying a few of those values below.

Kit Number	Name	Paternal Ancestor Name	Country	Haplogroup	DYS393	DYS390	DYS19	DYS391	DYS385		DYS426	DYS388	DYS439	DYS389i	DYS392	DYS389ii
Estes 10 - Abraham - Sylvester 1684-1754 Bertie and Granville Co., NC																
199378	Estes	George Washington Estes, abt. 1845 - 1923	United States	R-BY490	13	25	14	11	11	14	12	12	12	13	13	29
17420	Estes	Abe b 1647, Sylvester, Thomas, Thomas, Burroughs	England	R-M269	13	25	14	11	11	15	12	12	12	13	13	29
13805	Estes	Nathaniel Estes, b. 1770 and d. 1845	England	R-BY490	13	25	14	12	11	14	12	12	12	13	13	29
Estes 2 - Abraham - Elisha b <1700-1782 + Mary Ann Mumford, Henry Co., Va.																
B68177	Estess	William Estes, b. 1800 and d. 1889	United States	R-M269	13	25	14	12	11	14	12	12	12	13	13	29
14381	Estes	Uncertain - poss Thomas Este and Margaret Crawford	Unknown Origin	R-M269	13	25	14	12	11	14	12	12	12	13	13	29
249475	Estes	Nicolas Ewstas, b. 1495 and d. 1533/4	England	R-M269	13	25	14	12	11	15	12	12	12	13	13	29

As the volunteer project administrator, I've divided Estes testers into genealogical lines based on which son of Abraham, the immigrant, they descend from.

Let's use the values of two markers as an example.

All of the markers except DYS391 and the second value of DYS385, bracketed in red, match. Within the Estes family line, the matching marker values aren't of interest genealogically. The value is in the mismatching markers that will, hopefully, define lineages.

The testers mismatch on those two markers, so let's look for consistency between their values. Three men descend from Abraham's son, Sylvester, and three descend from his son, Elisha.

58 https://www.familytreedna.com/public/Estes?iframe=yresults

Kit #	Son of Abraham	DYS391	DYS385 (2nd value)	Comment
199378	Sylvester>George	11	14	
17420	Sylvester>Abe	11	**15**	Mutated to 15 once in both Sylvester's and Elisha's line
13805	Sylvester>Nathaniel	**12**	14	Value of 12 found in Elisha's line and once in Sylvester's line
B68177	Elisha>William	**12**	14	
14381	Elisha>possibly Thomas	**12**	14	
249475	Elisha>Joel	**12**	**15**	

For marker DYS391, the "normal" or ancestral value for the Estes DNA project[59], meaning found in the majority of Abraham's sons' lines, is 12. This marker appears to have mutated twice in Sylvester's line, through two different sons, to 11, but not in Sylvester's line through Nathaniel.

However, there's a problem.

- If Sylvester **himself** had a value of 11, then he would have given **ALL** three of his sons 11 copies. George and Abe received 11 copies, but Nathaniel's descendants have 12. Did Sylvester actually have a value of 11, and it back-mutated to 12 in Nathaniel's line?
- In the reverse situation, if Sylvester had a value of 12, then two of his sons' lines independently mutated to 11.
- Either way, this is not a dependable marker in this family.

We find the same type of situation for DYS426 where 14 is the Estes ancestral value, or norm, and a value of 15 has occurred twice independently in both Sylvester's and Elisha's lines.

This type of conflicting data makes it impossible to group men conclusively, especially those without proven genealogy, using STR values alone.[60] It's exactly this reason that genealogists have turned to the much more stable SNPs through the Big Y test.

---

59 https://www.familytreedna.com/groups/estes/dna-results

60 https://dna-explained.com/2022/11/05/the-ancestors-are-speaking-an-18-year-y-dna-study-that-led-us-home-52-ancestors-381/

Earliest Known Ancestors and Trees

Don't forget about the Earliest Known Ancestor (EKA) field and country locations. In addition to individual matches and projects, the Discover™ tool, Globetrekker, the Time Tree, and the Group Time Tree all use this information.

Abraham - Abraham Jr. c 1697-1759 + Ann Watkins and Elizbaeth Jeeter, Caroline Co., Va.			
92743	Estes		Unknown Origin
45614	Estes		Unknown Origin
46167	Estes	Abraham Jr 1697-1759 m Ann Clark, Phillip bef 1720	Unknown Origin
43144	Estes	Abraham Jr 1697-1759 m Ann Clark, Phillip bef 1720	Unknown Origin
51909	Estes	Thomas Estes	United Kingdom
49592	Estes	Abraham Jr 1697-1759 m Ann Clark, Samuel b 1727	England
Abraham - Elisha b <1700-1782 + Mary Ann Mumford, Henry Co., Va.			
14495	Estes	Abraham b 1647, Elisha d 1782 m Mary Ann Mumford	England
19696	Estes	Henry Estes b 1874 in Orange Co Va	Unknown Origin

For men who don't know the identity of their Estes ancestor[61], the EKA field of their matches, or trees, or a combination of both, can indicate exactly where they need to search.

TIP: The EKA and the tester's tree may not contain the same information. Some people complete one or the other, but not both. Always check both.

Of course, you can always email your matches and ask about their genealogy.

The EKA and trees are especially useful if a unique STR marker sequence or unique haplogroup defines their specific lineage.

Estes 2 - Abraham - Elisha b <1700-1782 + Mary Ann Mumford, Henry Co., Va.				
B8468	Estes	Robert Estes, b. 1475 and d. 1506	Engl[illegible]	R-P312
14495	Estes	abraham estes	England	R-DF49
19696	Estes	Henry Estes b 1874 in Orange Co Va	Unknown Origin	R-M269
201191	Estes		Unknown Origin	R-M269
235224	Estes		Unknown Origin	R-M269
14381	Estes	Uncertain - poss Thomas Este and Margaret Crawford	Unknown Origin	R-M269
29843	Coffey		Ireland	R-M269
244708	Estes	Nicholas Ewstas b 1495 Deal, Kent, England	England	R-BY490

Looking at the group for Elisha, son of Abraham, in the Estes DNA project, you can see that there are four haplogroups. R-M269 is colored red because it's predicted using STR results and not confirmed by SNP testing. The three haplogroups in green are more specific and are confirmed by SNP testing of some type. In this case, SNP testing could mean the purchase of one confirming SNP, an obsolete SNP-based test type that's no longer offered, a SNP Pack, or one of the Big Y tests. Now that the Big Y-700 test is available, we no longer recommend purchasing either individual SNPs or SNP Packs. Big Y test results are always the most specific and are automatically updated as new information is discovered.

61 https://dna-explained.com/2016/11/16/concepts-undocumented-adoptions-vs-untested-y-lines/

As the project administrator, I know that haplogroup R-BY490 is a result of Big Y-700 testing, but if a man matched kit 244708, he would be able to determine which test was taken by noting the "tests taken" beneath the name, or the "markers tested," on the Y-DNA matches page as shown below.

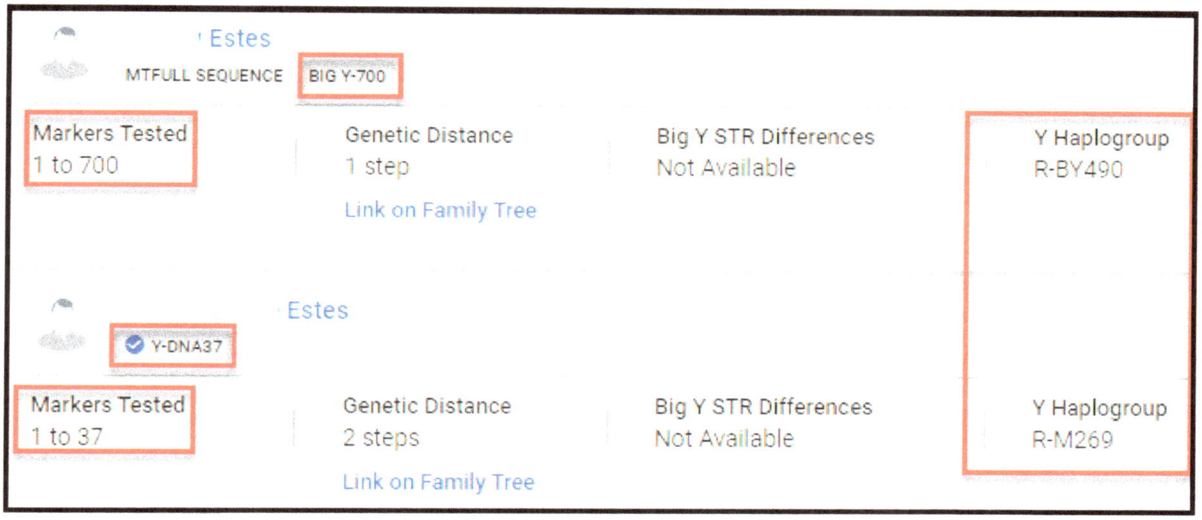
Estes
MTFULL SEQUENCE
BIG Y-700
Markers Tested
1 to 700
Genetic Distance
1 step
Link on Family Tree
Big Y STR Differences
Not Available
Y Haplogroup
R-BY490
Estes
Y-DNA37
Markers Tested
1 to 37
Genetic Distance
2 steps
Link on Family Tree
Big Y STR Differences
Not Available
Y Haplogroup
R-M269

The other two haplogroups that are confirmed, R-P312 and R-DF49, are below R-M269 on the haplotree, but far above R-BY490. These participants purchased SNP packs or individual SNPs many years ago.

Using the Discover™ Ancestral Path for Haplogroup R-BY490[62], focusing on the haplogroups shown in Elisha's project grouping, we can see the time difference in Big Y-discovered SNPs versus individually purchased and confirmed SNPs, as compared to STR-predicted haplogroups.

Haplogroup	Step in Tree	Haplogroup Age Estimate
R-BY490	1 (for this tester)	1650 CE
R-BY482 - Parent haplogroup for Estes men	2	1500 CE
R-DF49	12	2350 BCE (~4350 years ago)
R-P312	18	2850 BCE (~4850 years ago)
R-M269	23	4350 BCE (~6350 years ago)
A-PR2921 Y-Adam	49	232,000 BCE (~234,000 years ago)

If these R-M269 Estes men or those who have confirmed individual SNPs were to all take the Big Y-700[63] test, they assuredly would all fall, at minimum, into haplogroup R-BY490 or its upstream parent haplogroup. It's probable that some of them would form a new haplogroup within the Elisha Estes line based on their Private Variants, which are mutations that no one else in their line yet matches.

62 https://discover.familytreedna.com/y-dna/R-BY490/path

63 At some point in the future, the Big Y-700 may be replaced by a newer test. The Big Y-700 refers to the most current Y-DNA test available.

Haplotree and SNPs

The Haplotree & SNPs page displays a SNP tree similar to the Public Tree, including a Country and Surname Report.

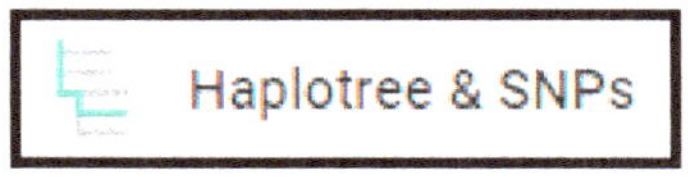

The difference is that this tree not only shows every SNP, but whether the tester is positive or negative for the reference value, or whether the SNP has no results.

TIP: If you have already taken the Big Y test, do NOT purchase a SNP Pack or individual SNPs if they are offered on this tree. Your entire Y chromosome has already been scanned. Before purchasing any individual SNPs, contact FamilyTreeDNA support to discuss your goals. The Big Y-700 is a much more cost-effective and useful product.

If you have not taken the Big Y-700 test, you're much better off taking or upgrading to a Big Y test which tests all SNPs instead of purchasing individual SNPs or bundles of SNPs that only move your test part way down the tree.

Furthermore, SNP tests only test known SNPs, while the Big Y is a test of discovery, revealing previously unknown SNP mutations that create new, individual haplotree branches.

The Haplotree & SNPs page shows:

- The tester's location on the haplotree, indicated by the grey bar
- Upstream and downstream branches
- The test results of each SNP
    - Positive (green)
    - Presumed positive (orange) because downstream SNPs are positive
    - Negative (red)
    - Presumed negative (grey) because SNPs above it are negative, or there are positive SNPs on collateral branch
    - Downstream (blue, at bottom) SNPs below your lowest positive result, but for which you were not tested, so they cannot be accurately presumed negative or positive
- Equivalent SNPs or Variants, at right, may one day become separate branches of the tree. Equivalent SNPS are the opposite of private variants where no one else matches that mutation. Equivalent SNPs occur when everyone in that haplogroup has the same multiple SNPs. The haplogroup is formed and named after one SNP location. Eventually, men with only some of these variants may split the branch.

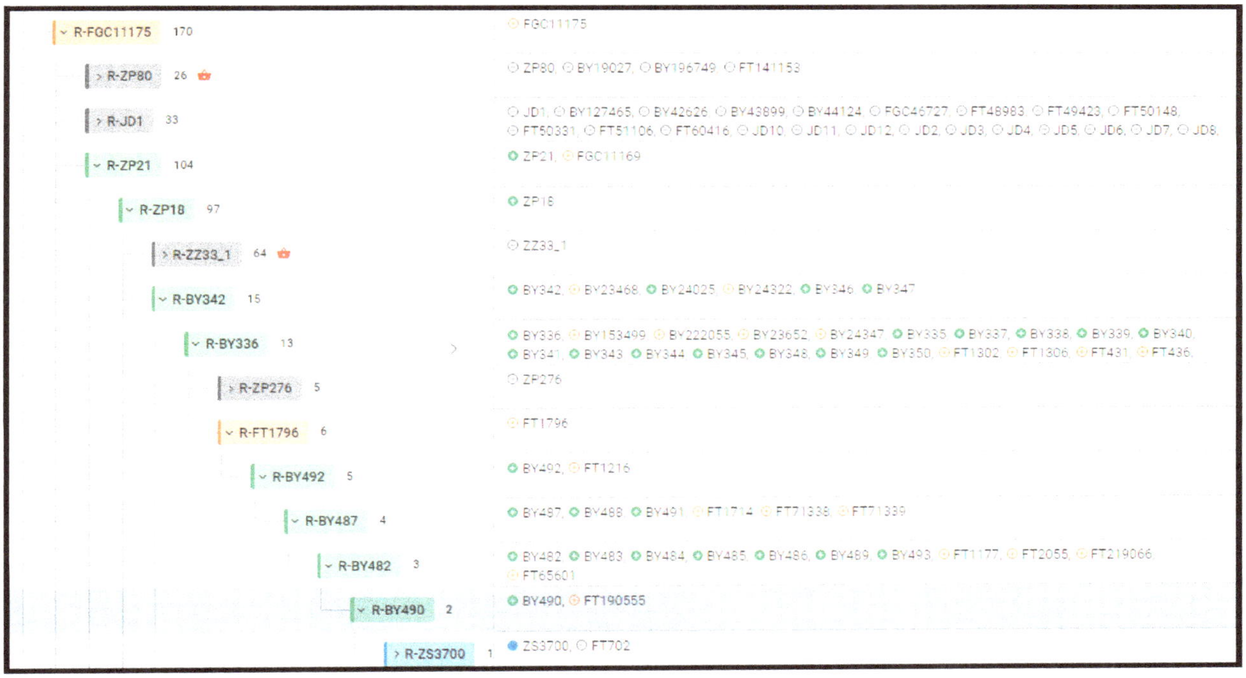

While R-BY490, above, has only two equivalent variants, R-M269, a very common predicted European haplogroup, shows 24,613 downstream branches and a total of 97 equivalent variants.

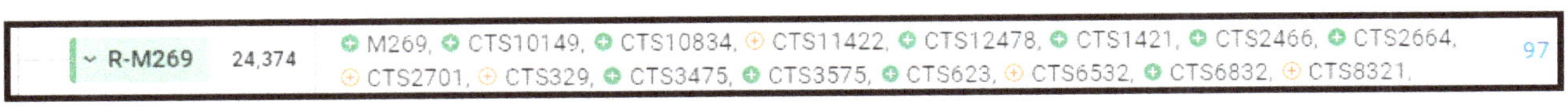

Those 97 equivalent variants are just waiting to become their own branch one day when a group of men emerge who have some of those variants but not others, or have additional, branch-defining variants.

Haplogroups are assigned in one of five ways:

- A high-level haplogroup is reliably predicted with any level of STR testing.
- Individual SNP testing
- A somewhat refined haplogroup can be obtained by purchasing SNP packs that test specific locations, although these have fallen out of favor with the advent of the much more specific Big Y tests. The tiny red baskets to the right of R-ZP80 and R-ZZ33_1 indicate that these SNPs are found in a SNP pack.
- Men who take the Family Finder test or upload autosomal tests from some vendors will receive[64] an intermediate-range haplogroup which cannot be used for Y-DNA matching. They would benefit from Y-DNA testing.
- Big Y tests scan the accessible region of the Y chromosome for all mutations, both known and unknown, facilitating the assignment of the most specific haplogroup possible.

64 This feature has been announced but not yet released as of October 2023.

Therefore, the haplogroups for some men won't match, but the mismatch is a function of the test type or level. They might not match exactly because there is one mutation difference, and it forms a new haplogroup with another man. Haplogroups do not have to match exactly to be meaningful and useful.

TIP: To see how closely related two haplogroups are, use Discover's haplogroup Compare tool that facilitates the comparison of any two haplogroups, providing the path between the haplogroups to a common ancestral haplogroup, as well as the time to the most recent common ancestor (TMRCA).[65]

Haplogroups of men in the Estes project might match if they tested at the Big Y-700 level. Testers can view the testing level of their matches on the Matches page.

In addition to the Variants view, the Haplotree & SNP page offers three other views by selecting the option in the dropdown menu in the upper left corner of the page.

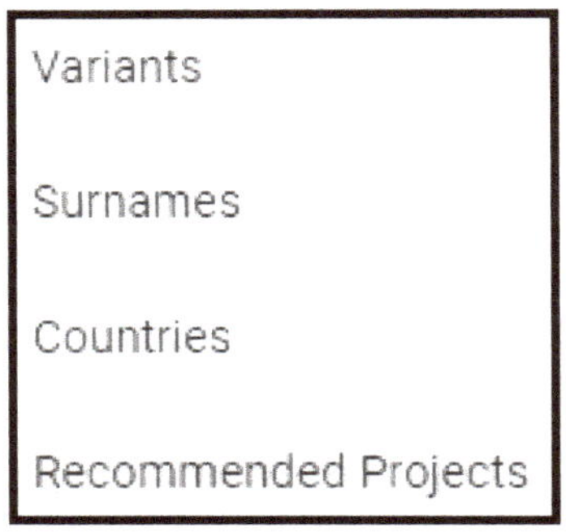

- Associated surnames (when public, and when two or more testers on the same branch have the exact same surname spelling)

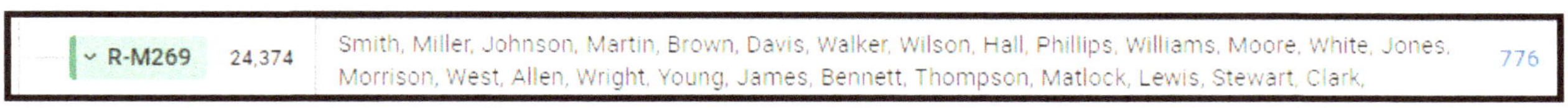

- Associated countries

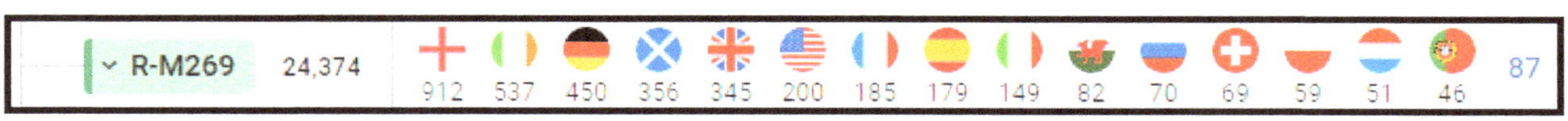

- Associated haplogroup projects listed at their proper place in the tree

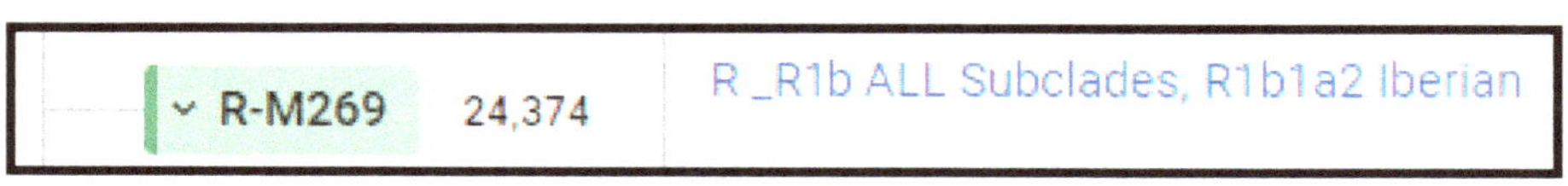

Of course, these large numbers in haplogroup R-M269, which is often predicted for STR testers, is exactly why people upgrade to the Big Y test – refinement!

Big Y testers will be tested for all known SNPs. Additionally, previously unknown mutations, called Private Variants, are often discovered, leading to new, more granular, and lineage-specific haplogroups. Private Variants are discussed in the Big Y section.

65 https://dna-explained.com/2023/10/11/new-discover-tool-compare-haplogroups-more-at-familytreedna/

SNP Data Download

To download your SNP results, navigate to the Haplogroup & SNPs page, where you can select "SNP Results" to view or download a file of your SNP test results. If you have done more than one type of SNP testing, the test type will be listed next to it, whether it was a test type no longer offered, a Genographic Project 2.0 transfer, an individual SNP or SNP pack, Big Y-500, or Big Y-700.

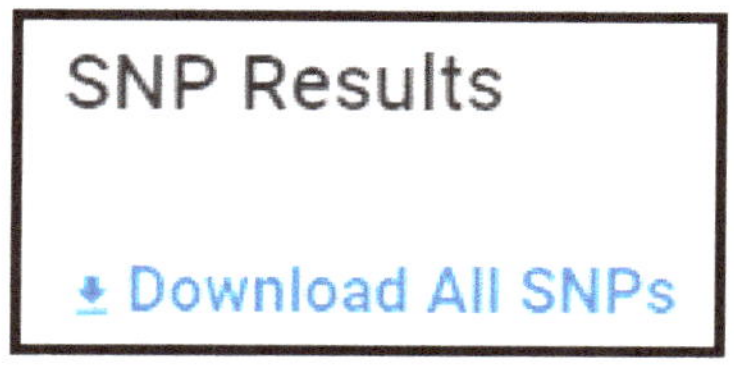

Public Y Haplotree

The Public Y haplotree is free for everyone at FamilyTreeDNA, whether you have tested there or not. The link can be found in the footer at the very, VERY bottom of every page

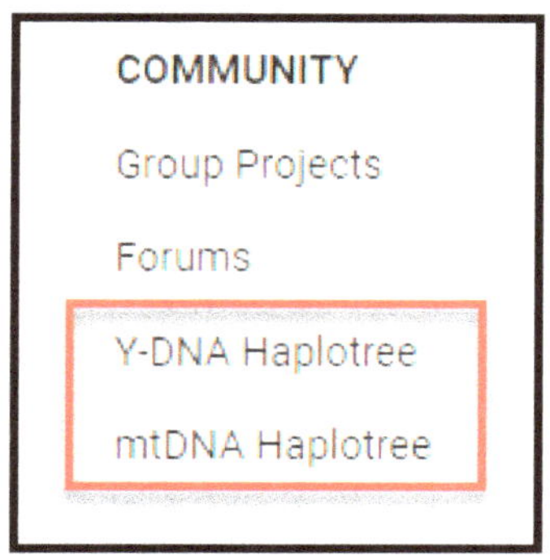

If you have taken a DNA test of any type, the Public Haplotree is also available on your personal page under "Other Tools."

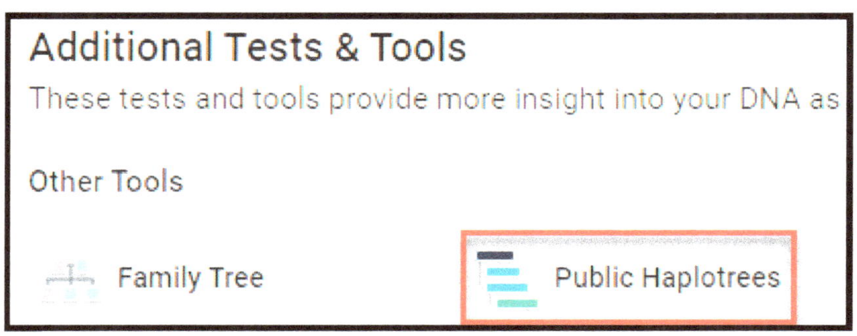

I particularly like the Public Haplotree,[66] because it includes:

- Information for everyone in a given haplogroup, not just the people you match.
- Country flags
- Country Report
- Surname Report

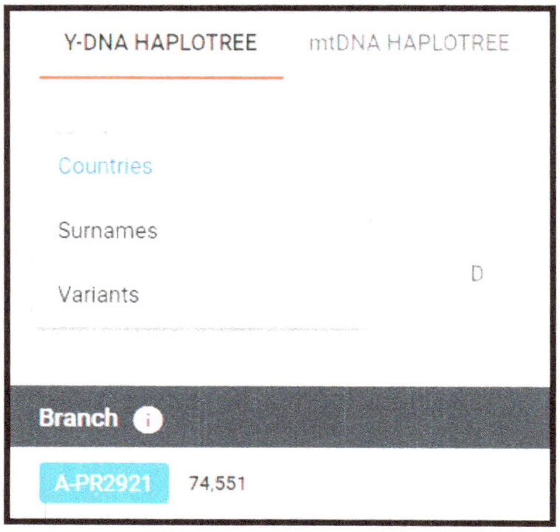

Use the dropdown menu in the upper left corner to choose the view you wish to see.

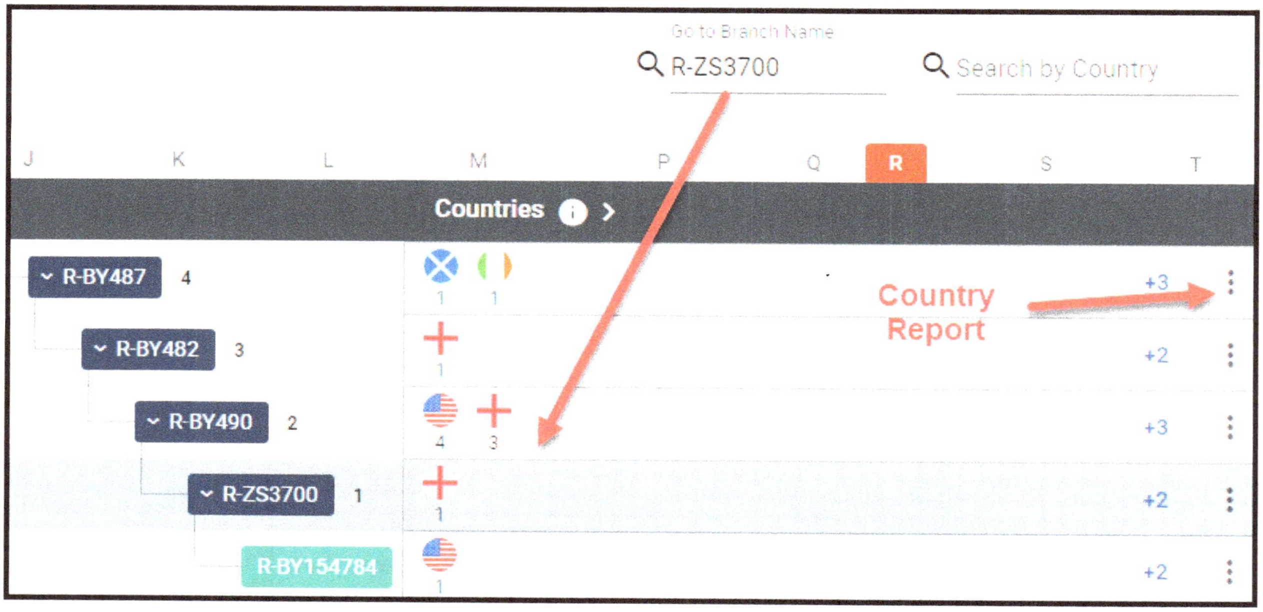

66 https://dna-explained.com/2018/09/27/family-tree-dnas-public-y-dna-haplotree/

The Public Tree includes self-reported locations, displayed as flags, for people assigned to that haplogroup based on their ancestor's earliest known location. At the tips of the haplogroup branches, there will be few men, comparatively speaking, but as you work your way up the tree, there will be many more people assigned within the parent haplogroups, and you won't match all of them on your personal page.[67]

"Walking" your haplogroup back in time in the tree suggests possible migration and settlement patterns. For Big Y testers, Globetrekker[68] literally does walk your haplogroup across the globe - tracing your ancestor's specific path.[69]

The Country Report is available on all views under the three dots (hamburger menu) with details about where that specific haplogroup is found, along with how many downstream branches exist.

The Surname Report provides a list of surnames when they are available, but keep in mind those surnames are ONLY for people with this specific haplogroup with two or more men bearing the same spelling of a surname. If there are three men on a branch, and each has a different variant spelling, none of those variants will appear. If two have the same spelling and the third doesn't, two will show with that specific spelling. For example, if one has Estes, one has Estis, and one has Estice, none of those variants will appear. If two have Estes and one has Estis, the Estes name will show.

If men have a more refined confirmed haplogroup, their surname is reported under their end-of-line haplogroup. The end-of-line haplogroup used to be called the "terminal SNP," meaning the SNP furthest down the tree for which the man has been predicted or tested positive, but that phrase has fallen out of favor.

TIP: The end-of-line haplogroup is the most refined, or closest in time to the present, haplogroup for a given man, based on his testing level. R-M269 could be the end-of-line haplogroup for a man who has only taken the STR tests, but his father or brother could have a much different, and much more recent haplogroup if they have taken the Big Y-700 test. The Big Y test provides the most refined haplogroup possible for any man's end-of-line haplogroup and Family Finder intermediate-level haplogroups fall someplace in the middle.

TIP: Remember, the Public Haplotree and Haplogroup & SNPs pages ONLY show SNP-confirmed testers. These haplotrees do not include people whose haplogroup is predicted, meaning they have only taken an STR test.

Keep in mind when viewing a SNP significantly above lower branches in the haplotree, like R-DF49, there's a good possibility that the people listed have not taken the Big Y test, so this is not representative of that entire surname branch. If you see a surname of interest, check the corresponding Surname Project to see if other related men have taken more comprehensive tests, and where they are placed on the tree.

67 Currently, you will match another Big Y tester if you have 30 or fewer mismatches. If you have more than 30 SNP differences, you will not match. The matching threshold could change in the future.

68 https://discover.familytreedna.com/y-dna/R-ZS3700/globetrekker

69 https://dna-explained.com/2023/08/04/globetrekker-a-new-feature-for-big-y-customers-from-familytreedna/

Surname Report: Y-DNA Haplogroup R-DF49

Surname	Participants	Distribution
Barriskill	4	14.29%
Hopkins	4	14.29%
Estes	3	10.71%
Mylrea	3	10.71%
Stewart	3	10.71%
Blair	3	10.71%
Kendall	2	7.14%
Davis	2	7.14%
Johnson	2	7.14%
Conkin	2	7.14%
Total	**28**	**100.00%**

* All surnames are self-reported by the participants and may not reflect accurate haplogroup ancestry.

** Two or more kits with public project profile sharing and the same surname spelling are required for a surname to show on the Haplotree.

For men with these surnames, R-DF49 is their terminal SNP, meaning the SNP furthest down on the tree that has tested positive for these men. Given the level of testing available today, it's very unlikely that any of these men have taken the Big Y test, and if they did, R-DF49 would assuredly NOT be their own personal end-of-branch SNP.

TIP: While the end-of-line is the closest or youngest SNP in time confirmed for a man, the end-of-branch SNP is the most refined SNP possible for him, were he to take the Big Y-700 test. A man with Private Variants may yet have a new haplogroup waiting in the wings, so today's end-of-branch haplogroup may not be tomorrow's end-of-branch haplogroup for men who take the evergreen Big Y test. Think of the end-of-branch haplogroup as your own personal leaf on your branch or twig of the tree.

Three Estes men are listed with a confirmed haplogroup of R-DF49 as a result of Family Finder haplogroup assignments.

If a man with a particular surname isn't shown with a specific haplogroup, like R-DF49, it could be because:

- Men who have only taken STR tests aren't shown because they have taken no SNP-confirmed tests.
- No men of that surname have purchased the R-DF49 SNP individually or in a SNP pack where R-DF49 was the terminal SNP.

- A minimum of two men have not taken a test that confirmed SNPs, tested positive for this SNP as their end-of-line SNP test, **and** opted in for public project display.
- Men by that surname have that SNP but have taken the Big Y test and are placed several branches further downstream.

Matches Maps

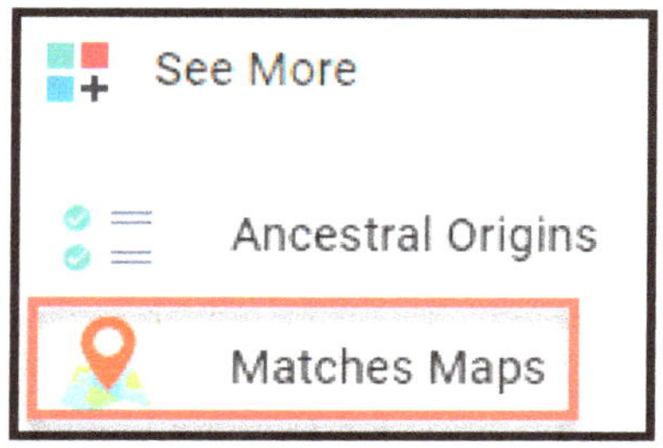

Match locations provide critical clues about common ancestors!

Your Matches Map is displayed by match level and includes matches who have entered geographic locations for their earliest known ancestors (EKA.)

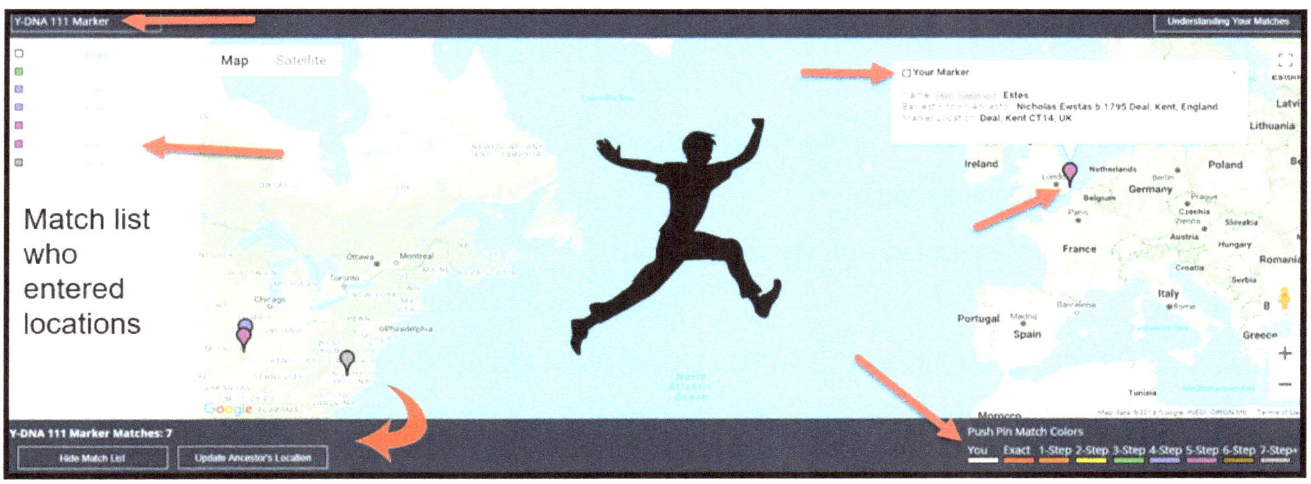

Your pin will be white unless it's obscured by matches in the exact same location, which is the case with the Estes matches in Deal, Kent, England.

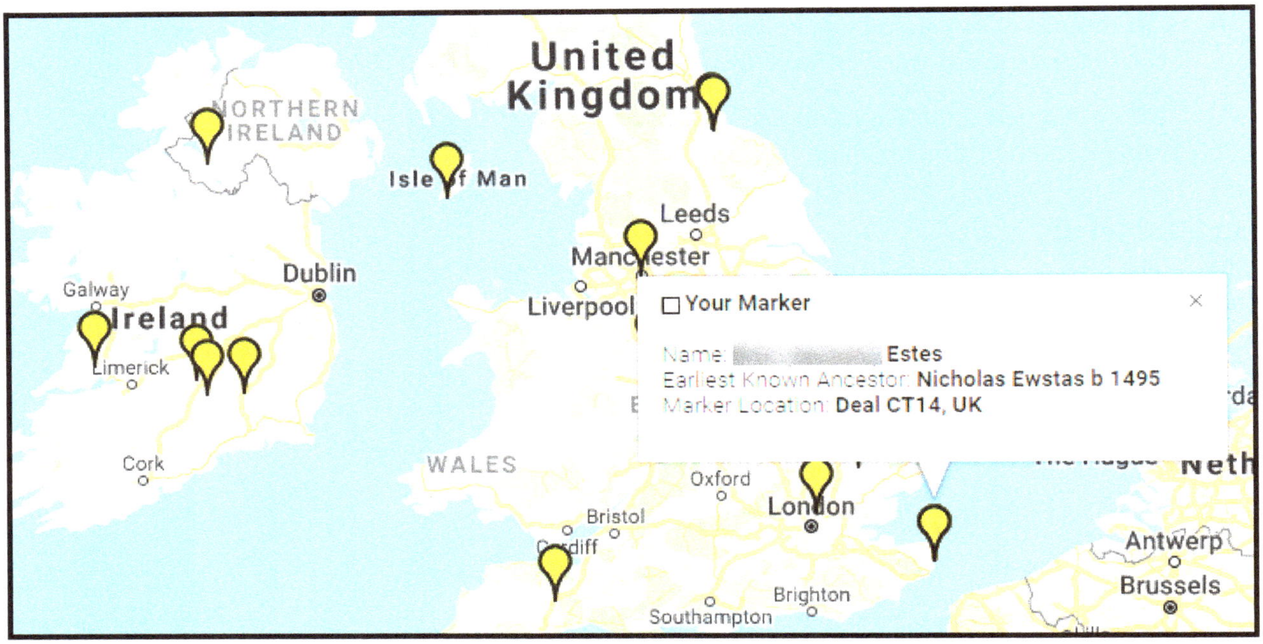

The pins are color-coded based on the number of mutations difference, or genetic distance. Exact matches, with a genetic distance of zero, are the closest.

Click on the name on the match list to "go to" their pin.

Of course, the first thing to ask is, "Who are the neighbors?" What might you have in common?

What other surnames do you match?

What history might be associated with those surnames?

Or locations?

Next, let's see what kind of hints we can find in Ancestral Origins.

Ancestral Origins

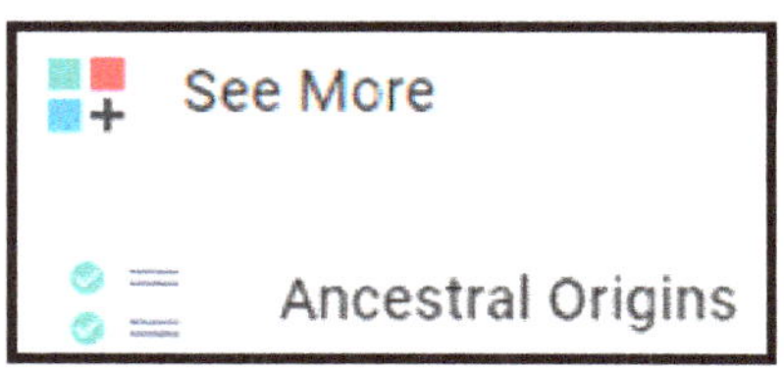

FamilyTreeDNA compiles the location information provided by your matches about their ancestors.

For some people, the information is fairly vanilla, but for others, it can be informative, especially any comments.

In this case, the comments indicate that several testers' ancestors from different locations were Ashkenazi. The fact that many testers provided the same information lends credence to this information, especially since people generally know if they are or their ancestors were Jewish, or not.

67 Marker

EXACT MATCH				
Country	Match Total	Country Total	Percentage	Comments
Hungary	1	586	0.2%	
Ukraine	1	1411	0.1%	Ashkenazi (1)
GENETIC DISTANCE -1				
Country	Match Total	Country Total	Percentage	Comments
Belarus	2	660	0.3%	Ashkenazi (1)
Lithuania	1	853	0.1%	Ashkenazi (1)
Poland	3	2673	0.1%	Ashkenazi (2)
Ukraine	1	1411	0.1%	Ashkenazi (1)

Sometimes, locations are more confusing.

United States	125	15602	0.8%	MDKO: United States (6)
United States (Native American)	9	1779	0.5%	MDKO: United States (2)

United States does NOT always mean Native American. Generally, it only means that people are brick-walled in the US. However, there is a United States (Native American), United States (Kānaka Maoli) along with a Canada (First Nations) and a Canada (Inuit) flag.

There weren't always specific "Native" or indigenous categories though, and people selected "United States" when they actually meant either "Native," or "unknown." You can't always depend on any particular interpretation of this tester-provided information.

It's not uncommon to discover "Native American" specified for clearly European or other haplogroups. People are recording what they were told, or maybe even just the "side," like "Grandpa's side was Native American." Testers seldom remember to go back and correct this information if they discover something different.

Ancestral origins can be very useful. Just use your judgment and retain your genealogical skepticism. Evaluate everything as pieces of evidence. European haplogroups are not Native American, and "United States" does not necessarily mean "Native American."

Haplogroup Origins

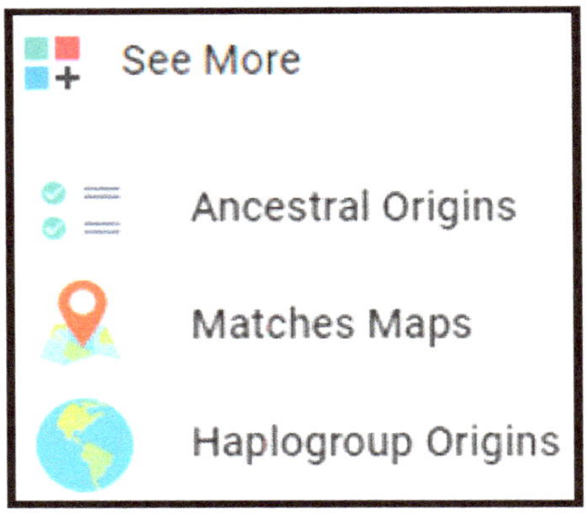

The Haplogroup Origins report provides a composite view of the haplogroups you match, and where they are reported to have originated based on tester-provided information.

111 Marker

Haplogroup	Country	Comments	Match Total
GENETIC DISTANCE -2			
R-BY490	England	-	1
GENETIC DISTANCE -3			
R-BY490	England	-	2
R-BY490	United States	-	1
GENETIC DISTANCE -4			
R-BY154784	United States	-	1
GENETIC DISTANCE -5			
R-BY490		-	1
R-BY490	United States	-	1
GENETIC DISTANCE -7			
R-M269	England	-	1
GENETIC DISTANCE -10			
R-BY482	England	-	1

Genetic Distance is not a predictor of haplogroup, in part, because STRs are much less stable than SNPs.

Haplogroup Origins can reveal location or cultural groups, providing clues as to where you might want to look for your ancestors.

This is particularly important when you have absolutely no idea where your ancestor originated.

These end-of-line/end-of-branch Big Y haplogroups suggest strongly that anyone matching these men should look in England and should also check their matches map!

Of course, our Estes tester has matches to men with R-M269 who have not tested above 111 markers. We know that because had they taken any kind of SNP test, they would have been placed someplace downstream of R-M269.

Big Y Results

The Big Y-700 is the top-of-the-line, highest-resolution explorer-level test for Y chromosome testing.

Like with all DNA tests, the power is in matching against the database, and the more people who test, the better and more refined the results will be for everyone.

You can upgrade from an earlier Y-DNA test to the Big Y, or you can order the Big Y-700 straight out of the gate.

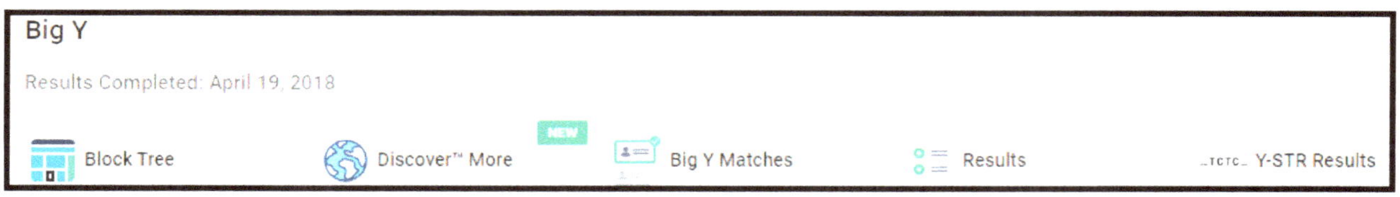

With the Big Y test, you receive:

- All STR features and tools previously described in the STR Results section, plus at least an additional 589 markers, equaling at least 700 STR markers.
- Block Tree – Your place on the haplotree of mankind, with your most refined matches displayed graphically, in tree format.
- Big Y Matches – Men you match with 30 or fewer SNP mutations, or mismatches.
- Results - Named Variants – SNPs that have been named and (probably) placed on the tree.
- Results - Private Variants – SNPs that are private to you, have not been named, so not yet placed on the tree. Private Variants are haplogroups-in-waiting, meaning waiting for another tester on your branch to have the same mutation.
- Results - Y-DNA Chromosome Browsing Tool
- Discover™ Haplogroup Reports – a variety of extensive Y-DNA reports.

Big Y Matches

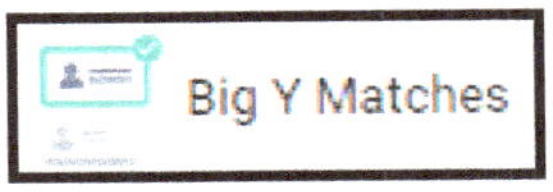

Big Y Matches are men who match you on the SNP portion of the Big Y test and are shown under Big Y Matches. They may or may not match you on the STR panels, depending on how recently your common ancestor lived and how many STR mutations you've each accumulated. STR marker matches are shown under the Y-DNA Matches button discussed previously.

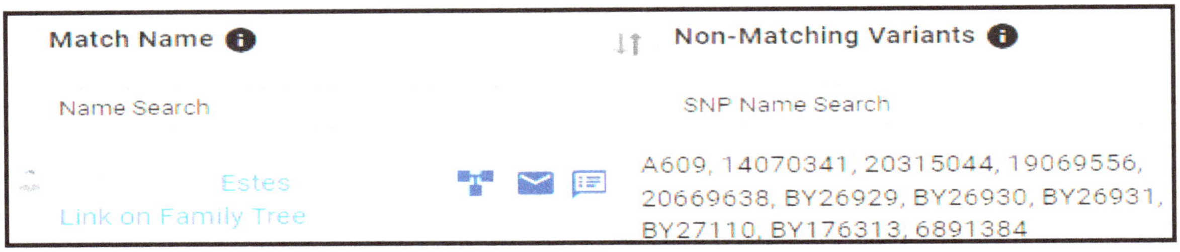

Your match list includes your match's name, a tree icon, the envelope to send an email, a notes field, and Non-Matching Variants, which are locations where you do NOT match these men. This means that you DO match the other SNP locations. Men with 30 or fewer non-matching SNPs will appear on each other's match list.

30 SNP differences equate to roughly 1500 years, which is generally further back than surnames but certainly still relevant.

Thankfully, FamilyTreeDNA curates this information into the Block Tree and into Discover.

Named Variants

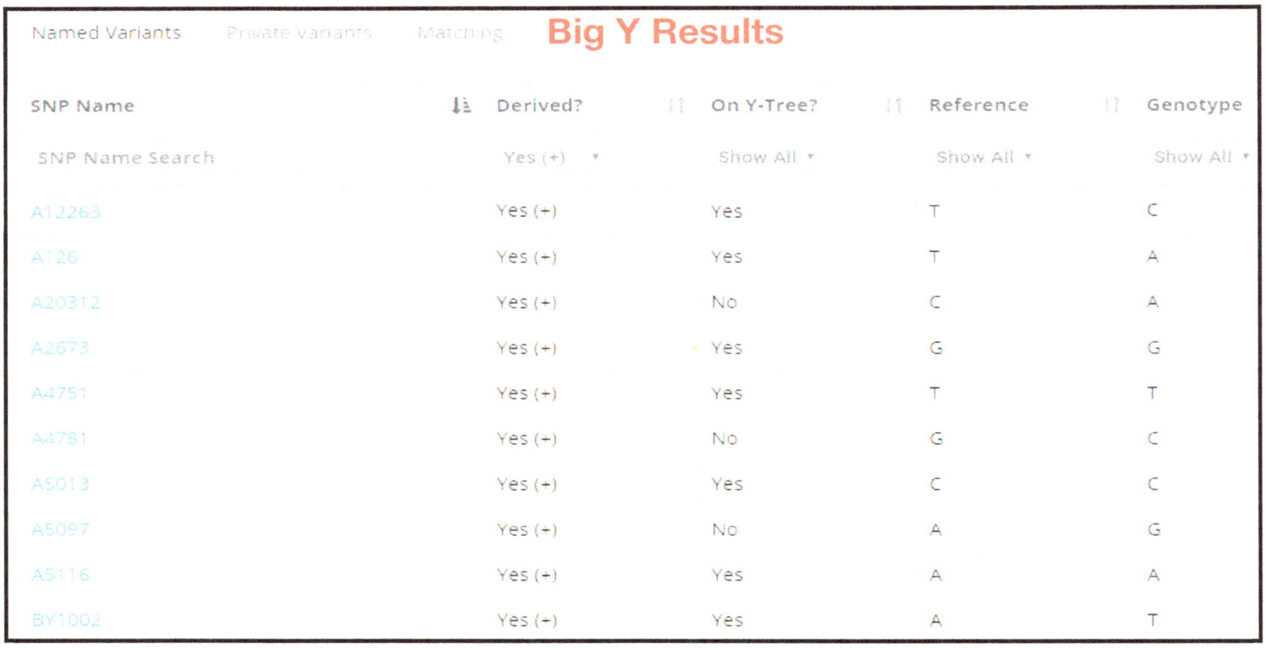

SNP Name	Derived?	On Y-Tree?	Reference	Genotype
SNP Name Search	Yes (+)	Show All	Show All	Show All
A12263	Yes (+)	Yes	T	C
A126	Yes (+)	Yes	T	A
A20312	Yes (+)	No	C	A
A2673	Yes (+)	Yes	G	G
A4751	Yes (+)	Yes	T	T
A4781	Yes (+)	No	G	C
A5013	Yes (+)	Yes	C	C
A5097	Yes (+)	No	A	G
A5116	Yes (+)	Yes	A	A
BY1002	Yes (+)	Yes	A	T

You can view your Named Variants under Big Y Results. Variants, meaning mutations or SNPs, are named when two or more men in the same lineage share that particular variant, assuming it's a quality read. When variants are named, they become potential haplogroup names and are placed on the tree if they pass a quality control review.

- Derived means that you have this mutation.
- Some SNPs are named but not placed on the tree because of quality issues, so don't be concerned if you see a named SNP but it's not on the tree. Since it has a name, it has been evaluated but did not meet the criteria for inclusion.
- The Reference value is the T, A, C, or G in that position in the human genome reference model, and the Genotype is the value you have at this location.
- Private Variants are mutations, or variants, that have not yet been named, either because no one else in this same line has that mutation, the line as a whole has not been reviewed recently, or it's unreliable.

Weeds Alert: In the interest of accuracy, I need to cover something at such a painful level of detail that it's very down-in-the-weeds. If you don't want to root around in the weeds, just skip this short Down in the Weeds section. Or keep reading, since you never know when you're going to need to know this for Trivia!

Down in the Weeds

Did you notice that some of the Named Variants, shown above, have the exact same nucleotides in both the Reference and Genotype columns? If you did, congratulations!

Big Y - Results

Named Variants   Private Variants   Matching

SNP Name	Derived?	On Y-Tree?	Reference	Genotype
SNP Name Search	Yes (+)	Show All	Show All	Show All
A12263	Yes (+)	Yes	T	C
A126	Yes (+)	Yes	T	A
A20312	Yes (+)	No	C	A
A2673	Yes (+)	Yes	G	G
A4751	Yes (+)	Yes	T	T
A4781	Yes (+)	No	G	C
A5013	Yes (+)	Yes	C	C
A5097	Yes (+)	No	A	G
A5116	Yes (+)	Yes	A	A
BY1002	Yes (+)	Yes	A	T

If you look in the Derived column, it says "Yes," which means the tester has this mutation. This is VERY confusing because there doesn't appear to be a mutation. If the Genotype and Reference are the same, it's not a mutation, right?

In other words, the genotyped value you have is exactly the same as the reference value – so this shouldn't be listed as a variant at all. Right?

You'd be exactly right, but there's a hitch – which is why we're down here in the weeds.

A haplogroup R man was used for the Y-DNA Human Genome hg38[70] [71] reference model, which is used by all scientists and researchers worldwide. Haplogroup R wasn't formed until about 26,000 years ago, some 200,000 years after Y-line Adam lived. Therefore, some named variants found in haplogroup R are in the reference model, but they are actually mutations when compared with Y-line Adam.

Haplogroups must be assigned taking into account the 200,000 years preceding haplogroup R, which is why you'll see some locations with the same value in both the Reference and Genotype columns. The haplogroup R man already had these mutations, but they were not present in Y-line Adam, represented by haplogroup A-PR2921[72]. Therefore, they actually ARE a mutation, it's the reference model that's incorrect.

Mitochondrial DNA has the same issue, which is why the original Cambridge Reference Sequence versions (CRS and rCRS) were updated in the RSRS, Revised Sapiens Reference Sequence in 2012. The CRS was based on a haplogroup H2a2a1 individual, and the RSRS model is based on Mitochondrial Eve.

Ok, we're done in the weeds now. Thank you for your attendance.

Y-Chromosome Browsing Tool

FamilyTreeDNA provides a Y chromosome browser that allows you to view the details of either a Named Variant or Private Variant, along with the quality of that result.

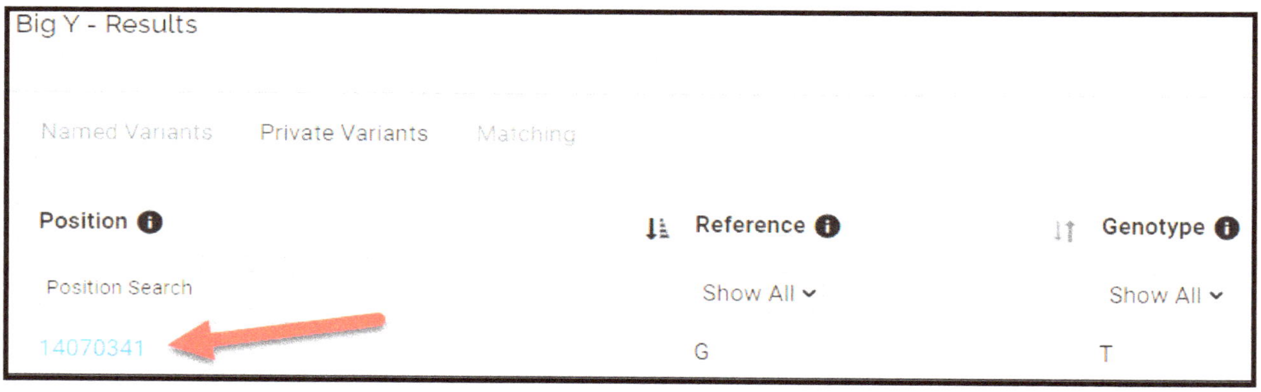

To view a specific location, click on the position for either a private or named variant.

A browser pops up with a small black divot aligned above the position you've selected.

70 https://gatk.broadinstitute.org/hc/en-us/articles/360035890951-Human-genome-reference-builds-GRCh38-or-hg38-b37-hg19

71 https://dna-explained.com/2018/01/12/working-with-the-new-big-y-results-hg38/

72 https://www.familytreedna.com/public/y-dna-haplotree/A

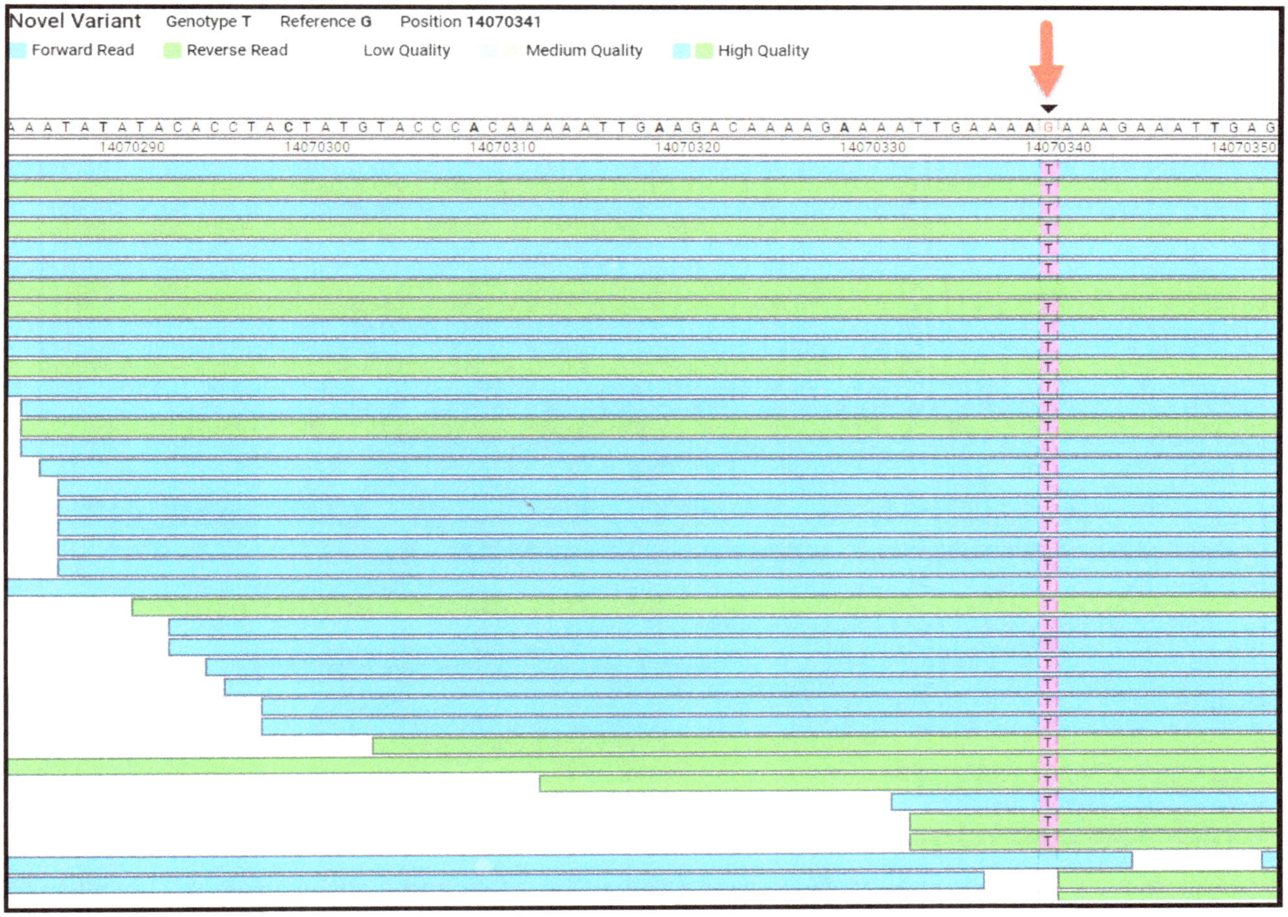

The blue and green rows represent reads, or scans, of the chromosome. Blue rows indicate that the read was on a forward strand of DNA's double helix, and green rows indicate it was on a reverse strand of the helix. The darker the color of the bar, the better the quality of the read.

The reference value is shown in red text in the bar at the top, right beneath the black divot, which is a G in this case. Beneath the reference value, highlighted in bright pink, your value is displayed if it's different from G. In this case, the scan found a "T" 34 times, representing a very consistent, high-quality read for a value of T.

In this example, G is the reference value - the value in the reference genome- T is this person's genotype, which is a derived value, meaning it is different from the reference value.

This is a very clean read, but some reads aren't consistent.

To be counted as an actual mutation, the mutated value must be found:

- In greater than five quality reads AND
- Not in a "messy" region

TIP: The Big Y test generally scans the Y chromosome at least 30 times, and often "as many times as it takes" to achieve a quality read.

What does a messy region look like? Great question.

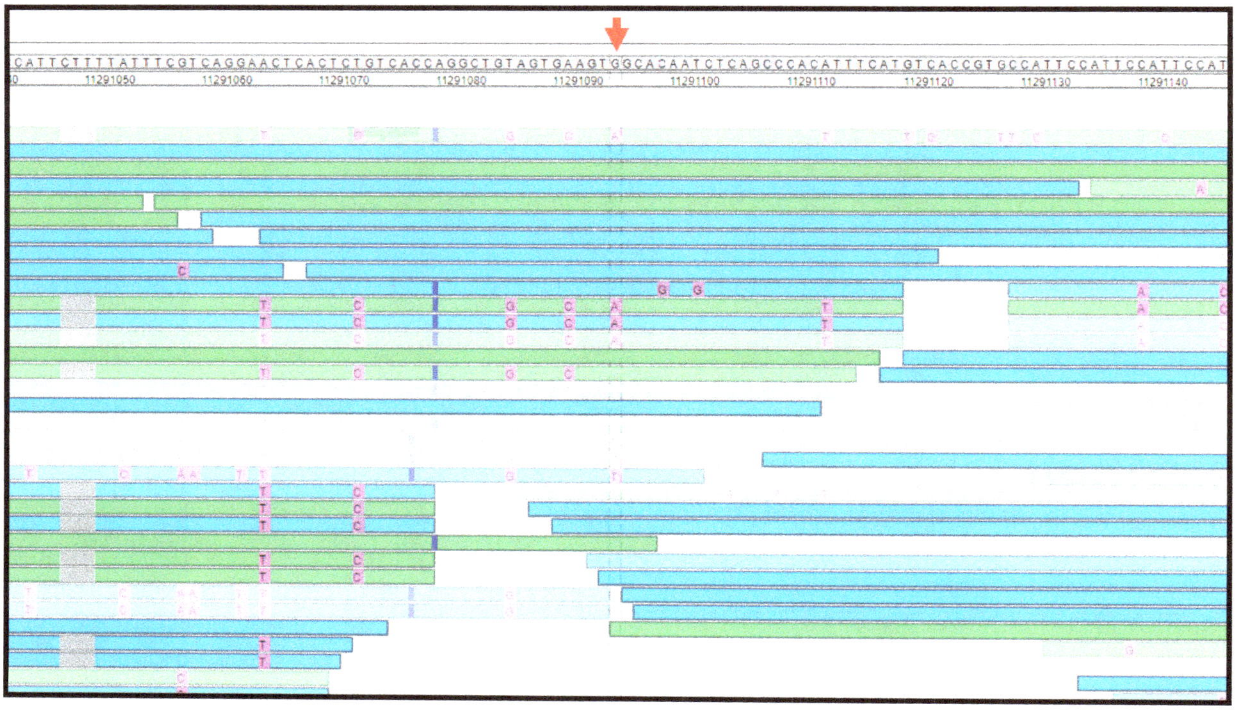

Here's an example of a poor-quality read in a messy area. The values found are inconsistent. The reference value is G, but both an A and a T are found three times each. Furthermore, low-quality forward and reverse reads are lighter, indicating poor quality. Quality reads are darker. Additional indicators of a messy region are shown by the other scattered, random pink mutations in this region.

These scan anomalies are not and should not be counted as mutations when they occur under these circumstances. This is also why every private variant match is reviewed by the phylogeneticist during the naming process. [73]

Big Y Block Tree

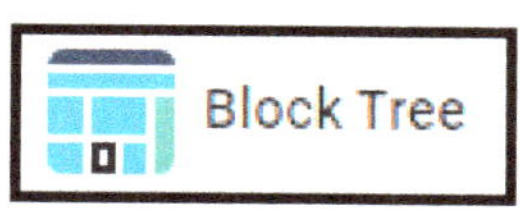

The Block Tree is a method of curating and displaying your Big Y matches on the haplotree to make it easier to visualize their positions in relation to each other.

Keep in mind that men who have not tested to the Big Y-700 level will also be displayed on the tree if they have taken the Big Y-500 and match within a genetic distance of 30 SNPs. If they were to upgrade to the Big Y-700, they might be placed on a more refined branch of the tree. The Big Y-500 lacks the granularity of the Big Y-700 and should be upgraded whenever possible.

73 https://blog.familytreedna.com/big-y-manual-review-lifetime-analysis/

In genetic genealogy, 30 SNP mutations difference on the Y chromosome equates to approximately 1500 years. SNP mutations occur approximately every 80 to 120 years in each lineage. The more data points available, meaning testers, the more refined the age estimates can be.

In each haplogroup branch, the names of your matches will be shown, along with the flag locations of their earliest known ancestor, if they entered that information.

I've removed the match names that would normally appear below the number of matches in this graphic. I've filled in the ancestral names and birth years of the men in whose lifetime these mutations occurred, according to proven genealogy.

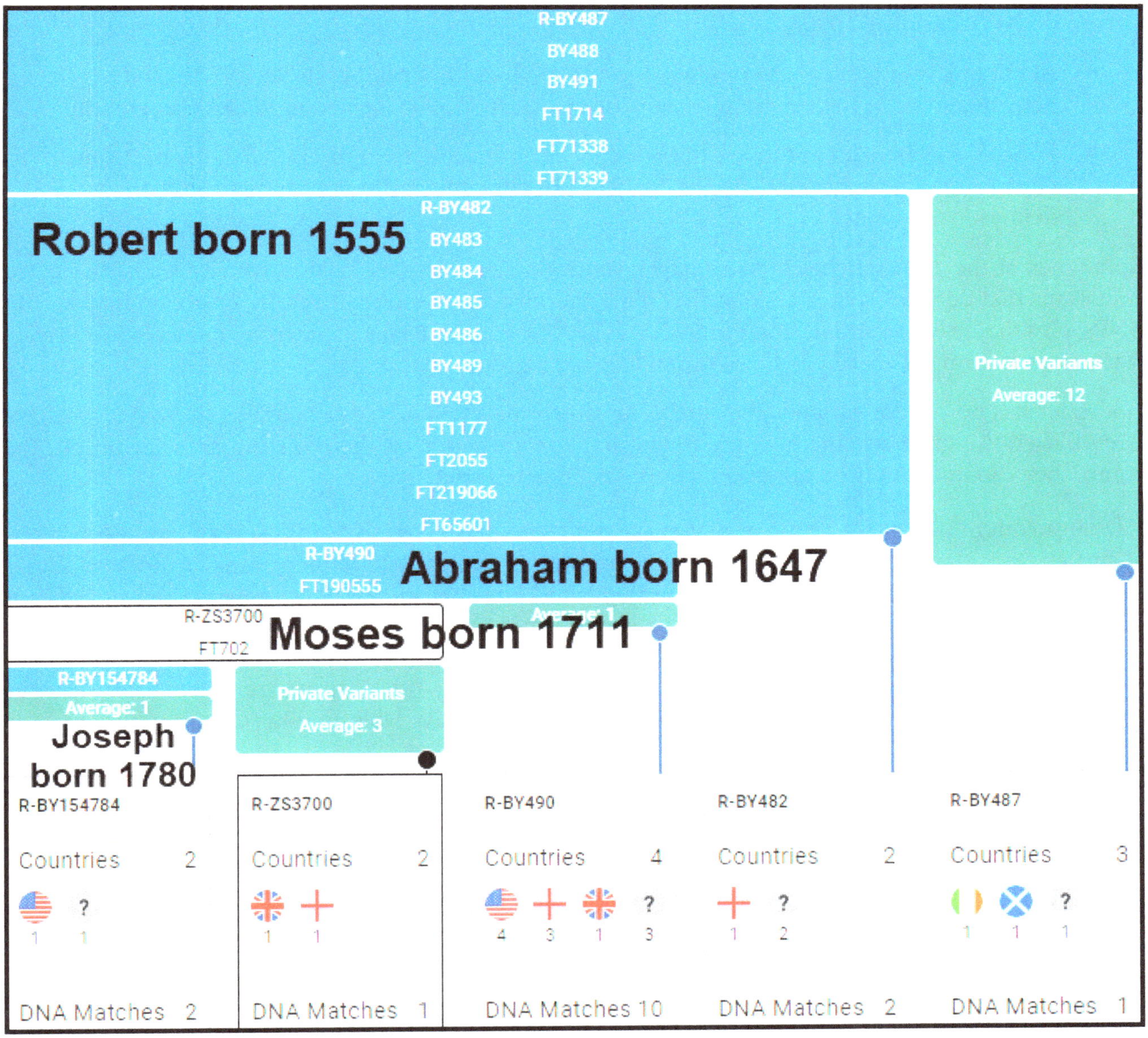

In the Estes line, we've been able to confirm the descendancy, along with the year the actual SNP mutation(s) occurred, by testing multiple men in each line.

- Haplogroup R-BY482 is the umbrella haplogroup that all Estes men carry, but is found in very few men with other surnames. We know approximately when it occurred, because all descendants of Robert born in 1555 have this mutation, so it occurred in 1555 or earlier.
- Abraham, the grandson of Robert born in 1555, was the Estes immigrant to the colony of Virginia. Abraham was born in England in 1647 to Silvester, born about 1600, and has the mutation that formed haplogroup R-BY490. We know that this mutation first occurred in his father, Silvester, because descendants of Abraham's uncle, also named Robert, born in 1603, do NOT have R-BY490
- Abraham's youngest son, Moses, was born in 1711 and has haplogroup R-ZS3700, but descendants of Moses's siblings do not. Therefore, R-ZS3700 formed in Moses's generation.
- Further downstream in Moses's line, Joseph, his grandson, born in 1780, had the mutation giving rise to haplogroup R-BY154784, and Joseph's siblings did not, so this mutation defines Joseph's line.

Some men at the end branches of these haplogroups do have Private Variants, which means they carry mutations that don't yet match anyone else. If another man tests and matches the upstream haplogroup SNPs, plus that private variant, a new branch will be formed with a new haplogroup name. I view Private Variants, sometimes also called Novel Variants, as haplogroups in waiting.

If a tester has no private variants, they are as far down the Y-DNA tree as possible, meaning they have been placed the most succinctly. If equivalent haplogroups exist on their branch, or upstream, in the future they can potentially be moved in the tree as branches split.

TIP: Equivalent haplogroups mean that every man who has tested so far has several mutations that, together, form their lineage. You can see an example of 11 equivalent haplogroups for Robert, above, two for Abraham, and two for Moses. If another man tests and doesn't have some of these equivalent haplogroups, the haplogroup, R-BY482 in this case, will be split into two.

While these tools are specific to men who have taken the Big Y test, there are public tools, such as the Public Y Tree[74] and the Discover™ Haplogroup Reports[75], available to everyone, that also provide significant value to Y-DNA testers.

Private Variants – Haplogroups-in-Waiting

Private Variants are unnamed SNPs discovered in individual testers which have not yet been found in other testers. A good place to compare Private Variants is in the Block Tree, seen below, where you see the average number of Private Variants for all the testers at the end of that branch. When another man has the same private variant in the same genetic line, that SNP location will be named, and those two men will form a new branch on the tree. Essentially, Private Variants are haplogroups-in-waiting.

74 https://www.familytreedna.com/public/y-dna-haplotree/A
75 https://discover.familytreedna.com/

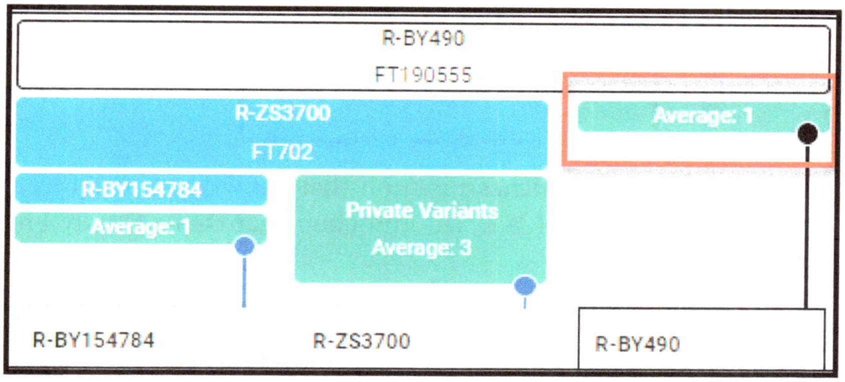

Viewing the block tree, our Estes tester at right has one private variant. When another man in the same line tests, if he has the same private variant, a new branch will be formed, and both men will then be assigned to the new haplogroup instead of R-BY490. When more than one man falls into a group, the number of private variants is averaged.

R-BY490 will always be the parent haplogroup of these three haplogroup branches, however, and possibly more haplogroups, as new downstream haplogroups are discovered and defined.

Some parts of the tree have several testers, so many haplogroups have been discovered and named, but other portions have a great deal of potential for new haplogroups and splitting branches. The testers at far right below, have 11, 12, and 13 private variants.

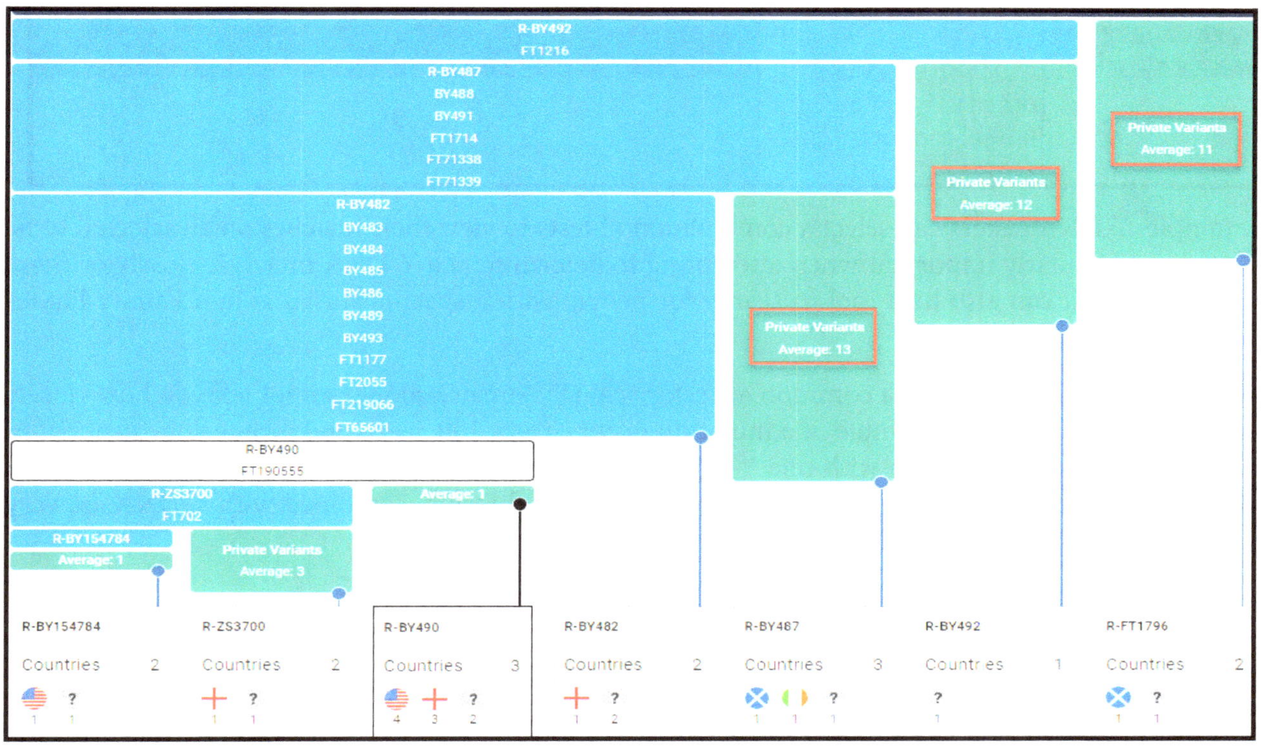

Another tool, the Public Y Tree, provides a different view of the haplotree.

Advanced Matches

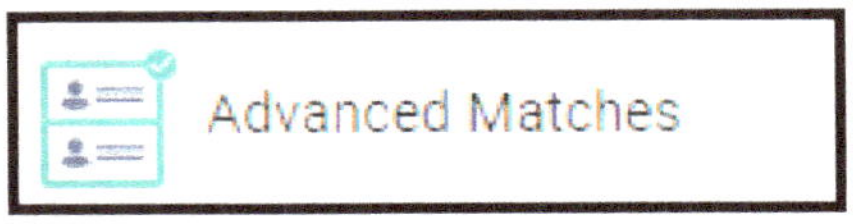

FamilyTreeDNA provides an Advanced Matches function that allows customers to combine different types of results, such as the various levels of Y-DNA, mitochondrial DNA, Family Finder, and X-DNA filtered by various surnames and projects.

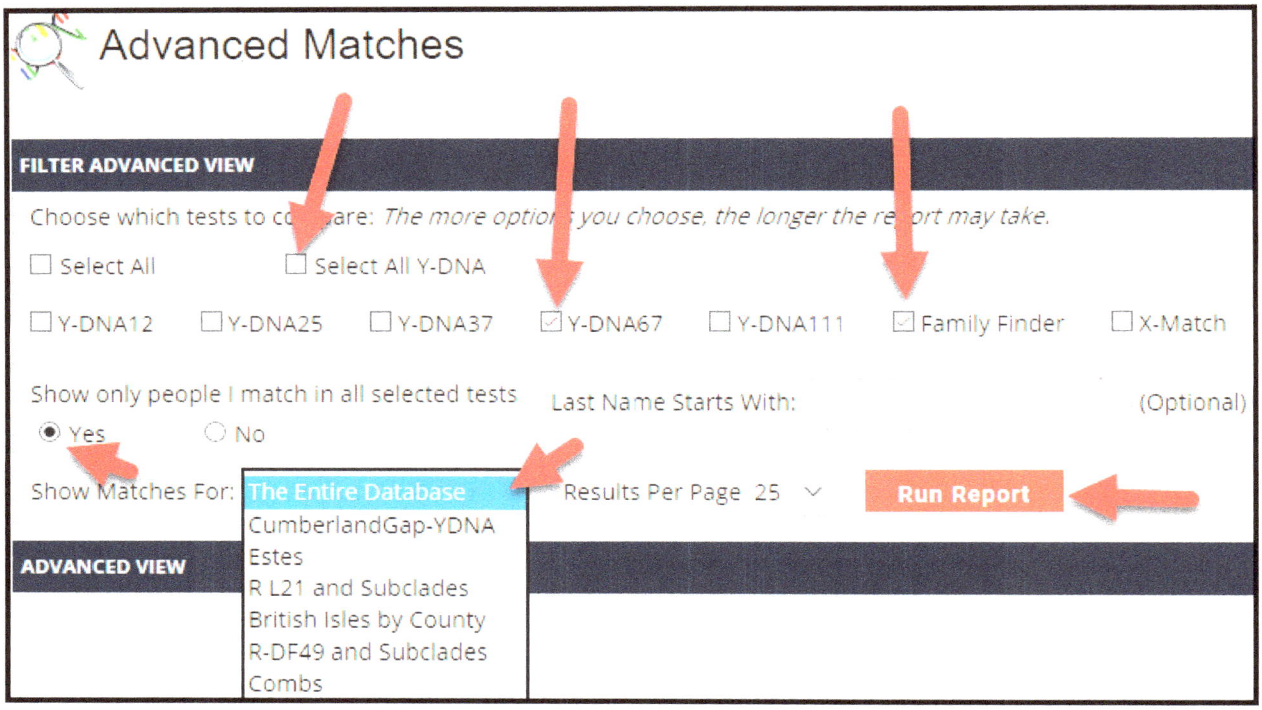

For example, Y-DNA testers can select a combination of tests to view their matches on all selected tests. This can be particularly important when attempting to determine if a Y-DNA match is closely or more distantly related. It can also be a tool to search for people with a specific surname in a Family Finder autosomal match list.

While Y-DNA matches indicate a common ancestor, a Y-DNA match alone cannot tell you how closely two people are related.[76] For example, if a mutation occurs every 100 years, and a genealogy generation is 25 years, on average, two men with one Y-DNA mutation difference could be related anyplace from one to 8 generations ago, on average. Family Finder autosomal results combined with Y-DNA are very informative and have the ability to refine the relationship distance.

76 Rare exceptions occur occasionally in men who are closely related and match on a SNP that has occurred in the last generation or so. In this case, the mutation narrows the possible relationships to "after" the mutation occurred.

By making the following selections, you can view people who match on all of the selected criteria:

1. Select any one, (**NOT** "All",) Y-DNA match level
2. Select Family Finder
3. Select "Yes" to "Show only people I match in all selected tests,"
4. Click Run Report

Selecting "All" means that another tester must match on all of the STR panels. That criteria will eliminate many testers. Only one mismatch at the 12-marker level is above the match threshold, so men won't be shown as Y-DNA matches if they have one mismatch at 12 markers and "all" is selected. I recommend selecting 111, the highest-level Y-DNA marker level test, running that report and then selecting other levels one by one.

TIP: The Advanced Matches tool allows testers to compare results against matches within individual Group Projects.

Group Projects are especially beneficial for Y-DNA testers, specifically surname projects. It's easy to join projects, and the Haplogroups & SNPs page, along with the Discover™ Haplogroup Reports, suggest projects that others with your Y-DNA haplogroup have joined.

Projects facilitate collaboration, allow you to work with others who have similar interests, and provide benefits such as the Group Time Tree.[77] [78]

Click on Group Projects at the top of your personal page, and then on either:

- "Manage Group Projects" to view or manage projects you've already joined
- "Join A Project" to join a new project

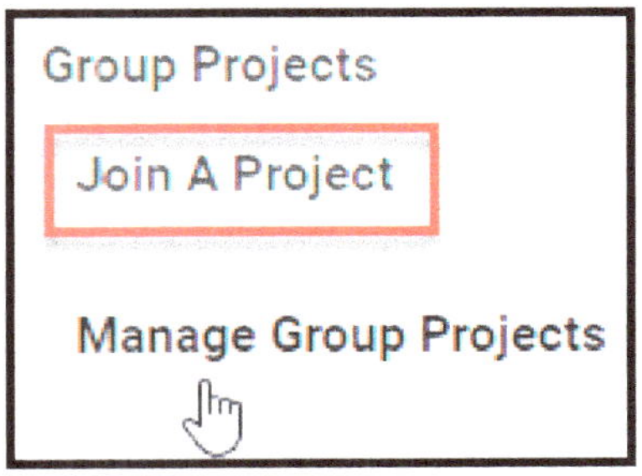

Public Tools

FamilyTreeDNA provides several public tools under two categories.

- The Discover™ Haplogroup Reports[79] – for Y-DNA only
- Y-DNA[80] and Mitochondrial DNA[81] Public Trees - found in the footer of every page

FamilyTreeDNA is planning to introduce a Discover™ Haplogroup Reports tool for mitochondrial DNA results after the new mitochondrial tree is released.

77 https://dna-explained.com/2023/01/13/sneak-preview-introducing-the-familytreedna-group-time-tree/

78 https://dna-explained.com/2023/01/17/project-administrators-how-to-prepare-your-project-for-familytreednas-new-group-time-tree/

79 https://discover.familytreedna.com/

80 https://www.familytreedna.com/public/y-dna-haplotree/A

81 https://www.familytreedna.com/products/mt-dna

Discover™ Haplogroup Reports Tools

In 2022, FamilyTreeDNA released the beta version of their new Discover™ Haplogroup Reports for Y-DNA.[82]

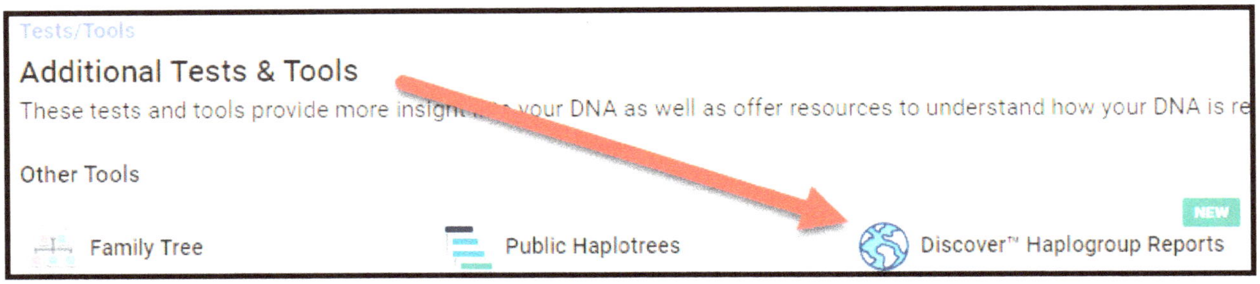

TIP: Discover™ is accessible from your Y-DNA account using the Discover™ Haplogroup Reports button located under Y-DNA, Big Y, and Additional Tests and Tools. Or, if you don't have a Y-DNA test, you can find it at discover.familytreedna.com.[83]

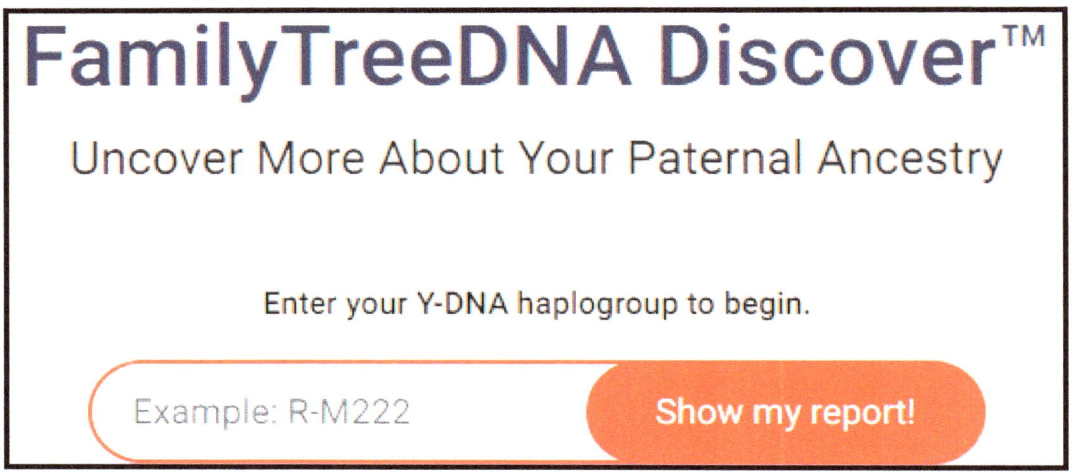

Discover™ is public and free, and you don't need to have tested with FamilyTreeDNA to use it. However, you'll have better and more relevant results if you have taken the Big Y-700 DNA test, or someone in your lineage has taken that test for the lines you're researching. Testers also have access to more Ancient Connections and Notable Connections, along with the Globetrekker tool that tracks your haplogroup from Y-Adam across the globe.

The Discover™ Haplogroup Reports tool is being enhanced regularly, so there will probably be more features available by the time you're reading this. Be sure to explore every tab. Tabs essentially equate to chapters in the book for each haplogroup.

---

82 Soon, the Discover™ tool will be enhanced to include mitochondrial DNA.

83 https://dna-explained.com/2022/06/30/familytreedna-discover-launches-including-y-dna-haplogroup-ages/

The Discover™ Haplogroup Reports tool includes several sections that enhance your testing experience and that many people share with family members.

Discover's Haplogroup Story

The Haplogroup Story tells you about the history of your haplogroup, interpreting the scientific data.

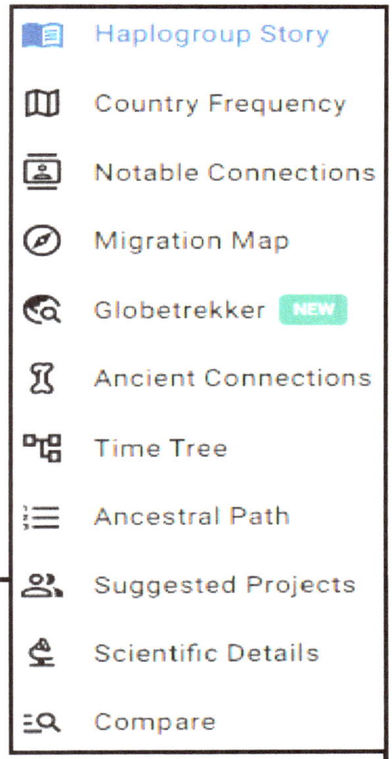

The story tells you when the branch was formed, meaning when the mutation occurred, the name of the parent branch, how many downstream, or child, branches exist, how many men are members of this haplogroup, and where their earliest known ancestors are from.

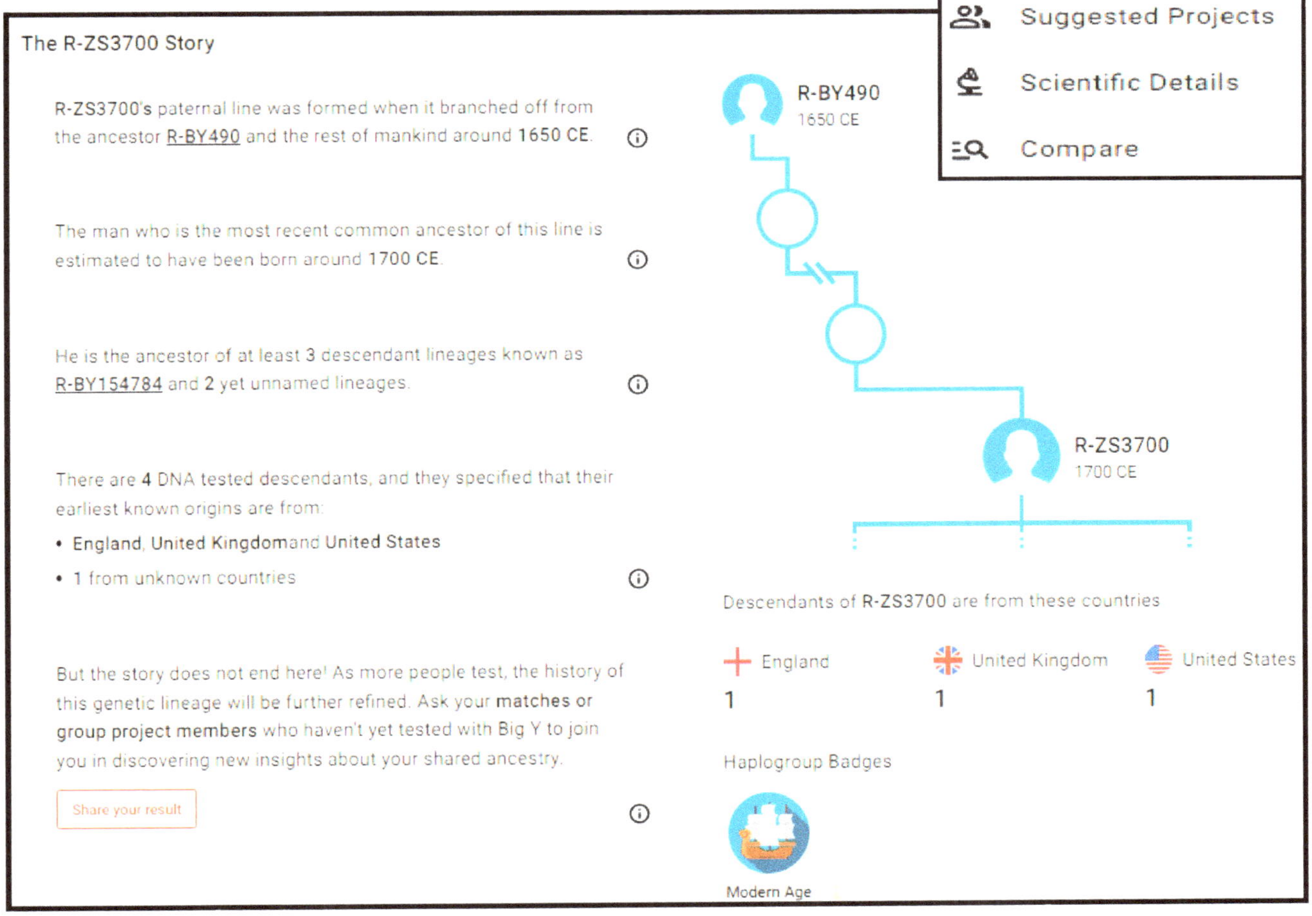

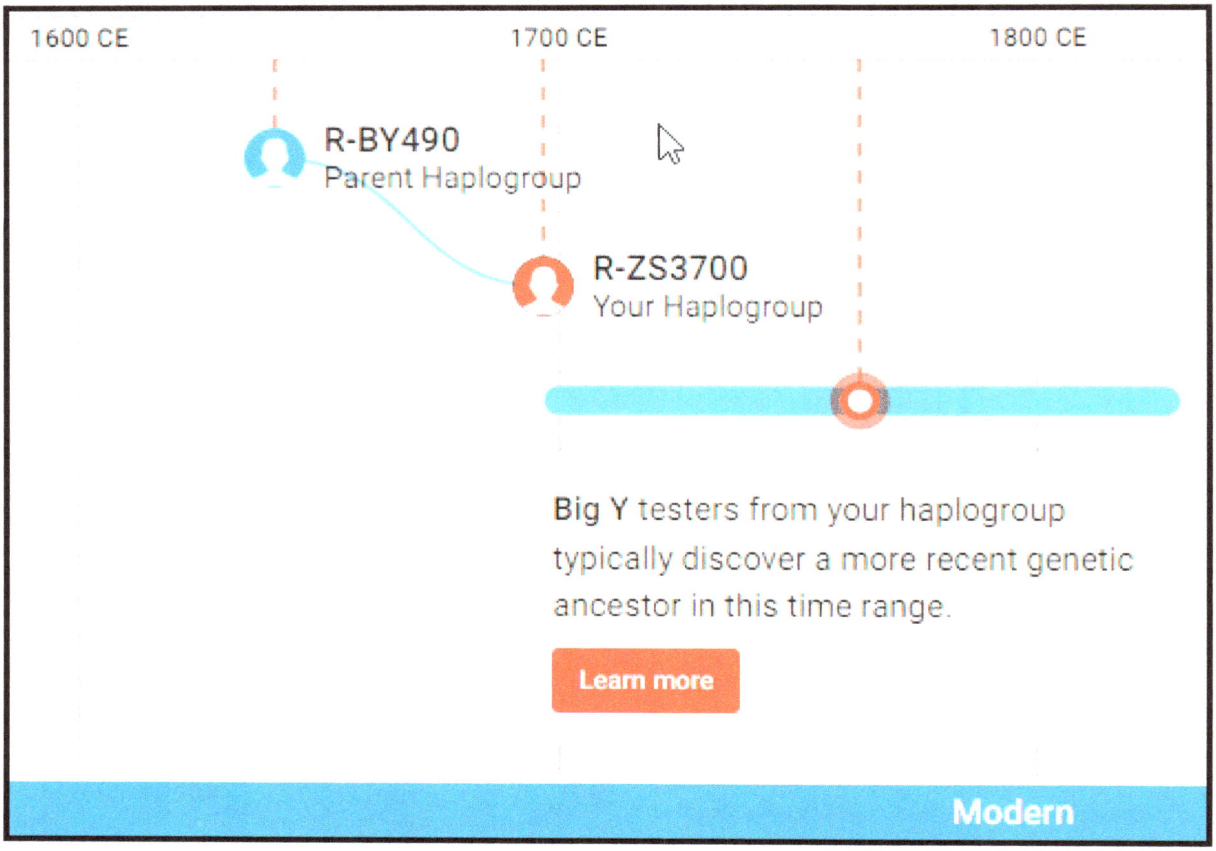

Haplogroup R-ZS3700 was born or formed in the Modern Era, sometime around 1700, when it split from R-BY490. We know that Moses Estes was born in 1711, and the R-BY490 mutation occurred at his conception, so the 1700 date is very close.

TIP: CE stands for "Common Era", which is functionally equivalent to AD, but expressed in a more widely accepted scientific format. If you were born in the year 2000, that's the same as 2000 CE or 2000 AD. BCE means "Before Common Era" which is functionally the same as BC.

Country Frequency

Country Frequency provides a heat map of the locations of the Earliest Known Ancestor for other testers whose end-of-line SNP is the haplogroup you're viewing.

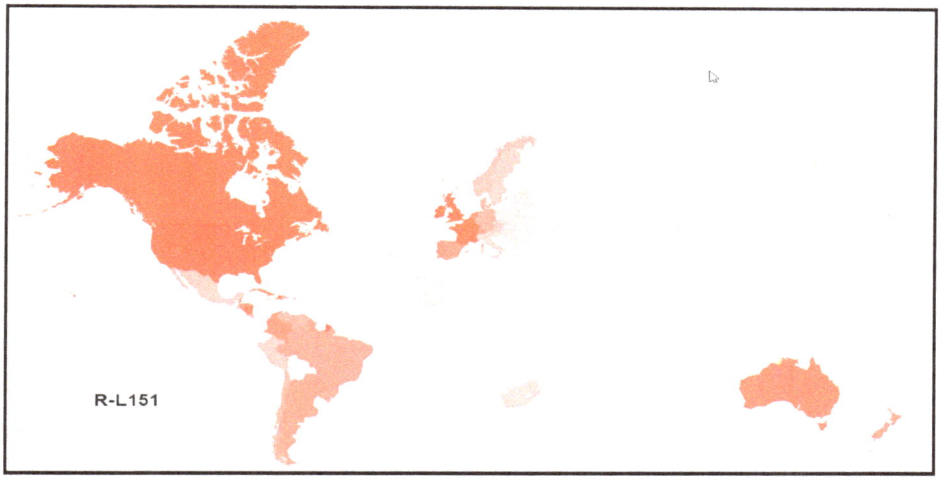

Ancestors of people whose end-of-line SNP is R-L151 are found in most of the world, except for portions of Africa and a few other locations. R-L151 is not the most refined haplogroup possible. In other words, R-L151[84], which was born about 3000 BCE, or 5000 years ago, has more than 28,000 descendant haplogroups in more than 160 countries.

Keep in mind that these locations reflect migration and sometimes where testers are brick-walled, like the United States, not necessarily original locations.

Notable Connections

Notable Connections is a fun section that displays notable people who share the same or upstream haplogroups.

You could match actors, politicians, musicians, scientists, royal families, ancient kings like Tutankhamun, and even Neanderthal Man. New entries are added regularly in both this section and Ancient Connections, so check back often.

Big Y testers who access Discover™ through their account may have 20 or more Ancient and Notable Connections, but public users accessing Discover™ through the free public interface or Y-DNA testers who have not taken the Big Y test are limited to about 11 connections in each category.

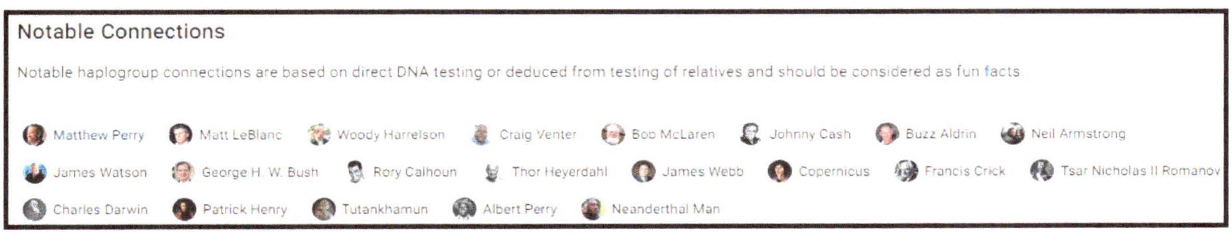

84 https://discover.familytreedna.com/y-dna/R-L151/story

Migration Map

The Migration Map displays the path out of Africa from about 230,000 years ago until about four thousand years ago.

The shovel icons indicate the locations of ancient DNA specimens.

TIP: Mousing over the shovel displays pertinent information, such as the specimen's name, age, location, and haplogroup.

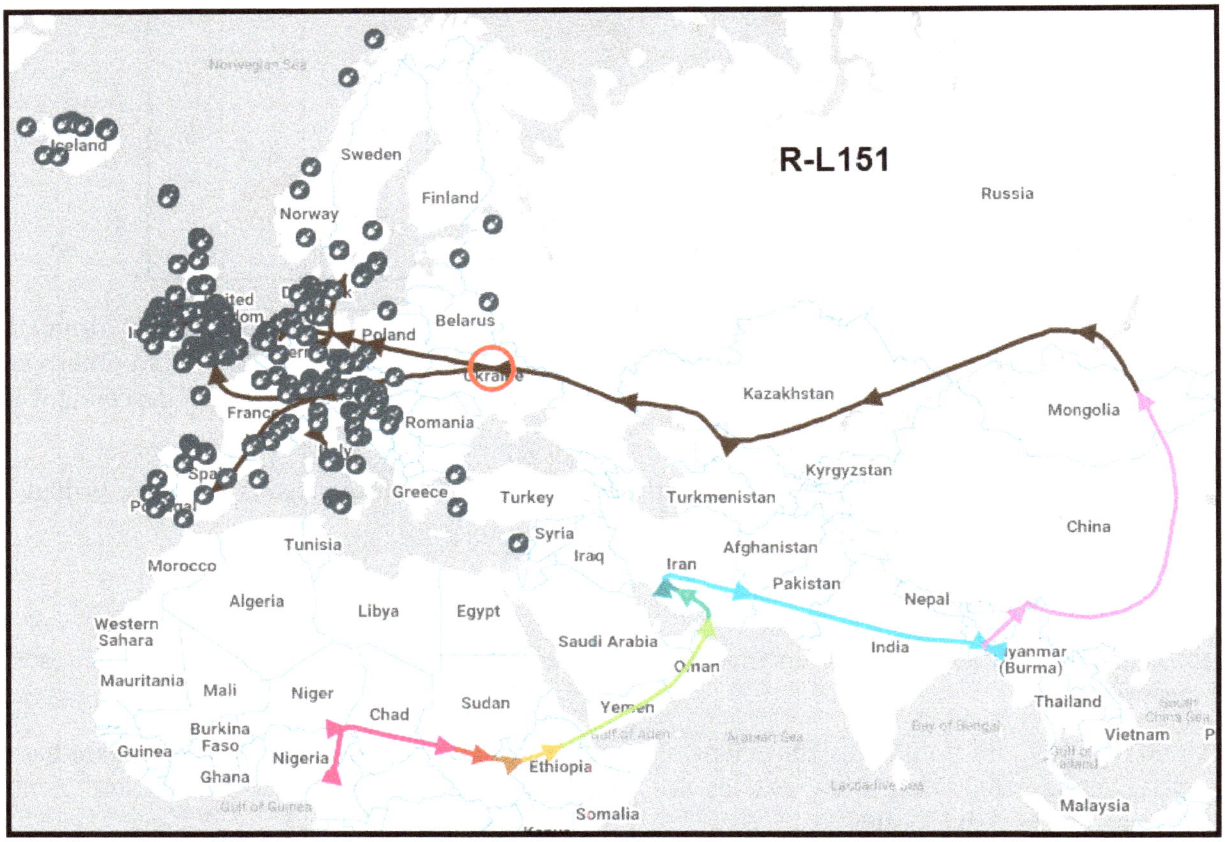

Globetrekker

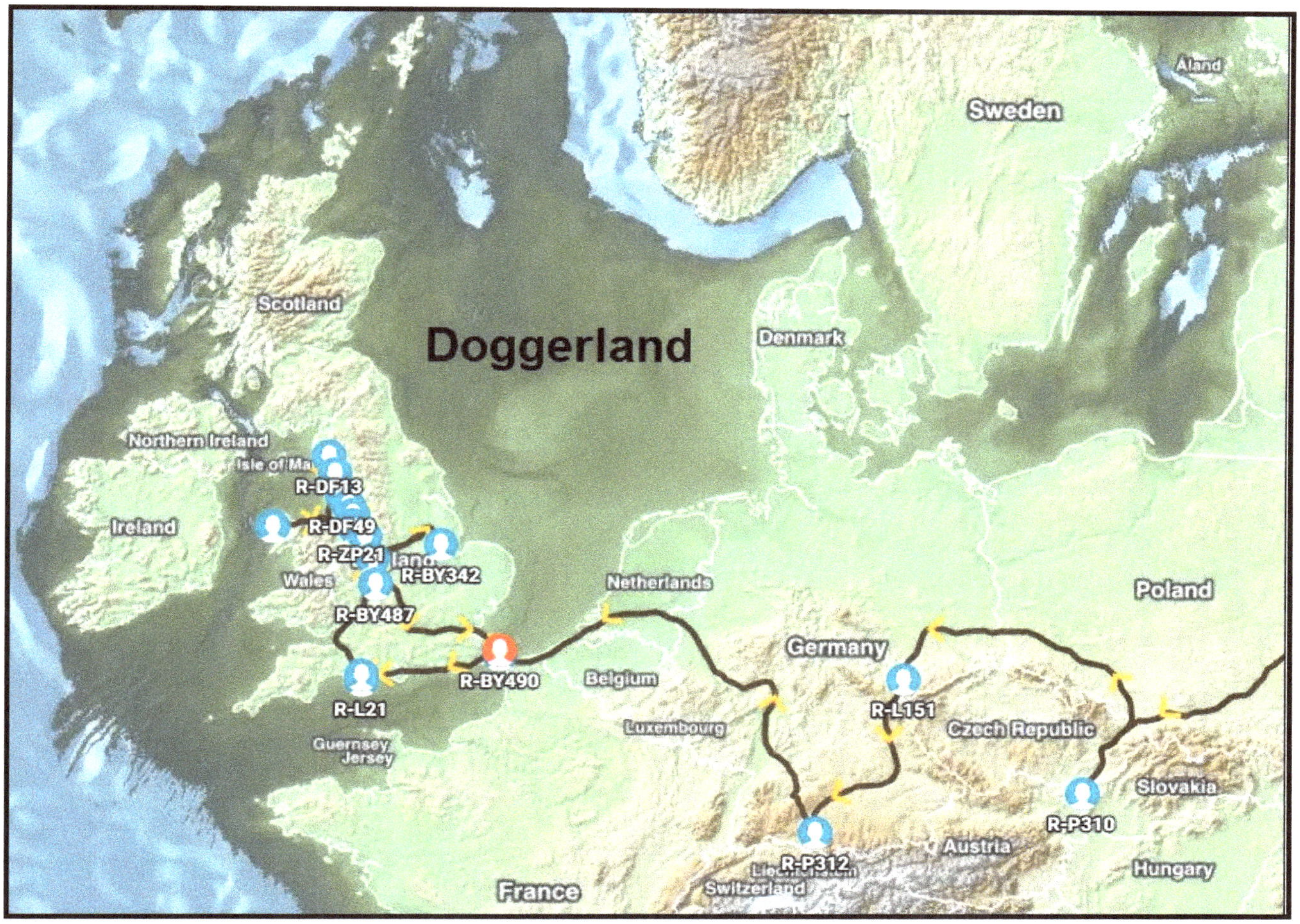

For Big Y testers, Globetrekker is a unique animated map, following the path and development of your haplogroup beginning with Y-Adam, then out of Africa to the location where it is currently found outside of the Americas, Australia, New Zealand, and other areas colonized during the European expansion era. At present, only indigenous Native American haplogroups are displayed in the Americas.[85]

---

85 https://dna-explained.com/2023/08/04/globetrekker-a-new-feature-for-big-y-customers-from-familytreedna/

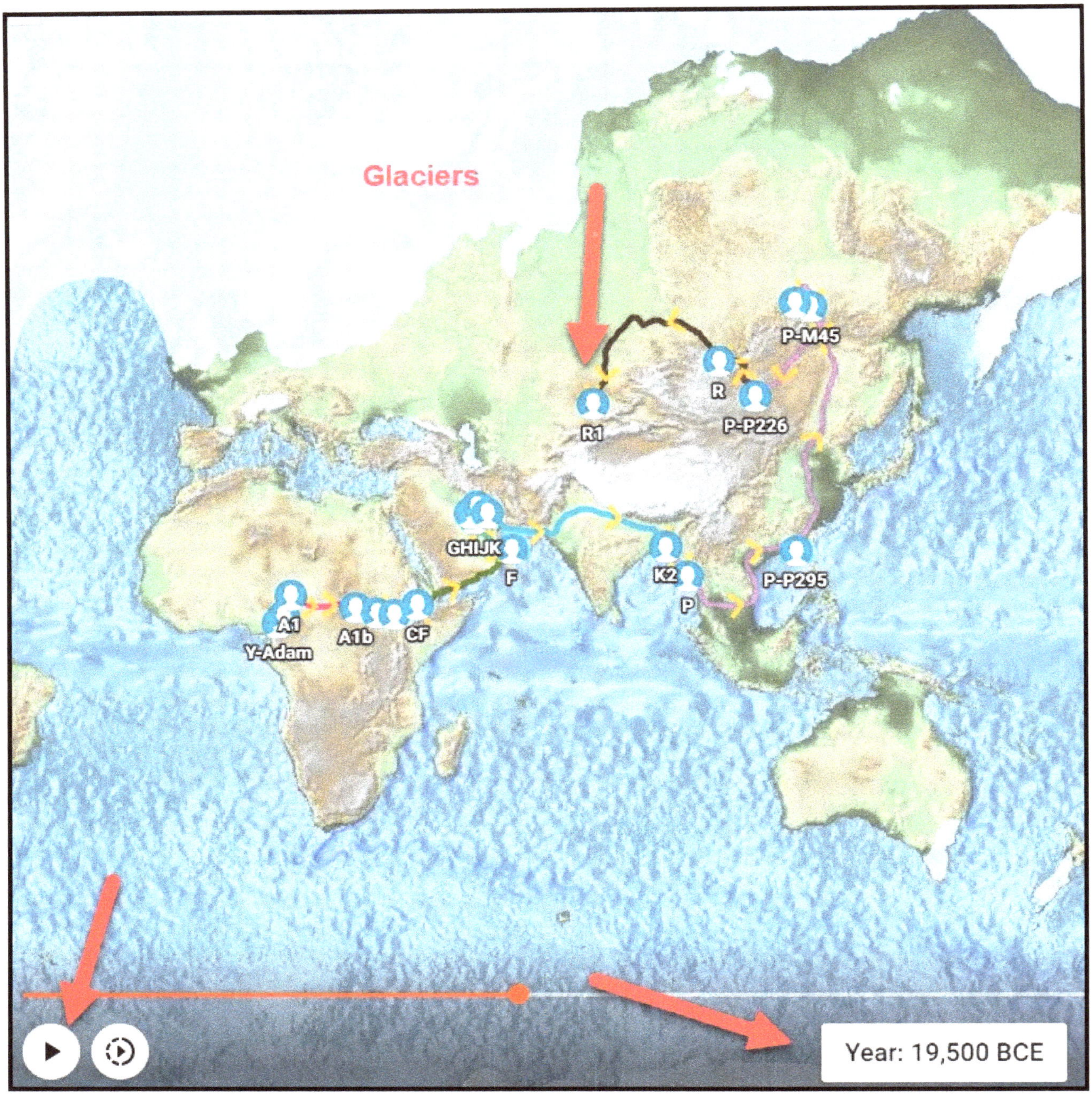

Terrain, elevation, sea level, currents, and even glaciation are taken into consideration when determining the most likely path for humans to have taken from place to place.

Globetrekker is a premium tool for Big Y testers only.

Ancient Connections

Ancient Connections display connections to your closest ancient samples.

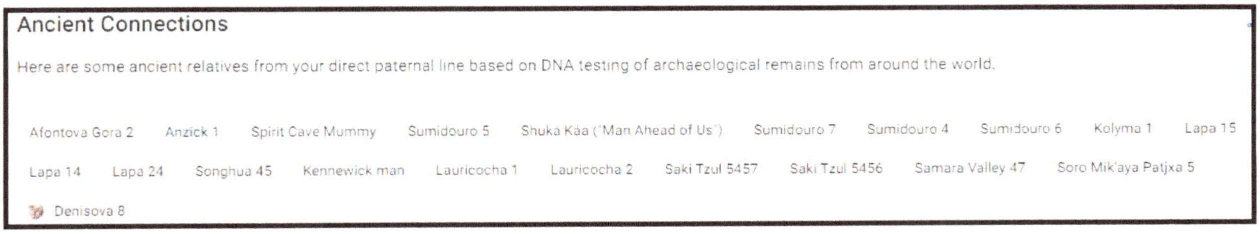

This haplogroup Q-M242 Native American customer shares a common paternal ancestor with the Anzick 1 Clovis burial in Montana.

Big Y testers who sign in through their account may receive 20 or more connections. Those who use the public version of Discover™ or who have not taken the Big Y test are limited to approximately 11.

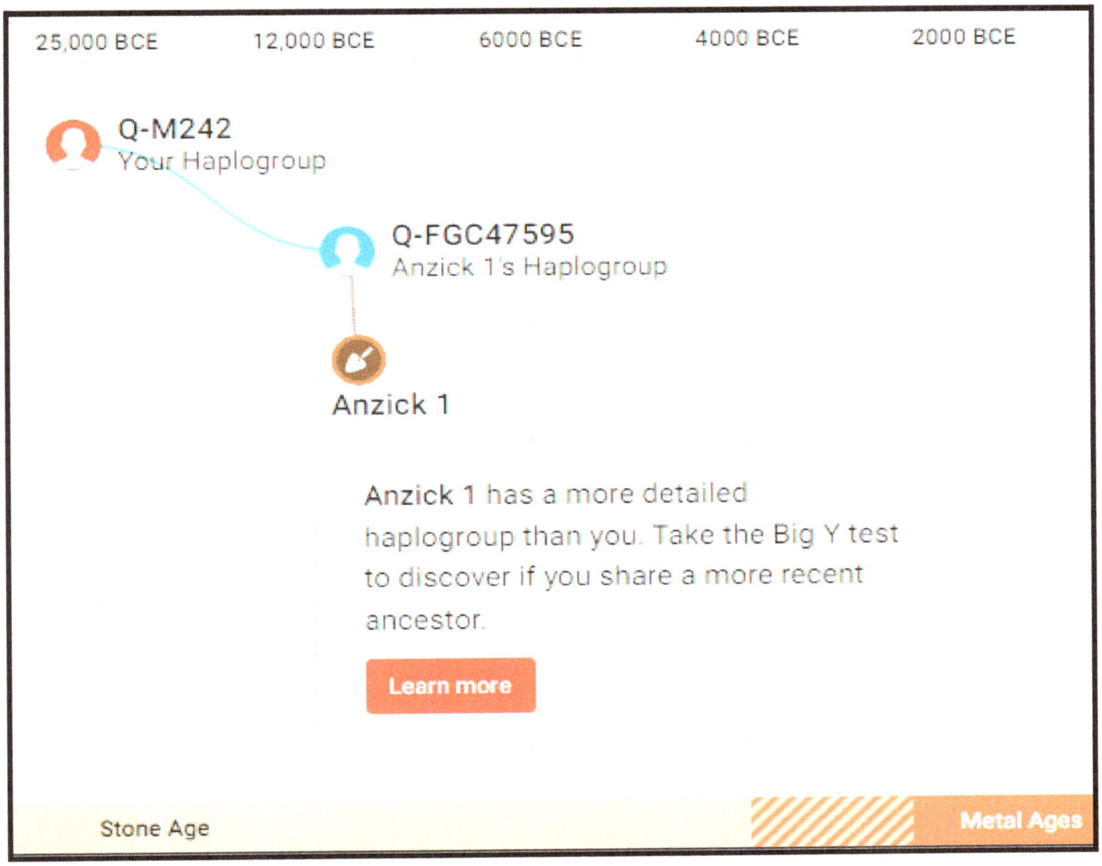

Upgrading to the Big Y test would provide this customer with a much more refined haplogroup than Q-M242, along with additional information.

TIP: BCE, Before Current Era, has the same meaning as BC. 1000 BCE is the same as 1000 BC, or approximately 3000 years ago.

Time Tree

The Time Tree shows a combination of the selected haplogroup, related haplogroups, Ancient Connections, Notable Connections, and Present-Day Testers (indicated by country flags,) depending on the options you select to display.

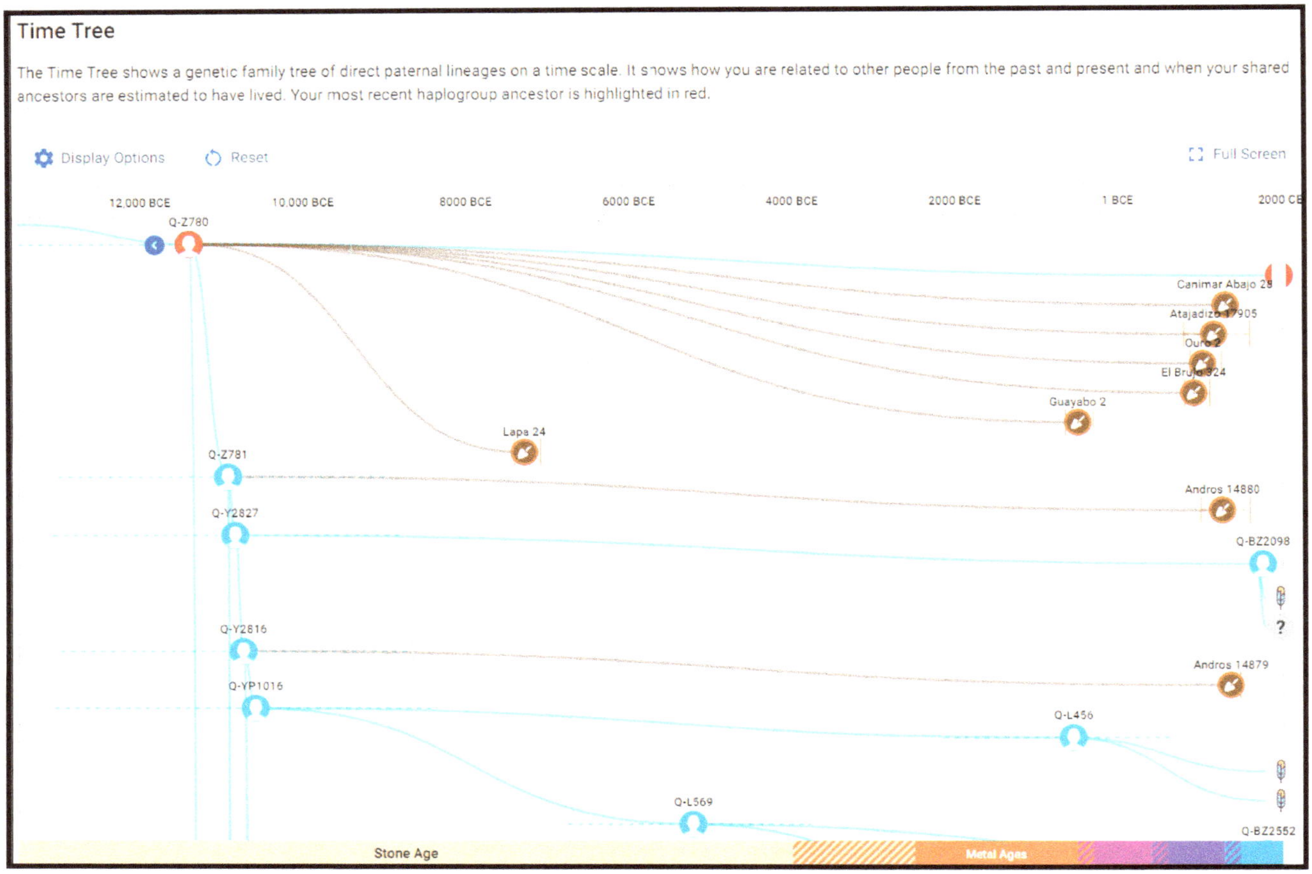

The estimated date when the haplogroup was formed, or when the person lived, is shown across the top. Mousing over any data point displays additional information, and clicking on any haplogroup takes you to that haplogroup's page.

The Time Tree uses tester information, along with ancient DNA samples and academic studies, to generate the Y-DNA tree and the Time Tree. You can help improve both by:

- Encouraging more testers, especially on your line, which will assist with calculating the time between mutations
- Specify birth year on all kits, especially the Big Y
- Link other testers to your family tree whenever possible so that Earliest Known Ancestor (EKA) information can be used for validation

Ancestral Path

The Ancestral Path walks your haplogroup back in time, beginning with the most recent haplogroups on the path and ending up with the Denisovan who lived before both Y-Adam and Neanderthal Man.

This example shows two of seven steps of the path from the selected haplogroup, Q-Z780, to the base of haplogroup Q, Q-M242.

TIP: Click the icon next to the string of SNPs under "Your detailed haplogroup path" to copy that sequence to paste anywhere you may need to include that information.

TIP: Click the header at the top of each column to sort by that column. For example, click "Tested Modern Descendants" to arrange the chart from most to fewest or fewest to most testers.

Suggested Projects

Suggested Projects are provided based on haplogroup, surname, and geographic projects that other men with this haplogroup have joined.

Ancestral Path

Every living man in the world shares a direct paternal line ancestor who lived around 230,000 years ago, and before that, our closest relatives are the Neanderthals and Denisovans. Each step represents a genetic ancestor on your direct paternal line. As more people test, this path will be further refined, and we will identify more steps on your ancestral line.

Your detailed haplogroup path is:
Q-M242>MEH2>M346>L53>L54>CTS3814>Z780

Steps	Haplogroup	Age Estimate	Archaeology Era	Time Passed	Immediate Descendants	Tested Modern Descendants	Ancient Connections
1	Q-Z780	11,000 BCE	Stone Age	2,000 years	2	243	15
2	Q-CTS3814	13,000 BCE	Stone Age	1,000 years	2	2,020	202

While all Y-DNA haplogroup projects are restricted to Y-DNA testers, that's not universally true for surname projects. And, while many geographic projects, meaning projects that are tied to a location or other binding cultural factors, are not restricted to either Y or mitochondrial DNA, some are specifically for either Y-DNA or mtDNA testers. Be sure to check the listing carefully to ensure you're joining the correct one.

The projects in the blue outlined boxes, at the top of the list, are haplogroup projects where the volunteer project administrators have configured this haplogroup as one of five that can be recommended for the haplogroup you are viewing.

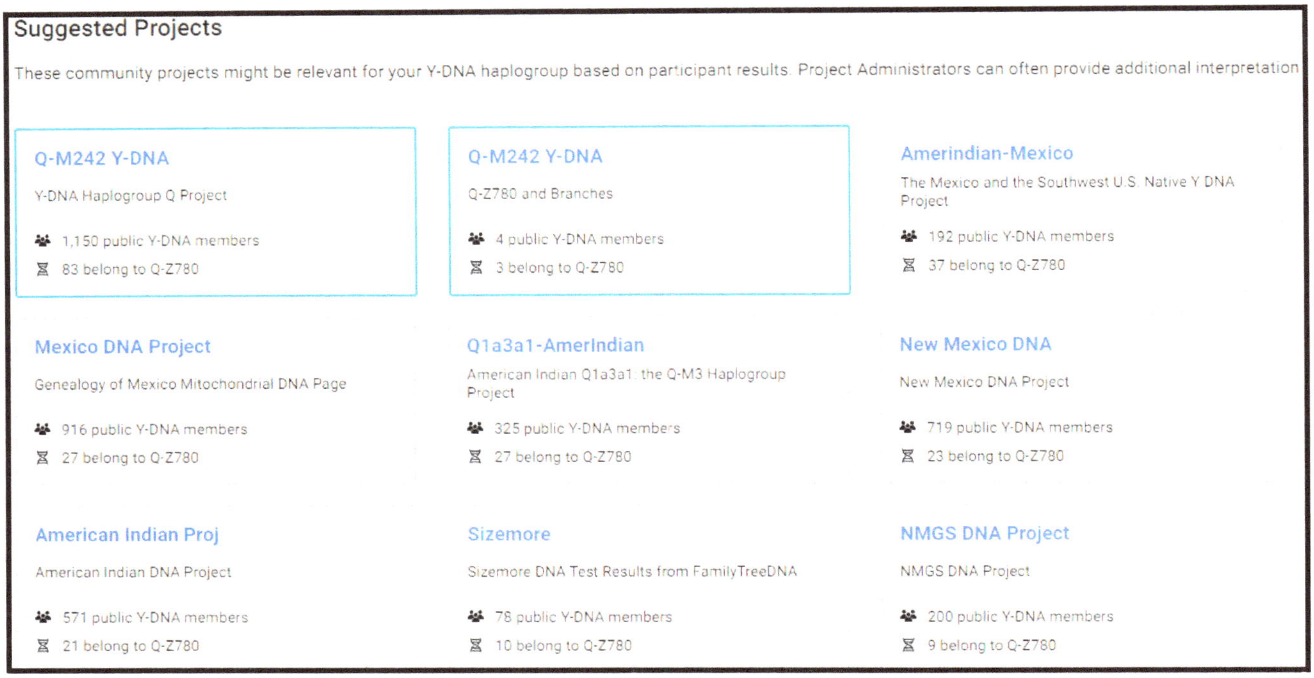

Scientific Details

Scientific Details contains two tabs. The first tab, **Age Estimate,** provides probability plots and confidence intervals for the age of the haplogroup you are viewing.

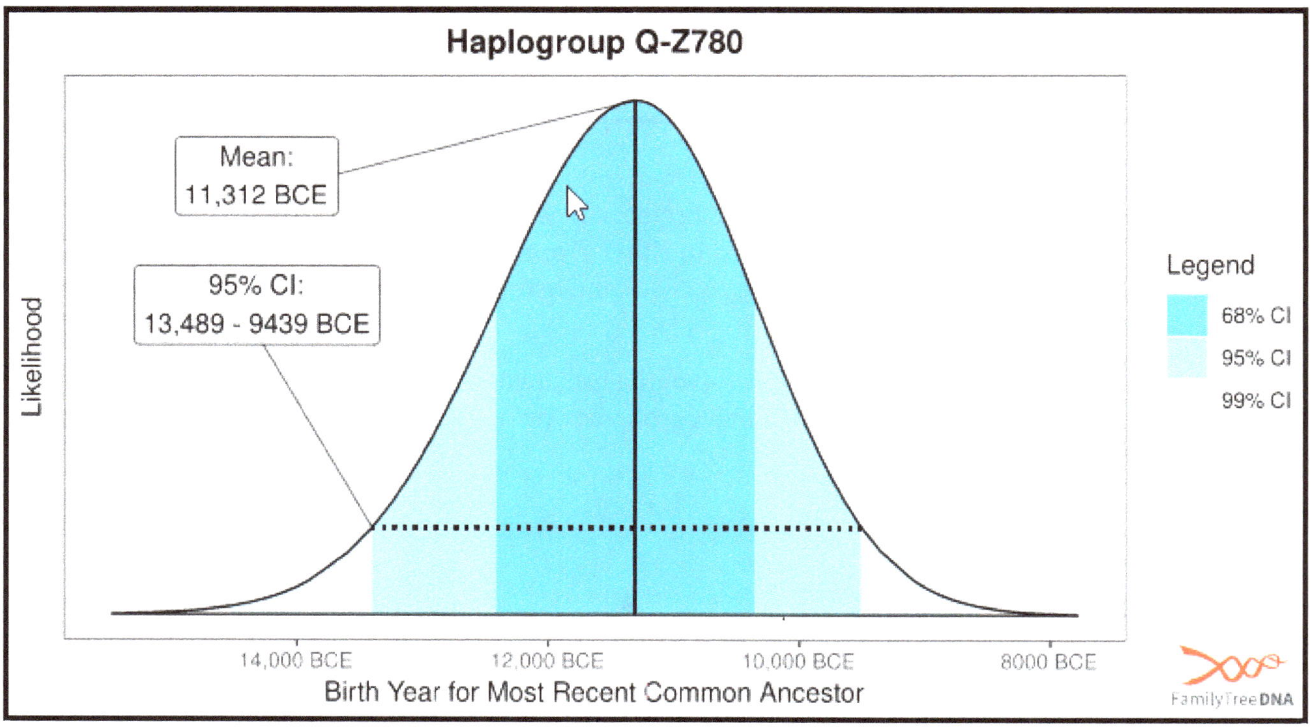

Statistic*	Years Before Present	Calendar Date
99% CI	16,644 - 10,509	14,622 - 8487 BCE
95% CI	15,511 - 11,461	13,489 - 9439 BCE
68% CI	14,433 - 12,379	12,411 - 10,357 BCE
Mean	13,334	11,312 BCE

** CI is the Confidence Interval for a given time range and Mean is the expected date.*

The second tab, **Variants**, shows the mutations, or variants that, taken together, comprise this haplogroup.

Age Estimate　Variants

These 28 Y chromosome mutations are shared by everyone in this haplogroup. They show a paternal lineage of father-son relationships that have accumulated mutations over time.

Name	Position (GRCh38)	Ancestral	Derived	Synonyms
Z780	8642499	C	T	M971
BY15623	11229136	G	A	

Compare

The Compare[86] feature allows you to compare any two haplogroups, providing information about where they reside on the tree relative to one another. Other interesting information is included about commonalities, such as locations which can be quite relevant for genealogists, or common types of connections, such as authors.

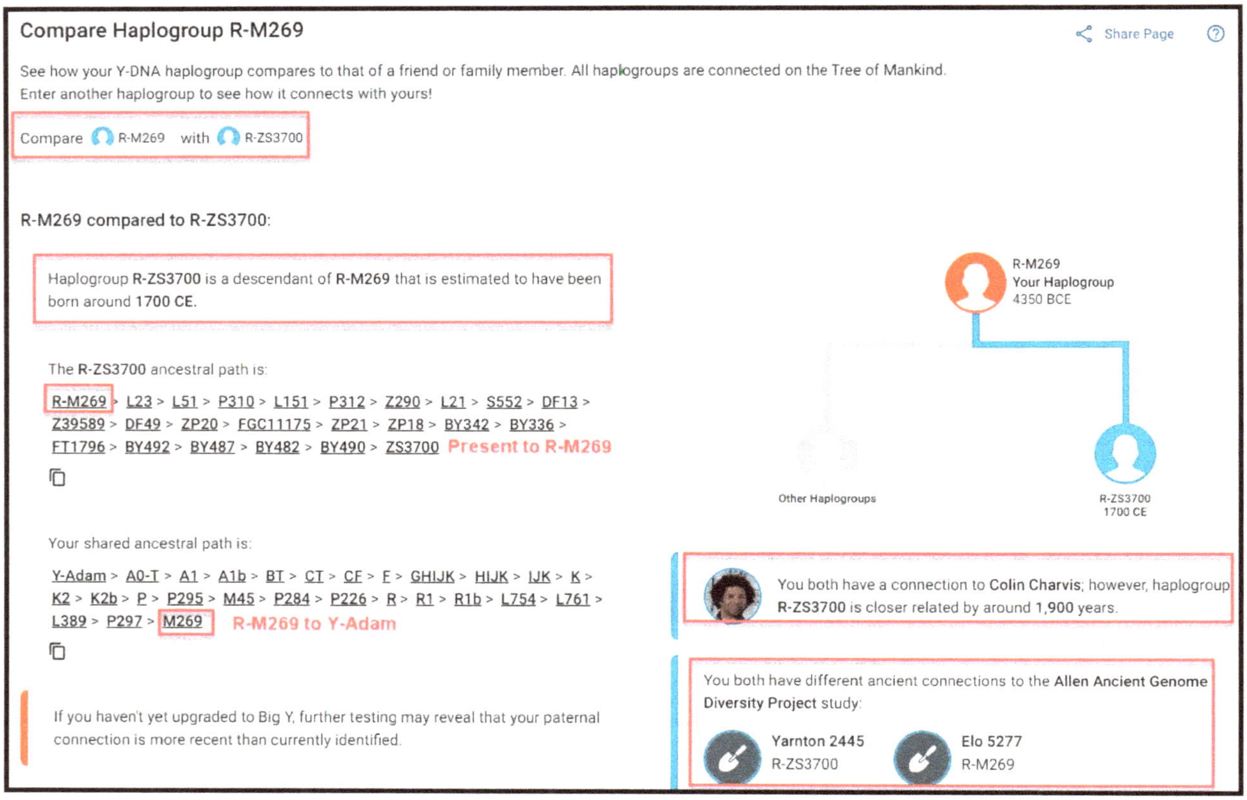

In addition to the description and lineage, the two haplogroups are displayed on the Time Tree.

About half of European men fall into the broad haplogroup R-M269, so you'll often see haplogroup R STR testers with a haplogroup prediction of R-M269. In this case, one of our Big Y-700 Estes testers is compared to men who have only taken the STR tests, with a haplogroup prediction of R-M269.

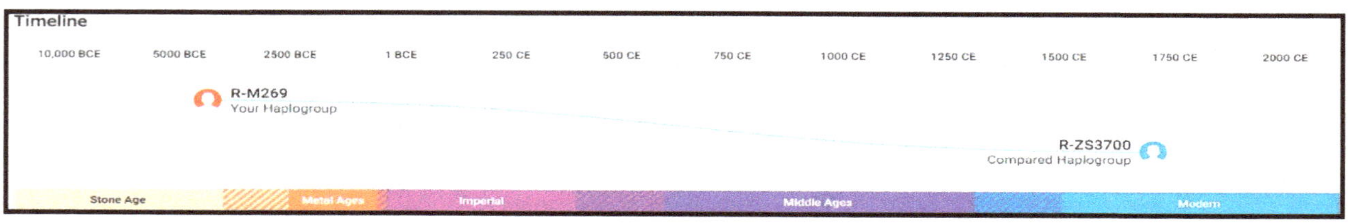

The Big Y-700 test moved this man's information from about 6350 years ago to about 1710 CE. That's HUGE! We can now reassemble entire family pedigrees, sometimes to the generation level, using Big Y-DNA tests.

86 https://dna-explained.com/2023/10/11/new-discover-tool-compare-haplogroups-more-at-familytreedna/

Public Y-DNA and Mitochondrial DNA Haplotrees

Both Y-DNA and mitochondrial DNA haplotrees are available:

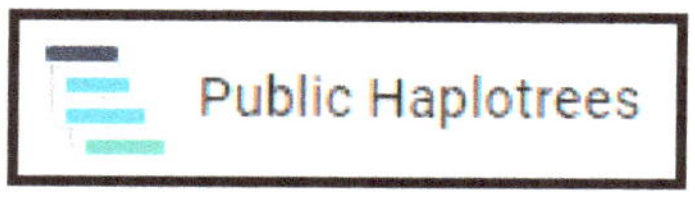

- By using the Public Haplotrees button under "Other Tools" on your FamilyTreeDNA account.

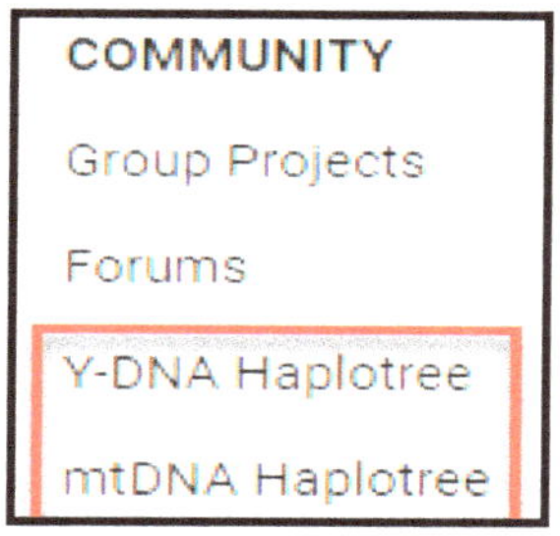

- By scrolling to the footer of the main FamilyTreeDNA page without signing in where they are available for free for everyone. They are also available in the footer when you are signed into your account.
- By using the direct web link for either the Y-DNA haplotree[87] or the mitochondrial haplotree[88].

For either tree, you will be taken to the oldest haplogroup, the tree's foundation, or root, which is the base of haplogroup A for Y-DNA and the branch above haplogroup L for mitochondrial DNA.

Both trees are searchable and display the countries entered by FamilyTreeDNA customers for their earliest known ancestors (EKA). While you will match some members of each haplogroup, it's unlikely that you will match all of the members of a specific haplogroup, unless it's at or near the tip of a branch of the Y-DNA tree.

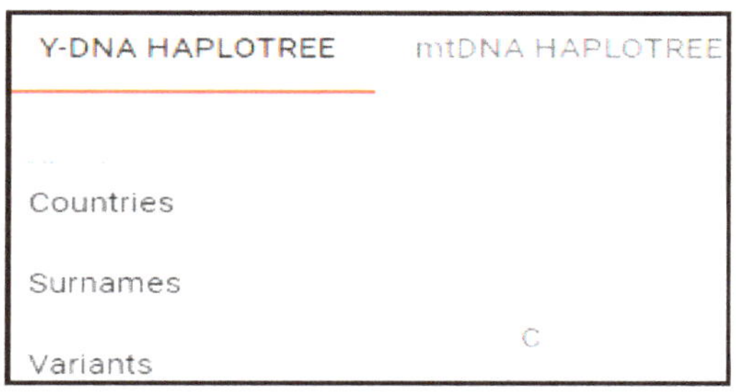

Y-DNA results are viewable by country, surname, and variants, but mitochondrial only includes countries and variants. Surnames change generationally with female lines, so listing surnames by haplogroup for mitochondrial DNA isn't useful.

---

87 https://www.familytreedna.com/public/y-dna-haplotree/A

88 https://www.familytreedna.com/public/mt-dna-haplotree/L

Country Selection

Selecting **Countries** displays the tree with the country flags for each haplogroup shown.

The countries where this haplogroup is found, according to the earliest known ancestor location data provided by testers, are shown by relevant flags.

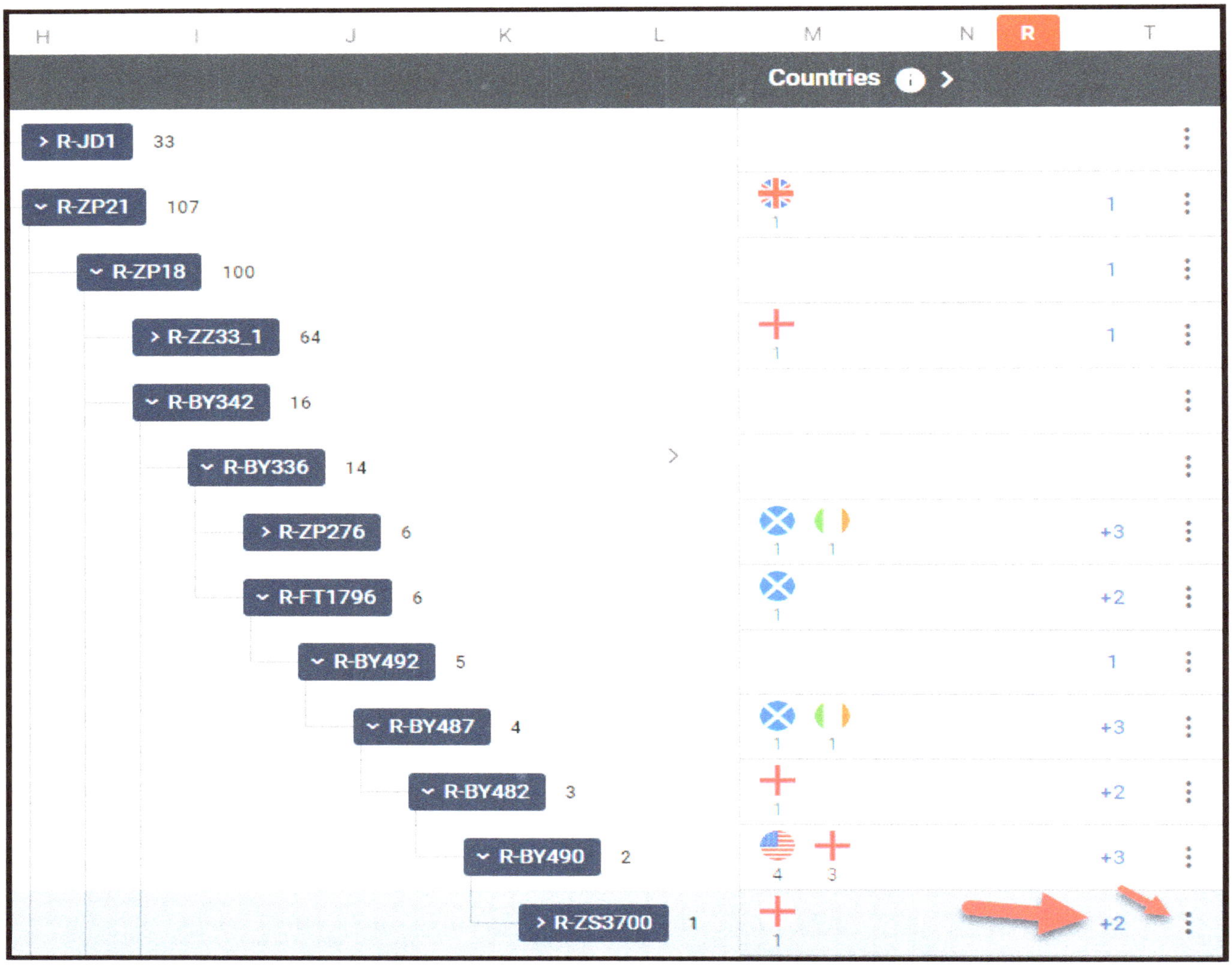

You may recognize the branches of R-ZS3700, R-BY490 and R-BY482 as Estes ancestors from Kent, England.

Haplogroups above that, beginning with BY487, reach back several hundred years before the 1490s, and testers are found today in Scotland and Ireland. To view the age of a haplogroup, enter that haplogroup into the Discover™ Haplogroup Reports tool.

Perhaps one of the most useful features of the public tree is the Surname Report, available by clicking on the 3 dots at right. Where a Surname Report is available, you will see it as one of two options, along with the Country Report.

Country Report: Y-DNA Haplogroup R-ZS3700

Paternal Origin*	Branch Participants R-ZS3700	Downstream Participants R-ZS3700 and Downstream (Excluding other Letters)	All Downstream Participants R-ZS3700 and Downstream (Including other Letters)	Distribution
England	1	1	1	50.00%
United States	0	1	1	50.00%
Unknown Origin	1	2	2	**
Total	**2**	**4**	**4**	**100.00%**

Items per page: 10 0 of 0

* All origins are self-reported by the participants and may not reflect accurate haplogroup origins.

** Unknown Origins are not included in the calculated distributions.

The Country Report, also available under the three dots, shows the total number of testers on this branch, number of branches, testers on all branches, and distribution percentages.

Surname Report: Y-DNA Haplogroup R-BY490

Surname	Participants	Distribution
Estes	6	100.00%
Total	**6**	**100.00%**

* All surnames are self-reported by the participants and may not reflect accurate haplogroup ancestry

** Two or more kits with public project profile sharing and the same surname spelling are required for a surname to show on the Haplotree.

The Surname Report displays the surnames of testers for each haplogroup who have opted to allow their surname to be displayed publicly, and where there are two or more testers with the same surname spelling.

Surname Selection

Selecting surnames on the public tree displays the surnames that tested positive for this haplogroup, but only for men who have either taken the Big Y test, received a Family Finder haplogroup[89], or purchased a SNP test. STR testers whose haplogroup is predicted as opposed to confirmed are not shown on the haplotree.

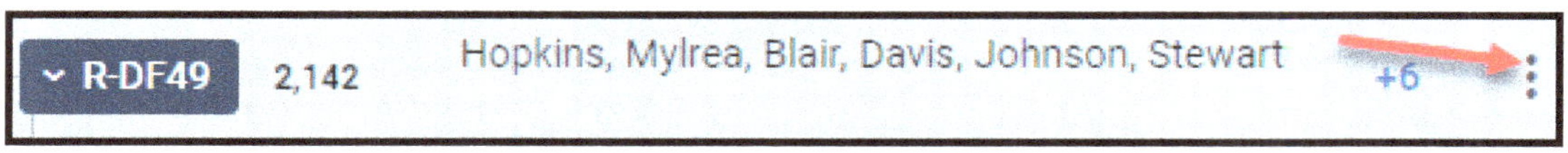

The Surname Report, available under the three dots, includes all surnames that have more than one tester with the same variant spelling and who have authorized public participation. The haplogroup shown is their haplogroup furthest down the tree that has been tested and is positive. For example, when clicking on the three dots, R-DF49 shows 16 people with 6 surnames. For non-end-of-branch haplogroups like

89 Only haplogroups derived from Family Finder autosomal tests, MyHeritage DNA tests or Vitagene tests, which are all run in the Gene by Gene lab are included in haplogroup statistics. The accuracy of the haplogroup information cannot be verified in files uploaded from other vendors.

R-DF49, keep in mind that this SNP probably was purchased individually, in a SNP pack, or assigned as a result of Family Finder testing, and these people would likely have a more refined haplogroup if they were to take the Big Y test.

Surname Report: Y-DNA Haplogroup R-M269

Surname	Participants	Distribution
Smith	41	1.40%
Miller	32	1.09%
Johnson	29	0.99%

For example, selecting haplogroup R-M269, the most common European haplogroup, produced a surname list of 776 SNP-confirmed names, headed by Smith with 41 participants. Of course, this information is much more useful for more refined haplogroups, further down the tree.

An individual tester's surname is only shown once, in their most refined haplogroup. In other words, if Estes men are shown under R-ZS3700, those men won't be shown on haplogroups higher in the tree, parent haplogroups, where other Estes men who purchased individual SNPs, an SNP pack, or have a Family Finder haplogroup may be appearing. If an Estes man has purchased the R-M269 SNP but does NOT have a confirmed SNP further down the tree, his surname will be shown under R-M269.

For more detailed information about various testers of a particular surname, refer to Surname Group Projects.

Variant Selection

Selecting to view the public tree by **Variants** shows the variants, also known as SNPs or mutations, unique to this haplogroup. Variants are passed from father to son, so variants are cumulative. In other words, every man in haplogroup R-S3700 also has the SNP mutation in R-BY490 and the mutations in R-BY482, and so forth, on up the tree.

The small numbers to the immediate right of the haplogroup indicate the number of "son" branches beneath that haplogroup. R-BY482 has three descendant or "son" branches, beginning with R-BY490, which has two descendant branches, and so forth.

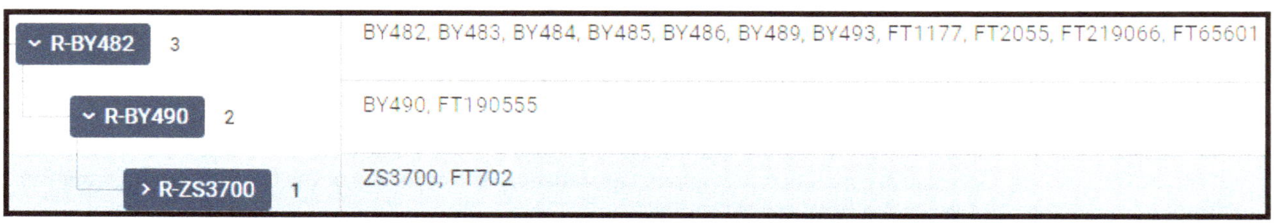

Haplogroup R-BY482 is defined by the presence of 11 different mutations that have been named and are associated with R-BY482. The 10 mutations shown to the right of BY482 are currently synonymous with BY482, although, in the future, some testers may be found without some of these mutations, which would split this haplogroup into two branches – one branch with the men having all the mutations, and the other branch with men missing one or more of those mutations.

Men who are members of haplogroup R-BY490 have all of the mutations contained in R-BY482 **PLUS** R-BY490 and its equivalent, R-FT190555.

R-ZS3700 men have all of the upstream SNPs, plus R-ZS3700 and its equivalent, R-FT702.

Y-DNA Projects

While FamilyTreeDNA offers multiple types of projects, both surname and haplogroup projects are particularly appropriate for Y-DNA testers.

Because Y-DNA descends from father to son, without mixing with any DNA from the mother, it's found essentially unchanged, except for occasional mutations, generation after generation. In Western culture, this means that the Y chromosome typically follows the paternal surname, which means that men of the same surname who share a common paternal ancestor will match at some level.

Both STR and SNP mutations accrue slowly, so, generally, the more distantly you're related, the greater the number of mutation differences, or genetic distance (GD), will be found between two men who share a common paternal ancestor.

Said another way, on the Estes surname line, one would expect my father to match his father either exactly or, since mutations can happen anytime, in any generation, maybe with one or two mutations. My father would match other men descended from Abraham Estes, born in 1647, eight generations up the tree, more distantly, probably with multiple STR and SNP mutations separating their lineages.

DNA projects provide a vehicle for people with common ancestors to collaborate and compare their DNA to a known ancestral population, meaning their relatives on the surname line.

Volunteer project administrators create, monitor, and control DNA projects by defining their goals, and determining who is eligible to join.

Some surname projects are for males only who carry that surname. Others are more inclusive and welcome other testers who descend from an ancestor with that surname, whether it's their direct paternal line or not.

There is no right or wrong policy. Projects vary based on their goals.

In the Estes surname project[90], we welcome all Estes descendants, but I only group Estes Y-DNA participants on our public web pages[91].

90 https://www.familytreedna.com/groups/estes/about/background

91 https://www.familytreedna.com/public/Estes?iframe=yresults

Presuming the project administrator has made the project publicly viewable, has enabled the Paternal Ancestor Name column in the public project display, and the testers have entered their Earliest Known Ancestor, you'll be able to view the information in any project that they've joined.

Kit Number	Name	Paternal Ancestor Name	Country	Haplogro
Estes 1 - Abraham - Abraham Jr. c 1697-1759 + Ann Watkins and Elizbaeth Jeeter, Caroline Co., Va.				
46167	Estes	Abraham Jr 1697-1759 m Ann Clark, Phillip bef 1720	Unknown Origin	R-M269
43144	Estes	Abraham Jr 1697-1759 m Ann Clark, Phillip bef 1720	Unknown Origin	R-M269
51909	Estes	Thomas Estes	United Kingdom	R-M269
49592	Estes	Abraham Jr 1697-1759 m Ann Clark, Samuel b 1727	England	R-M269
Estes 10 - Abraham - Sylvester 1684-1754 Bertie and Granville Co., NC				
199378	Estes	George Washington Estes, abt. 1845 - 1923	United States	R-BY490
17420	Estes	Abe b 1647, Sylvester, Thomas, Thomas, Burroughs	England	R-M269
13805	Estes	Nathaniel Estes, b. 1770 and d. 1845	England	R-BY490

Interested parties who have not signed up for a project or haven't taken a DNA test at FamilyTreeDNA can find projects in three ways.

Googling the term "Estes DNA Project" provides a link to the project. I often utilize this method to see if there is a surname project for the surname of an ancestor that I'm researching. However, that technique may not find alternative spellings.

The second way to locate projects publicly is found on the main FamilyTreeDNA page, without signing in.

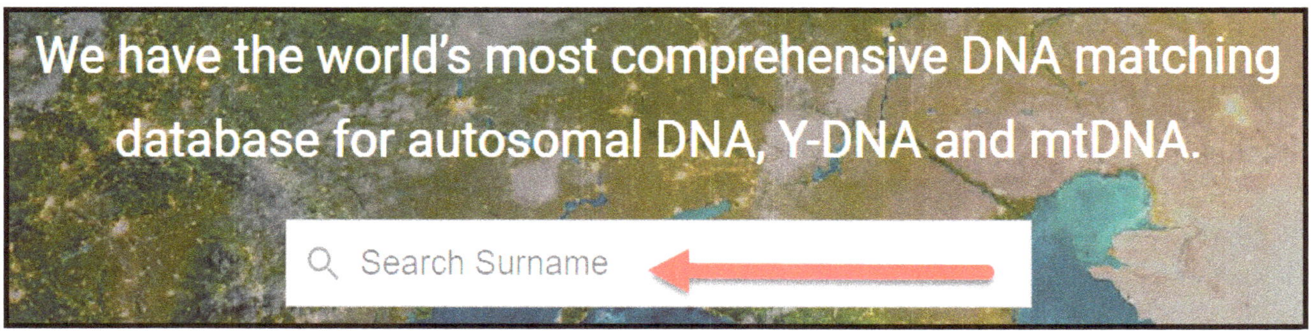

Scroll until you see the search box. By entering the desired surname and selecting the "Surname" project type, you can see how many projects include your surname of interest, and as a bonus, how many other people have tested with that surname.

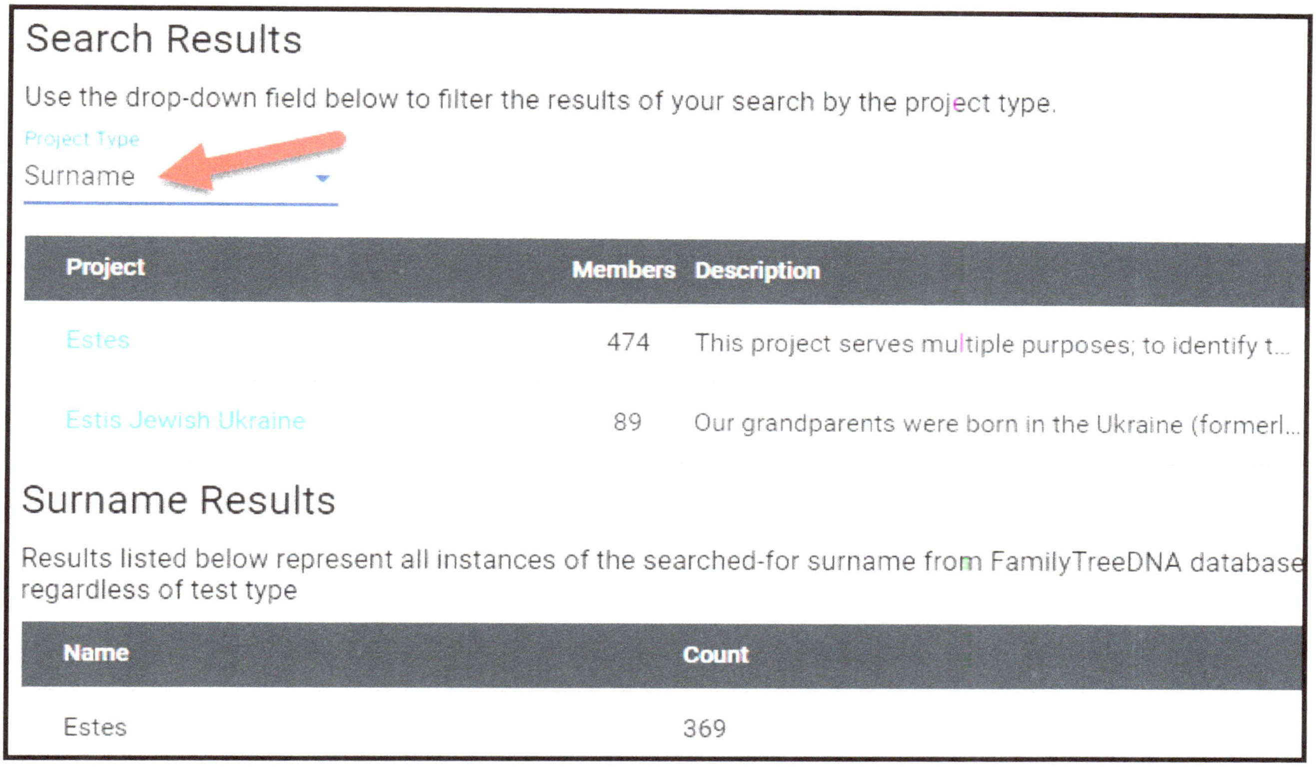

Project administrators include surnames in their project descriptions. For example, if you hunted for a derivative of Estes, such as Estis, the Estes surname project would be displayed because, as the administrator, I added Estis as a keyword, as did another project.

People can click through from here for more information, or to order a test and join a project directly from their personal page.

The third way to find projects is to scroll to the bottom of any FamilyTreeDNA page and click on "Group Projects."

Joining a Y-DNA Project From Your Personal Page

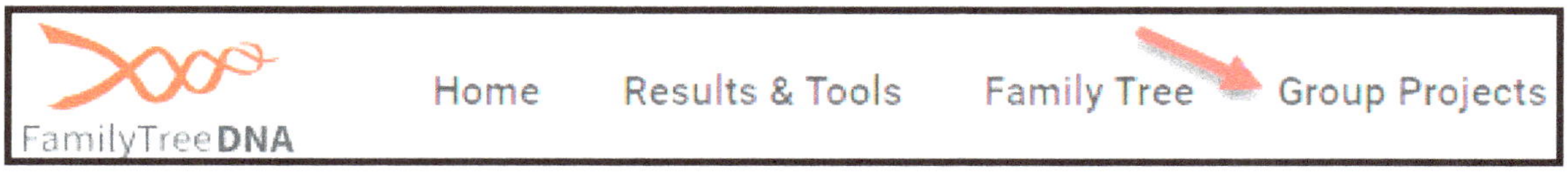

You can join a project directly from your personal page by signing on, then clicking on Group Projects at the top of the page.

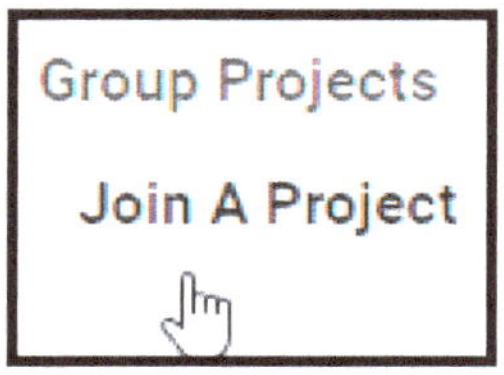

When you click on "Join a Project," FamilyTreeDNA displays a list of:

- Projects that match your surname or
- Projects where the administrator has entered your surname as a search term, indicating that some people with your surname may be interested in that project.

TIP: If the surname on your test is not the one you want to search for, just enter that surname in the Search box.

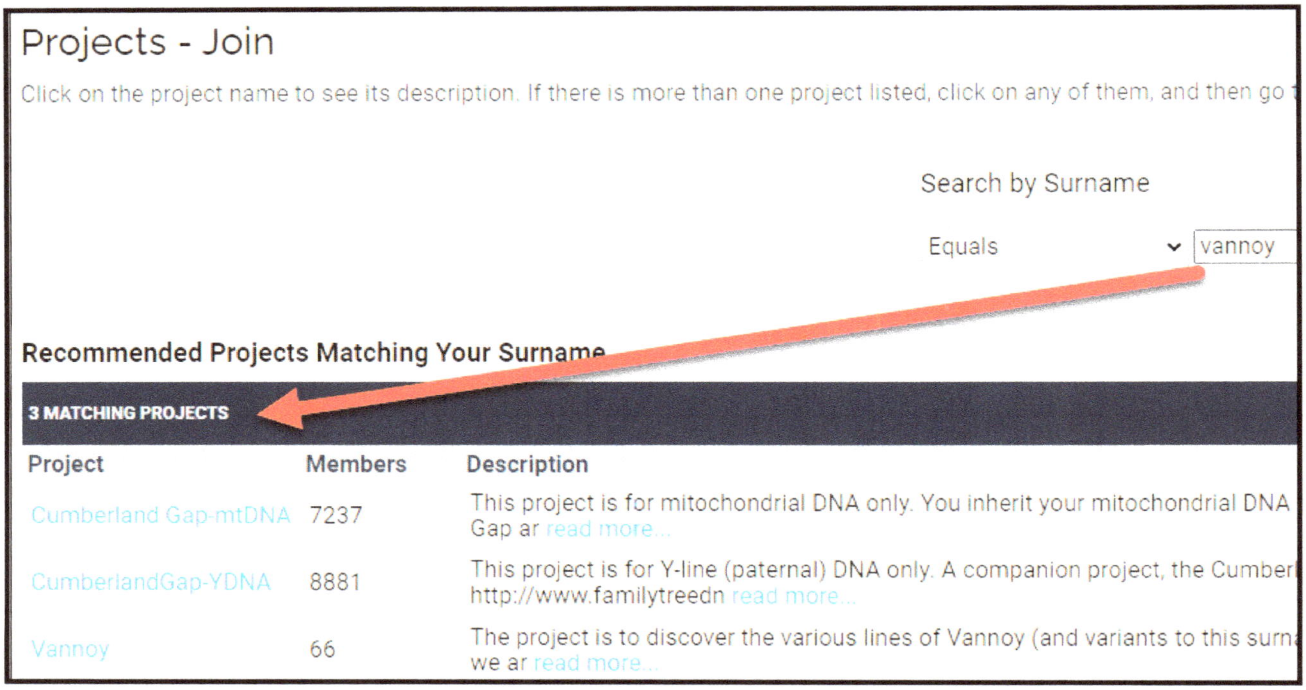

The projects displayed will include surname projects as well as geographic projects such as the Cumberland Gap project, mitochondrial DNA projects, or sometimes haplogroup projects.

This is NOT to indicate that any or all of these projects are a good fit for your situation, but they are projects where the administrator has indicated that people with a specific surname may be interested – essentially extending an invitation to consider.

We will discuss haplogroup and other types of projects more specifically in the Projects section, but the best way to find a relevant Y-DNA haplogroup project easily is by using the Discover™ Haplogroup Reports tool, entering your Y-DNA haplogroup and clicking on the Suggested Projects tab.

Group Project Time Tree

The Group Time Tree is similar to the Time Tree but displays only Big Y testers in a specific project. It also displays the Earliest Known Ancestors (EKA) entered by testers, which is one reason why completing this information is crucial.

In a publicly displayed project, click on DNA Results.

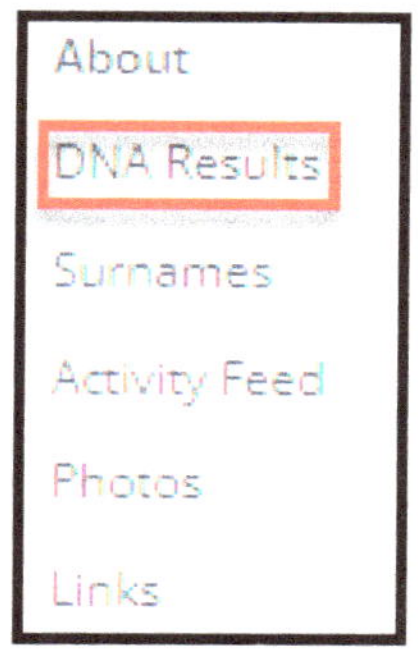

Then, under Y-DNA, select Group Time Tree.

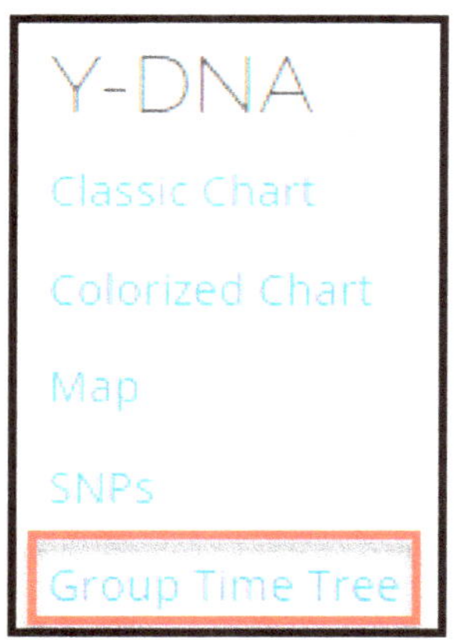

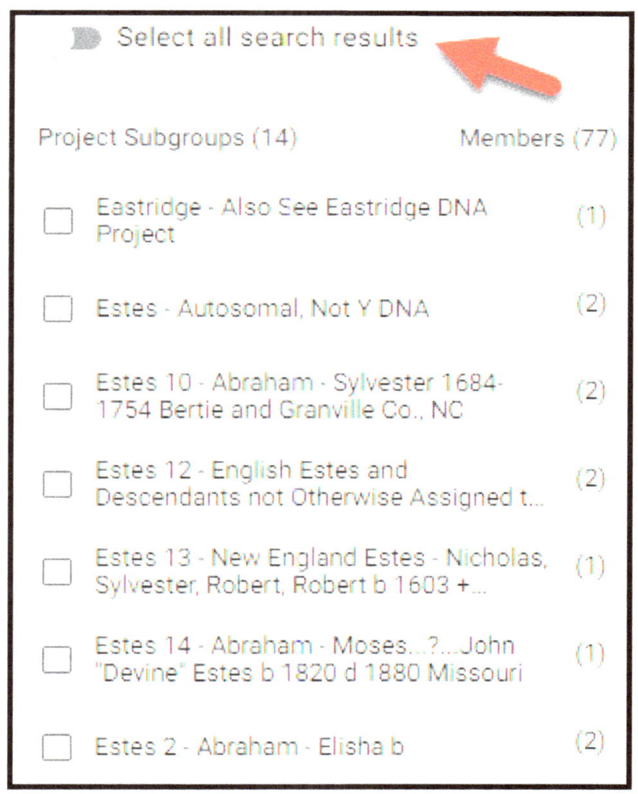

How the tree is displayed depends on how the project administrator has grouped the participants. Selecting the "Select all search results" results in all of the Big Y participants in the project being shown in one view of the tree.

This includes all Big Y-tested men in the project, even those who may have joined because they are related autosomally to this lineage. It also displays all groups within the project. For example, in the Estes project, the Eastridge line is not the same as the Estes line. Making that determination was one of the goals of Y-DNA testing.

You can select groupings that are relevant to you.

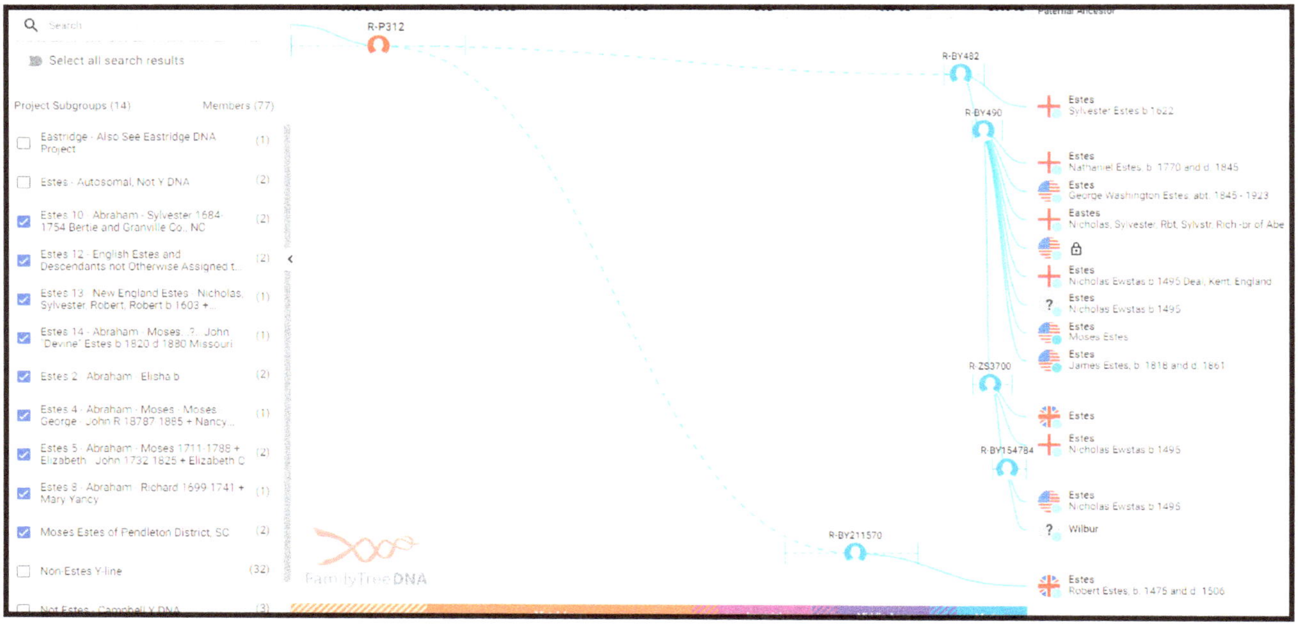

It's easy to tell by looking at the tree structure, alone, that one of the testers does not descend from the BY482 Estes line, given that their common ancestor descends from R-P312 about 2,800 years ago.

Removing that group from the display shows a closely related group of men and their earliest known ancestors.

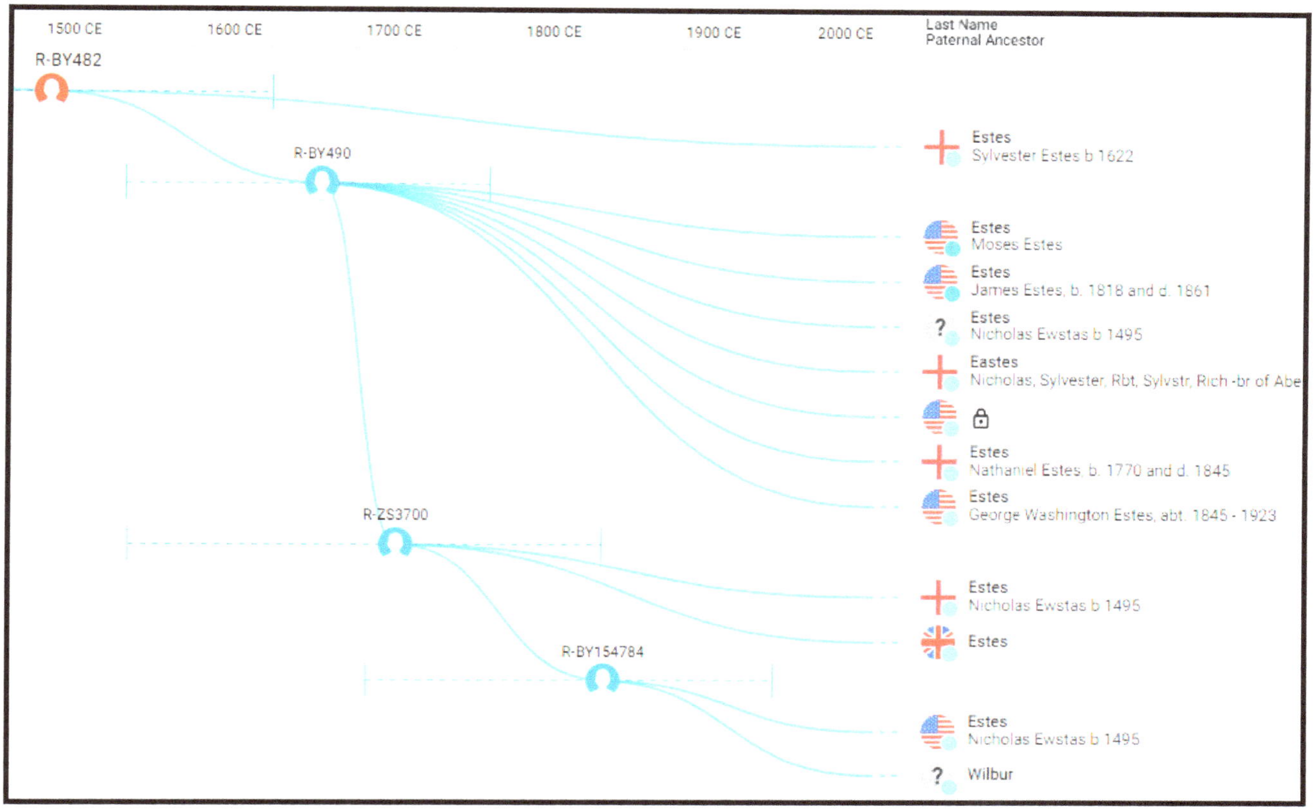

Only participants who have opted in for public sharing are shown. I wrote more about how the Group Time Tree works in the article *Sneak Preview: Introducing the FamilyTreeDNA Group Time Tree*[92] and *Project Administrators: How to Prepare Your Project for FamilyTreeDNA's New Group Time Tree.*[93]

Y-DNA Case Studies

Y-DNA testing is particularly useful for:

- Testing to determine a probable surname line
- Determining where you fit in a particular surname line, meaning which ancestor and ancestral branch you descend from
- Ruling out ancestral lineages
- Utilization in conjunction with autosomal and advanced matching tools to determine relationships

---

92 https://dna-explained.com/2023/01/13/sneak-preview-introducing-the-familytreedna-group-time-tree/

93 https://dna-explained.com/2023/01/17/project-administrators-how-to-prepare-your-project-for-familytreednas-new-group-time-tree/

Y-DNA Case 1 – Speak to Me!

For many years, genealogists had only STR markers for organizing and grouping men in paternal genealogical lineages.

The Big Y tests have changed that. Today, the Big Y-700 scans the entire "gold standard region" of the Y chromosome, reporting SNP mutations. SNP mutations occur every 80-120 years, or about once in every 2 or 3 generations, on average. Unlike STR markers, SNPs very rarely back-mutate and are much more stable, meaning the resulting grouped lineages are significantly more reliable.

In the article, *Y-DNA Genealogy Case Study: SNPs, STRs, and Autosomal – Why the Big Y-700 Rocks*[94], I provided a project-based analysis.

As of November 2022, the Speaks DNA group project had a total of:

- 105 autosomal testers
- 32 Speak (and similar surname) Y-DNA testers
- 8 Big Y testers

Genealogically, the Speak (Speaks, Speake, Speakes) family has experienced significant record loss in England, Maryland, North Carolina and Tennessee, both prior to and during colonial times and after the Revolutionary War. This unfortunate cascade of record-loss events has made it virtually impossible to tie later families to their earlier ancestors.

We knew, through Y and autosomal DNA testing, that these families were related, but exactly how eluded us due to multiple generations of at least partially missing records.

We also didn't know where the family originated in Europe, although there had been an assumption. Based on the emigration location, Maryland in the late 1600s, the origin was believed to be England. But where in England, if England?

In 2010, a Speak man from New Zealand took a Y-DNA test and matched the US immigrant group. The bonus was that he knew where in England his grandfather had lived. That information provided us with a Lancashire location to focus our research. During a genealogy visit, we met with 5 Speak men who lived in the area and who believed they were unrelated.

They took Y-DNA tests, and all matched each other as well as our immigrant line and the New Zealand cousin, ultimately leading our research trail to three villages and a hamlet within 11 miles of each other in the Lancashire countryside.

STR markers were inconsistent due to independent mutations and back-mutations in multiple lines over the intervening 500 years, but SNP mutations discovered during Big Y testing succeeded in dividing the men into groups that could be confirmed based on the genealogy we did know.

94 https://dna-explained.com/2022/11/14/y-dna-genealogy-case-study-snps-strs-autosomal-why-the-big-y-700-rocks/

Genetic groups of men, divided and clustered by both SNPs and genealogy were:

- The Lancashire group who never left, including our New Zealand tester
- The US "Thomas the Immigrant" group through his son, Bowling
- The US "Thomas the Immigrant" group through his son, John

We were very fortunate that "Thomas the Immigrant" had a SNP mutation that the Lancashire group does not have, and one of Thomas's sons, Bowling, had a SNP mutation that the other son, John did not have. This allows every Speaks man who takes the Big Y-700 test to immediately know whether he's in the resident Lancashire line, the Thomas-Bowling line, or the Thomas-John line based on their haplogroup.

Given that there are many disconnected Speaks families in regions of the US that were settled in later colonial years and after the Revolutionary War, the Big Y test immediately tells us which line the tester descends from, allowing us to set our sights on connecting with the appropriate target ancestor and his descendants.

For example, Aaron Luckey Speak was first found in 1787 in Iredell County, NC, and again three years later on the 1790 census. There were two known Speak males living there at that time who were candidates to be his father. Assuming they have been identified accurately through genealogy, they are both Bowling Speak's grandsons.

Two descendants of Aaron Luckey Speak took the Big Y-700 test, and he does descend from Bowling Speak, based on Bowling's haplogroup-defining SNP, as shown on the Block Tree, below.

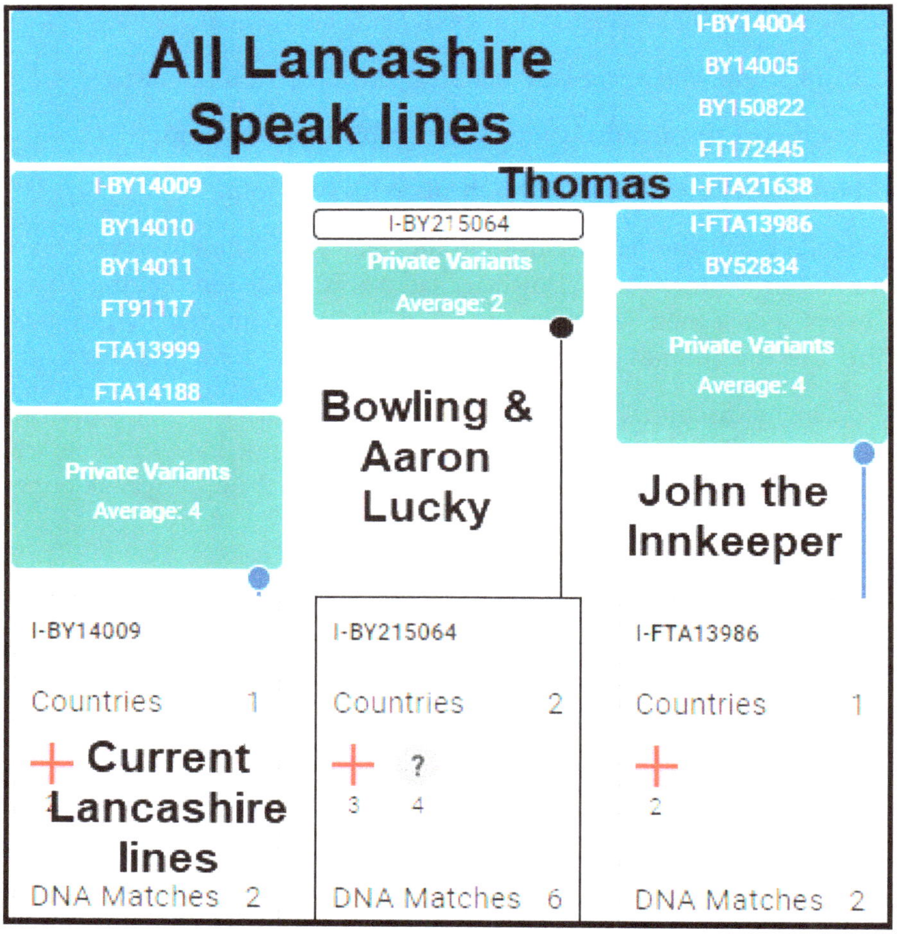

Based on genealogical records, we can eliminate some candidates, leaving both of Bowling's grandsons who migrated to Iredell County. Additional Big Y testers may split branches of the tree and ultimately provide even more granular information.

Unfortunately, STR markers could not assist with this lineage, nor could autosomal DNA. STRs are too unreliable, and these ancestors are too far back in time for autosomal to be useful in this particular case, not to mention we were trying to differentiate between two lines of the same family. SNPs, however, were exactly what we needed.

Y-DNA Case 2 – Found Father

Several years ago, a man we'll call John didn't know who his father was. He took a Y-DNA test with the hope of identifying his paternal surname line. He matched the group of our Speak males at 67 markers, which was all that was available at the time, and reached out to me as the project administrator. Based on who John matched most closely, we were able to identify a candidate line of Speaks males, some of whom just happened to live in the region where John grew up.

Autosomal testing had not yet entered the marketplace, but between John's Y-DNA test, local records, and proximity in the critical month and year of his conception, we were able to narrow the candidates to two men.

John hesitated at that point, concerned about what might follow. No one wants to face rejection, or unintentionally upend someone's life. We clearly didn't know the circumstances, or even if we were right. How to proceed, if at all, was a decision only John could make.

Several months later, I heard from John again. He had delayed writing the letter or making the call, but when he eventually did, he connected with a man who agreed to speak with him. The man said, "I'm not your father," and John's heart sank, but then the man continued, "…but I know who is." As it turned out, John's father had recently died, but the man he was speaking with was his uncle, and knew that his brother had dated John's mother. John's uncle and the rest of the family welcomed him with open arms.

Y-DNA testing is a crucial resource for all males.

Another case study illustrates why.[95]

Y-DNA Case 3 – When the Y-DNA Doesn't Match, But You're Still Related in the Same Generation…Wait? What???

My ancestor, Marcus Younger [96] (c1740-1815), was always presumed to be the son of Thomas Younger (c1707-1791). That word, "presume," is dangerous in genealogy, but in this case, that presumption was so old that I don't think modern genealogists knew they were working with an assumption. Maybe they weren't. Maybe it was an oral history of sorts or a family secret. Who knows?

The age difference was about right. Marcus and Thomas lived nearby and were found together in many documents in Halifax County, Virginia, where they had moved from Essex County on the border with King and Queen County. Thomas Younger was the son of Alexander Younger.

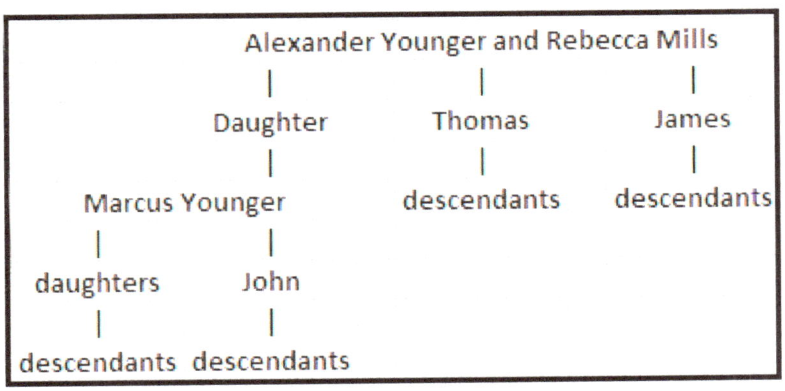

However, in a surprising turn of events, Y-DNA revealed that Thomas and Marcus were not paternally related, which clearly explains why Marcus was not in Thomas's will, but was instead a witness. Thomas

95 https://dna-explained.com/2013/11/17/proving-men-whose-y-lines-dont-match-are-related/

96 https://dna-explained.com/2014/06/08/marcus-younger-c1740-1816-mystery-man-52-ancestors-23/

and his brother James Younger's male descendants' Y-DNA matched each other, but neither matched Marcus. Not even close. This was baffling, though, because autosomal DNA showed clearly that Marcus's descendants triangulated with segments of Thomas's descendants as well as his brother James' descendants. So, they were related, but how is this possible given that their Y-DNA is in completely different base haplogroups?

After significantly more research, we discovered that several years after Alexander Younger's death, in 1732, Thomas was appointed as the guardian of his four sisters. One sister married, but the others dropped out of the records altogether, including estate distribution. Marcus was the correct age to belong to Thomas's sister through an illegitimate birth, which would explain how these people are related autosomally, carry the same surname, and were clearly very close, yet the Y-DNA doesn't match. Thomas probably raised Marcus after his sister's death.

Y-DNA Case 4 – Process of Elimination & a Cautionary Tale

Unfortunately, Moore is a very common surname. The James Moore[97] line of Halifax County, Virginia, has been the topic of genealogy research for decades. We know he was born about 1718 and was first found in Amelia County as an adult. Despite research by many genealogists, he has never been tied to any earlier Moore line. Even more frustrating, James doesn't appear to be connected to other Moore lines in either Amelia County or the part that became Prince Edward County, nor in Halifax County, where he eventually settled.

I had one theory after another, including the Moore family, who lived just down the road, literally within sight, who also came from Amelia County, but Y-DNA testing would prove all of those theories wrong. How about the Moore line who settled a couple miles in the other direction? Nope, and they aren't related to the other Moore family either. So frustrating.

Based on autosomal matches, we may be dealing with another unknown father situation, but that's impossible to determine, because we don't know what other lines James might share with neighboring, but paternally unrelated, Moore lines.

Today, I'm still willing to sponsor DNA testing scholarships for potential Moore lines, but I've just about run out of lines that haven't already been tested. I keep waiting for a DNA match on one of our Moore line testers – hoping for something, anything, from colonial America or across the sea. In the meantime, I'll just continue to watch for colonial Virginia lineages that haven't yet been tested in the hope that one of these Y-DNA tests will be the clue we need. At least testing those numerous lines has prevented us from drawing "reasonable" conclusions, especially considering autosomal matches, but that would clearly be wrong and would cause us to bark up the wrong tree.

---

97 https://dna-explained.com/2019/08/04/james-moore-c1718-c1798-westward-to-amelia-county-52-ancestors-249/

Chapter 4

MITOCHONDRIAL DNA – YOUR MOTHER'S STORY

Mitochondrial DNA (mtDNA) tracks your mother's direct matrilineal line. While only males can take a Y-DNA test, everyone inherits mitochondrial DNA from their mother and can take a mitochondrial DNA test.

Like Y-DNA, mitochondrial DNA is never mixed with the DNA of the other parent, so you inherit your mother's mitochondrial DNA intact, except for occasional mutations that make mitochondrial DNA useful for genealogy.

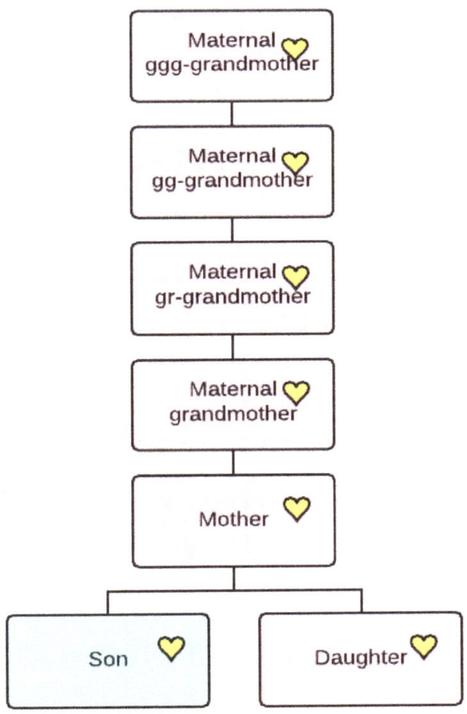

Everyone receives mitochondrial DNA, but only females pass it on, meaning that you receive your mother's mitochondrial DNA, who received it from her mother, who received it from her mother, and so forth, on up the maternal side of your tree.

The great news is that in the current generation, males and females can both test because everyone inherits mitochondrial DNA from their mother.

The biggest challenges with mitochondrial DNA are that:

- The female's surname historically changes in every generation, making the genealogy more challenging.
- Misinformation, especially on social media, leads people to believe that mitochondrial DNA isn't useful.
- As a result, fewer people test, inhibiting the growth of the database which in turn results in fewer matches.

If more people tested, people would receive more matches, some of which would lead to common ancestors, and people wouldn't discourage others from testing. Mitochondrial DNA provides information not available from any other source.

I have provided a free Mitochondrial DNA Resource page[98] that includes education, instructions for understanding and using mtDNA, plus case studies.

Mitochondrial DNA Goals

Mitochondrial DNA testing goals may include:

- Breaking down brick walls in the direct matrilineal line
- Learn about the genesis of the family line through your haplogroup
- Confirm that a female ancestor is the mother of your ancestor by target testing
- Confirming descent from a particular ancestor or ancestral family
- Confirm or refute Native American heritage and oral history
- Discovering who you do, or don't, match
- Delving into your matrilineal history before the advent of surnames
- Determine the source of your matrilineal lineage, meaning Native American, European, African, Asian, Jewish, etc.
- Understanding your ancestor's migration path
- Learning what you don't know, which may be different than what you think you know

98 https://dna-explained.com/mitochondrial-dna/

Mitochondrial DNA is NOT X-DNA

Sometimes people confuse mitochondrial DNA with X-DNA.

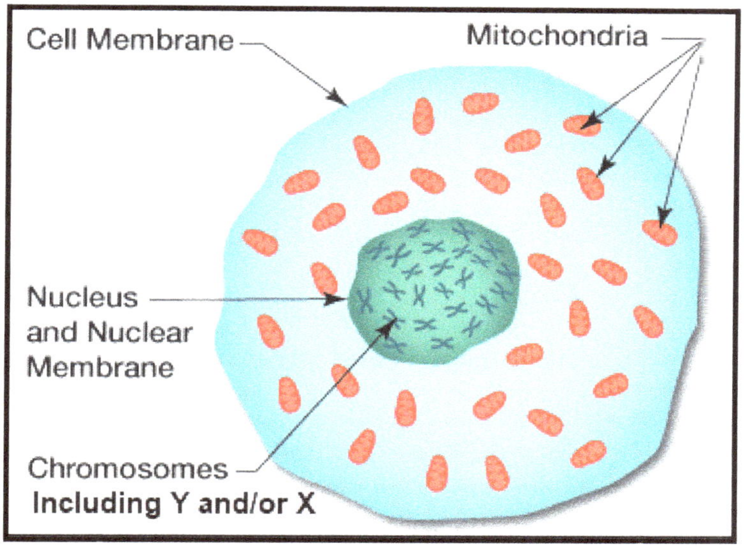

Mitochondrial DNA is comprised of 16,569 base pairs, and the double helix they form is arranged in a circle found outside the cell nucleus. Y-DNA, autosomal DNA, and X-DNA are located inside the cell nucleus.

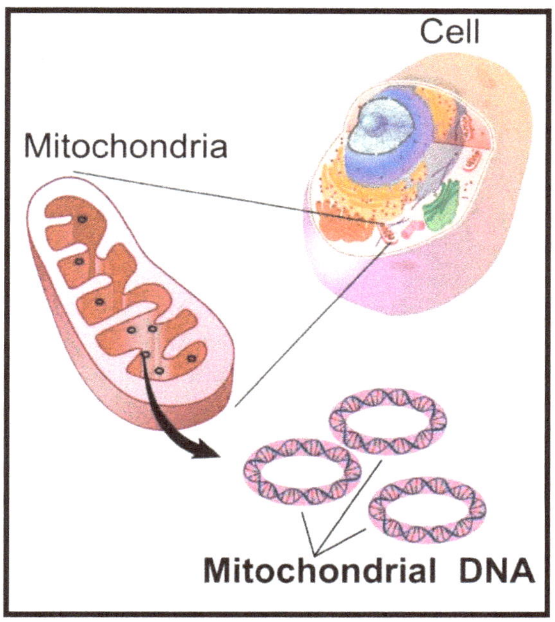

Each cell contains many copies of mitochondrial DNA, which produces energy to power every cell in our bodies.

Everyone receives mitochondrial DNA from their mother, and only their mother.[99]

The X chromosome, on the other hand, is one of the sex-determining chromosomes and has a unique inheritance path. Men only receive a copy of their X chromosome from their mother, because they receive a copy of their Y chromosome from their father, which is what makes males male.

Females receive an X chromosome from both their mother and their father, just like the other 22 autosomes.

I wrote about this in the article, *X Matching, and Mitochondrial DNA is Not the Same Thing.*[100]

We'll discuss the X chromosome further in the X-DNA Matching section.

Mitochondrial Regions

Mitochondrial DNA is a circular organelle that is divided into three regions for matching purposes.[101]

You might think about mitochondrial DNA as a clock face.

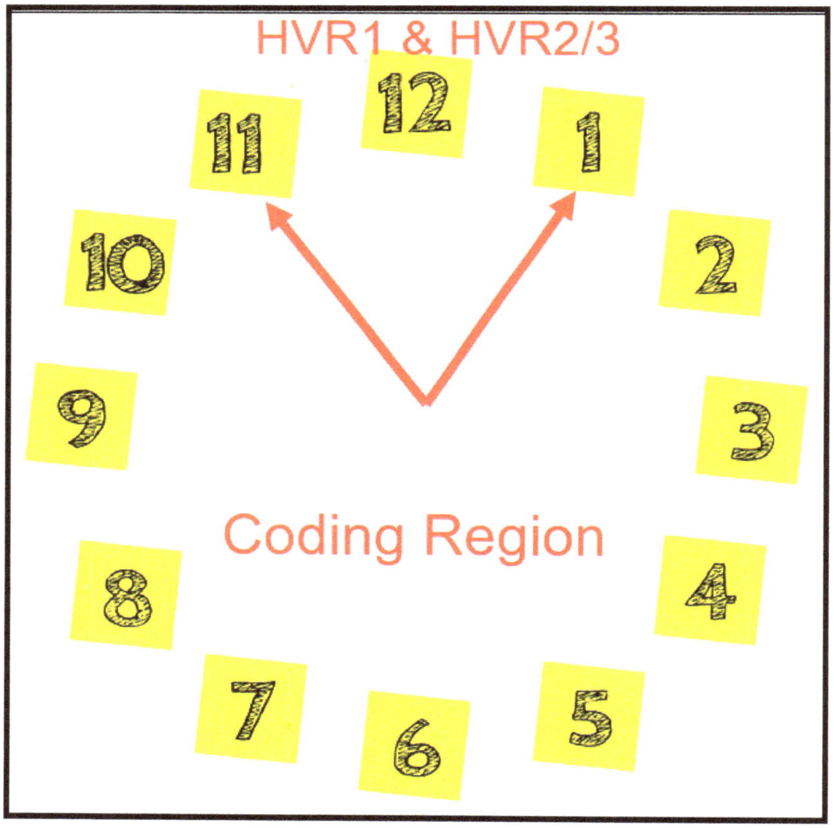

99 https://en.wikipedia.org/wiki/Paternal_mtDNA_transmission

100 https://dna-explained.com/2017/07/26/x-matching-and-mitochondrial-dna-is-not-the-same-thing/

101 https://www.familytreedna.com/understanding-dna.aspx

- HVR1 (Hypervariable Region 1) includes about 500 locations of your mitochondrial DNA and spans the space between 11 and 12.
- HVR2 (Hypervariable Region 2) combined with HVR3 (Hypervariable Region 3) includes approximately another 575 locations and spans from 12-1.
- The Coding Region contains the balance of the 16,569 locations extending from 1-11

A few genes are located in the Coding Region, meaning that mutations in that region are less common because organisms experiencing mutations in the region occupied by genes may not survive. On the other hand, HVR1 and HVR2 experience more mutations more often, because no genes exist in that region, so mutations don't cause genetic damage. Hence, the name "hyper-variable region."

Just like Y-DNA began with a 12-marker test, mitochondrial DNA for genealogy began with the HVR1 test, then progressed to the HVR2 test, then a full sequence test.

Today, the full sequence test (mtFull) that includes all 16,569 locations costs far less than the original HVR1 test. We can thank advances in technology for that.

Only the mtFull test can be purchased today, but you will still see people on your match list who only took the HVR1 or HVR1+HVR2 (mtPlus) test in the past and never upgraded.

TIP: Don't ignore those low-level matches, because even if they haven't tested all of the available locations, their genealogy might still hold the key that breaks down that brick wall.

Mitochondrial Model Versions

The mitochondrial DNA reference sequence known as the Cambridge Reference Sequence (CRS) was first published in 1981 using mainly the DNA of a volunteer in Cambridge, England.[102] That sequence was subsequently updated to correct errors in 1999 and is designated as the rCRS, or revised Cambridge Reference Sequence.

However, there was an "under the hood" problem.

Any difference from that model was considered to be a mutation. However, the problem was that this haplogroup H2a2a1 individual was European, meaning that mutations that occurred in the time between when Mitochondrial Eve lived some 140,000-150,000 years ago in Africa, and when that volunteer was born were considered to be mutations, when, in fact, they are the foundation of the tree before H2a2a1. H2a2a1 is not the center of the mitochondrial universe, but a branch that sprouted between 1,700 and 5,900 years ago.[103]

In 2012, Dr. Doron Behar et al changed that dynamic and shifted the analysis to a model whereby Mitochondrial Eve, the first woman who survived to have descendants today, is the base of the tree. The new Reconstructed Sapiens Reference Sequence (RSRS) is now the base of the tree, with 5,468 descendant branches.[104]

102 https://genome.cshlp.org/content/24/4/xi.full

103 https://www.ncbi.nlm.nih.gov/pmc/articles/PMC3322232/ and supplemental information

104 https://www.familytreedna.com/public/mt-dna-haplotree/L

FamilyTreeDNA reports the results for both models.

TIP: There's an easy trick to determine immediately whether someone is using or referring to rCRS or the later RSRS values:

- 16069T – rCRS results only list the position followed by the mutated value, omitting the leading value, which is the reference or original value
- C16069T – RSRS results list the reference value before the location, then appends the mutated value at the end

Mitochondrial Eve

Mitochondrial Eve is somewhat of a misnomer since the name suggests a Biblical person.

Mitochondrial Eve is defined as the first woman who survived AND has living people who descend from her through direct matrilineal descent, meaning the entire line of descent is female to female to the current generation, which can be male.

Mitochondrial Eve is the matrilineal common ancestor of all humanity. So yes, that means that we are all related. It's only a matter of how far back in the tree.

There were other women who lived, both during and before the lifetime of Mitochondrial Eve, but people who descend from those women matrilineally do not exist today. In other words, those lines died out, but Eve's line did not.

As more is learned and new testers are found who carry previously unknown mutations, such as the L7 lineage discovered in 2022[105], the timeframe in which Mitochondrial Eve lived may shift somewhat as our knowledge becomes even more refined.

Mutations

Let's talk about mutations. Some mitochondrial DNA mutations are used differently than for either autosomal or Y-DNA.

- Some mutations are used for haplogroup definition
- Some mutations are considered "extra" or "missing" and are used for matching to other testers
- Some mutations are unstable and are reported, but ignored for both haplogroup definition and matching
- Not all mutations are created equal

105 https://dna-explained.com/2022/06/25/mitochondrial-eve-gets-a-great-granddaughter-african-mitochondrial-haplogroup-l7-discovered/

Haplotree Branch Definition

Mitochondrial DNA haplogroups and descending branches are defined by specific mutations.

Generally speaking, once a mutation occurs, it's inherited by the descendants of the individual in which the mutation occurred.

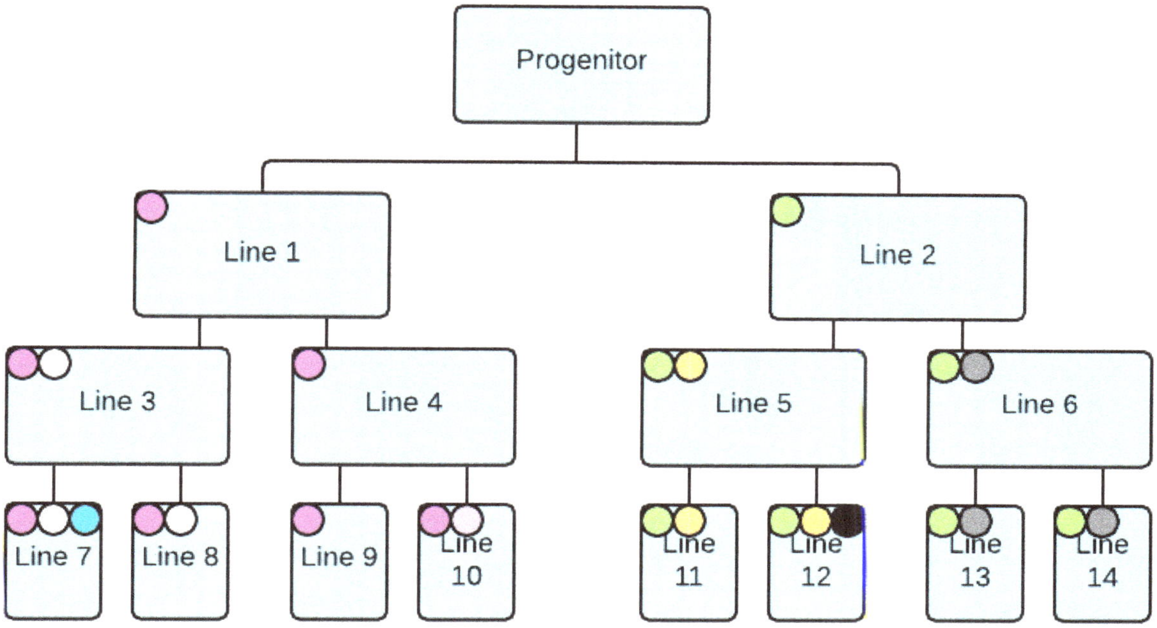

For example, in this graphic, we see that our progenitor has "no" mutations, and each of her children has one mutation. Line 1 has a magenta mutation, and Line 2 has a green mutation. As one moves down the tree generationally, each generation has the same mutation as the preceding generation, and may, or may not, accrue additional mutations.

In reality, mutations aren't going to happen in every generation, but the concept of accrual is what's important.

This person's results show that they have "extra mutations" which means those mutations aren't haplogroup-defining.

Extra Mutations	G185A	G228A	315.1C	522.1A	522.2C
Missing Mutations					

Matching occurs by comparing the results of two individuals to each other, which means taking into consideration their haplogroup-defining mutations, followed by both their extra and missing mutations, if any, with some exceptions. Make note of mutation 315.1C. You'll see this again a little later.

New haplogroup branches are defined by newly discovered mutations within the same line, causing the line to split into two branches.

Most new mutations are discovered in more recent generations, like our progenitor example, but not always.

In some cases, especially where the population has been under-sampled, new base haplogroups or older branches are discovered. This happened recently with haplogroup L7 [106], a 100,000-year-old lineage that was identified by the Million Mito Team in a few people with roots in Africa.[107] It's an older branch, far up the tree, but it's also the base for several other branches.

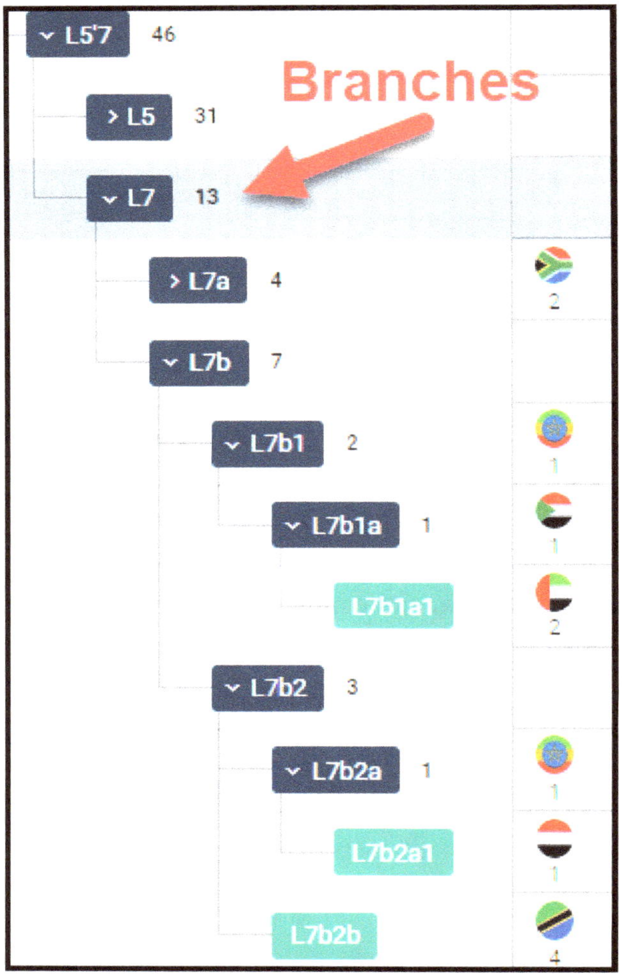

106 https://www.nature.com/articles/s41598-022-13856-0

107 https://dna-explained.com/2022/06/25/mitochondrial-eve-gets-a-great-granddaughter-african-mitochondrial-haplogroup-l7-discovered/

The new L7 branch created a split high in the tree. There are many more branches awaiting discovery as increasing numbers of people test, and more analysis is performed on existing samples. The fact that ancient DNA results are being tested and reported in prodigious numbers is quite helpful too.

While the Y-DNA tree is updated on an almost daily basis at FamilyTreeDNA, the mitochondrial haplotree is not. At least not yet.

There was never an official academic public consensus tree for Y-DNA as that tree grew[108], but there was for mitochondrial DNA, and it was called PhyloTree. After the last PhyloTree update in February 2016[109], the tree began to languish, and no new branches were added.

In 2018, FamilyTreeDNA published a free, enhanced mitochondrial haplotree,[110] with six times the number of samples as PhyloTree, and in a friendlier format.[111] They also added flags for locations, so it's easy to see where any specific haplogroup is found around the world.

Believing that the curator of PhyloTree would add and refine haplogroups in a future release, FamilyTreeDNA did not define and add new haplogroups as they have with their Y-DNA tree.

However, over time, it became clear that PhyloTree was no longer being updated.

In 2020, the Million Mito Team was formed to explore updating the mitochondrial reference tree. The initiative was announced at RootsTech[112], with the team consisting of Göran Runfeldt, Head of R&D for FamilyTreeDNA, Dr. Paul Maier, Population Geneticist at FamilyTreeDNA, Dr. Miguel Vilar, Lead Scientist for National Geographic's Genographic Project, and me.

The construction of the mitochondrial tree involves first reconstructing the original Phylotree using automation in order to provide consistency and transition within the community, from old to new. Unfortunately, the earlier curator never published his methodology, so we had to begin from scratch and reconstruct the existing tree by trial and error. In 2022, the team provided an update and a description of the challenges being faced.[113] We have discovered, among other things, that there is no research or academic software that can handle the magnitude of data available today so that software is being created.

---

108 https://genome.cshlp.org/content/18/5/830

109 https://www.phylotree.org/

110 https://dna-explained.com/2018/10/10/family-tree-dnas-mitochondrial-haplotree/

111 https://www.familytreedna.com/public/mt-dna-haplotree/L

112 https://dna-explained.com/2020/03/17/the-million-mito-project/

113 https://dna-explained.com/2022/04/13/million-mito-project-team-introduction-and-progress-update/

Today, you can view the current public tree[114] with two display options; Countries, and Variants, which is another word for mutations.

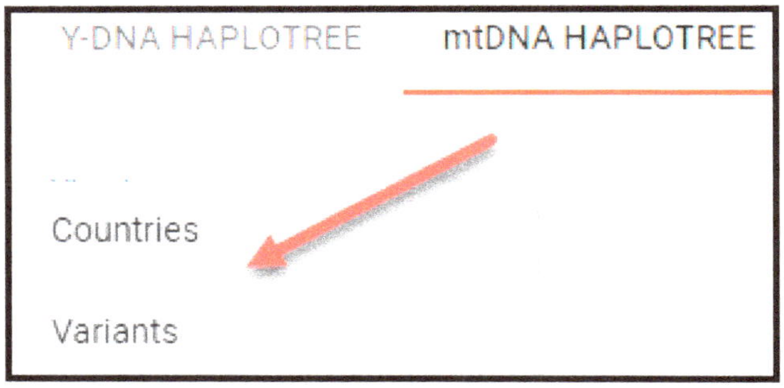

When selecting the **Variant** view, you'll see the tree with the mutations that define each haplogroup branch.

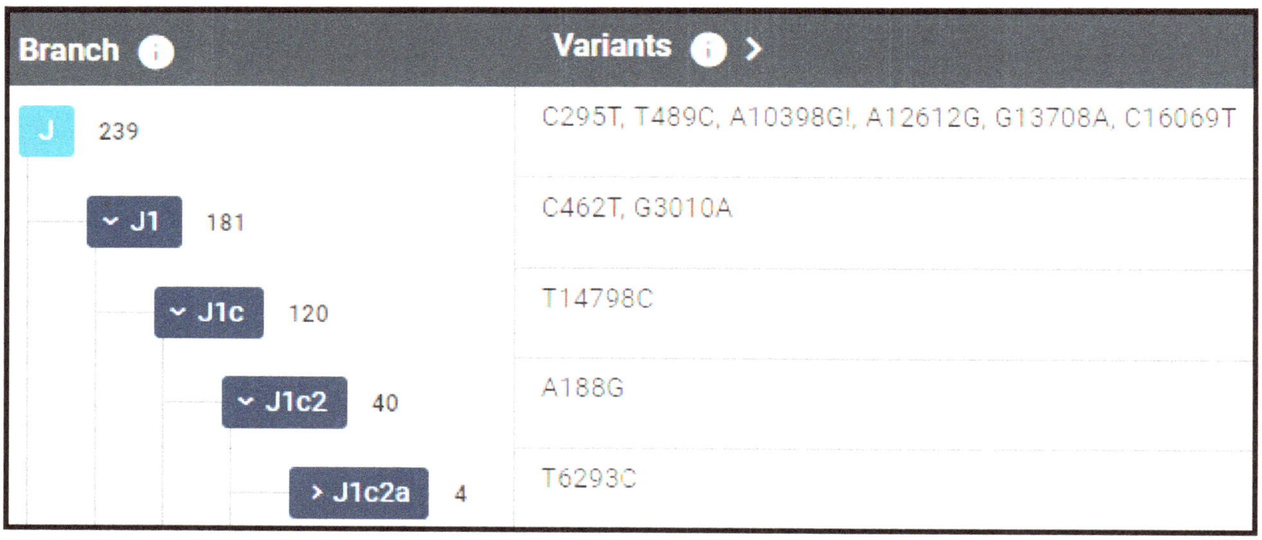
Branch
Variants
J 239
C295T, T489C, A10398G!, A12612G, G13708A, C16069T
J1 181
C462T, G3010A
J1c 120
T14798C
J1c2 40
A188G
J1c2a 4
T6293C

In this example, haplogroup J1c2a is defined by mutation T6293C, meaning J1c2a has this mutation in addition to the mutations accumulated in the parent haplogroups, shown above J1c2a. J1c2a also has 4 descendant branches, not pictured.

The parent haplogroup of J1c2a is J1c2 which is defined by mutation A188G, and J1c is defined by T14798C. The accumulation of mutations continues like a trail of breadcrumbs, leading back in time to the common ancestor of all humanity, Mitochondrial Eve, born in Africa approximately 140,000 years ago.

Switching to the **Country** view provides the ability to see where your haplo-relatives are from, which may provide insight into where your ancestors came from, both recently and further back in time.

114 https://www.familytreedna.com/public/mt-dna-haplotree/L

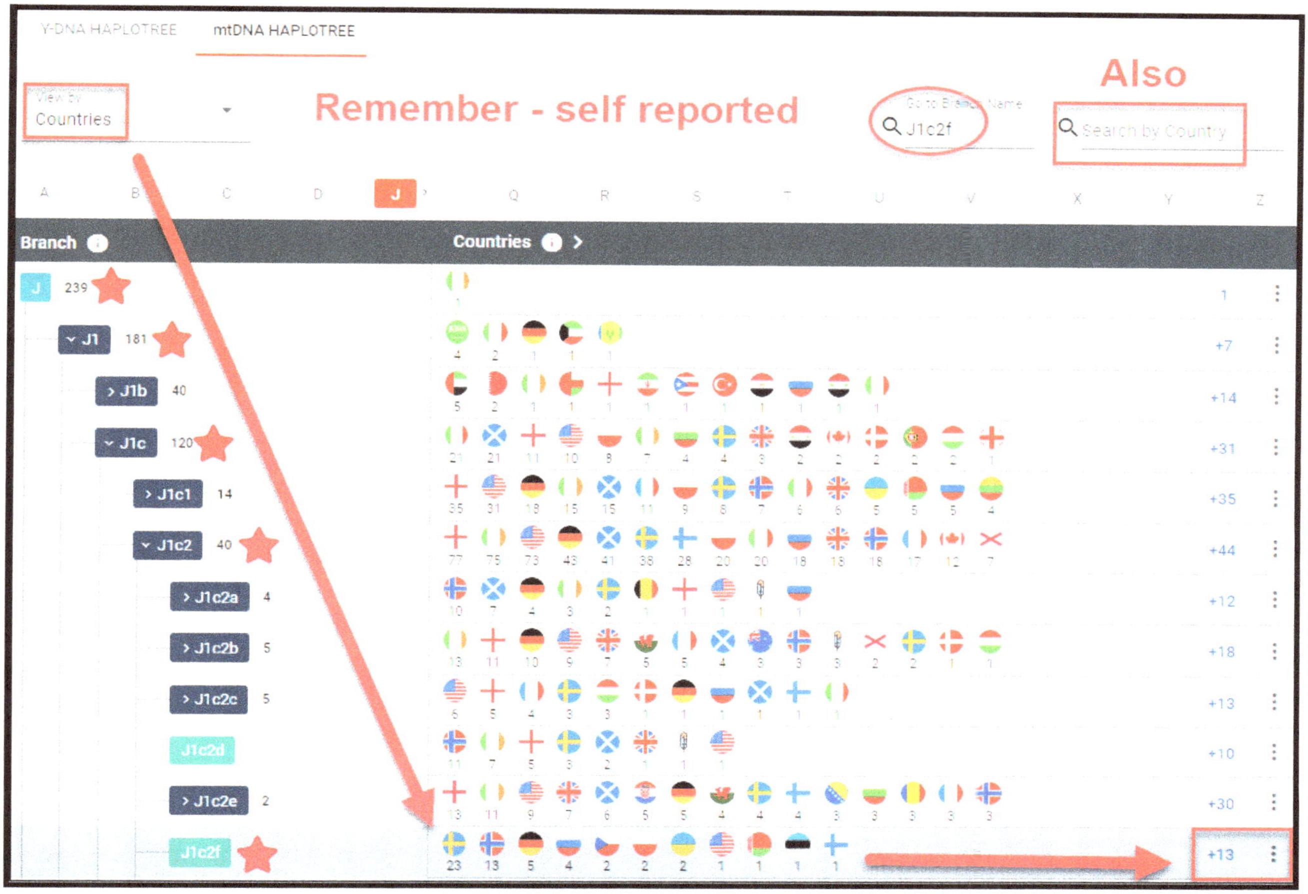

Several sibling branches are shown immediately above J1c2f. Parent/child branches are noted with stars.

TIP: Clicking on the three "hamburger" dots at the far right provides a report by country for each haplogroup.

Country Report: mtDNA Haplogroup J1c2f

Maternal Origin*	Branch Participants J1c2f	Downstream Participants J1c2f and Downstream (Excluding other Letters)	All Downstream Participants J1c2f and Downstream (Including other Letters)	Distribution
Sweden	23	23	23	41.82%
Norway	13	13	13	23.64%
Germany	5	5	5	9.09%
Russian Federation	4	4	4	7.27%
Czech Republic	2	2	2	3.64%
Poland	2	2	2	3.64%
Ukraine	2	2	2	3.64%
United States	1	1	1	1.82%
Belarus	1	1	1	1.82%
Estonia	1	1	1	1.82%
Finland	1	1	1	1.82%
Unknown Origin	20	20	20	**
Unknown Origin	14	14	14	**
Total	89	89	89	100.00%

Be sure to check these reports because it's unlikely that on your personal page, you will match everyone else in your haplogroup, so this is the only place you'll see that information.

Testing yourself, your father, your maternal grandfather, and your paternal grandfather will provide you with the mitochondrial DNA of all four of your grandparents and four of your great-grandparents too. Of course, if those specific relatives are not available to test, you can follow the mtDNA line to living relatives who would provide the same information. For example, for your grandfathers, their sisters could test, or daughters of those sisters - but not daughters of your grandfathers, as they received their mtDNA from their respective mothers.

Different Types of Mutations

Think of mutations as special-delivery messengers from your ancestors.

Different types of mutations mean different things scientifically, as well as how they pertain to genealogy. If you're satisfied with working with your matches, that's fine, and you can skip to the Mitochondrial DNA Dashboard section.

However, the type of mutation and who has it may affect matching. Plus, science is interesting, right?

Travel Buddy Mutations

Sometimes haplogroups are defined by multiple mutations.

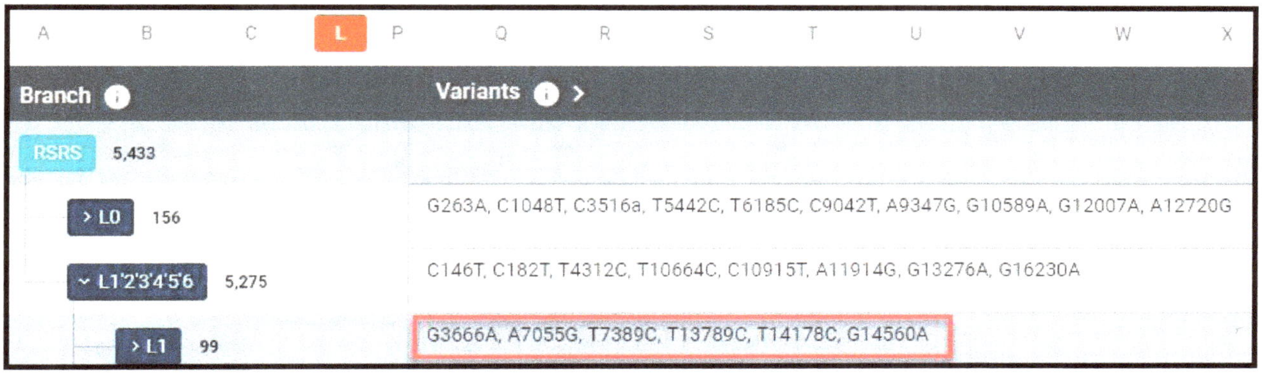

For example, you can see that haplogroup L1 is defined by 6 mutations, meaning all people in haplogroup L1, or any of its 99 subclades, have those mutations.

At some point in the future, a group of people may test who have a subset of the multiple mutations that form haplogroup L1, which would divide L1 into two (or more) branches.

Similar to Private Variants and Equivalent SNPs in Y-DNA tests, multiple haplogroup-defining mutations are also haplogroups in waiting.

Haplogroup Mutation Inheritance

Mutations that define haplogroups are generally inherited by every downstream haplogroup. Notice the word generally.

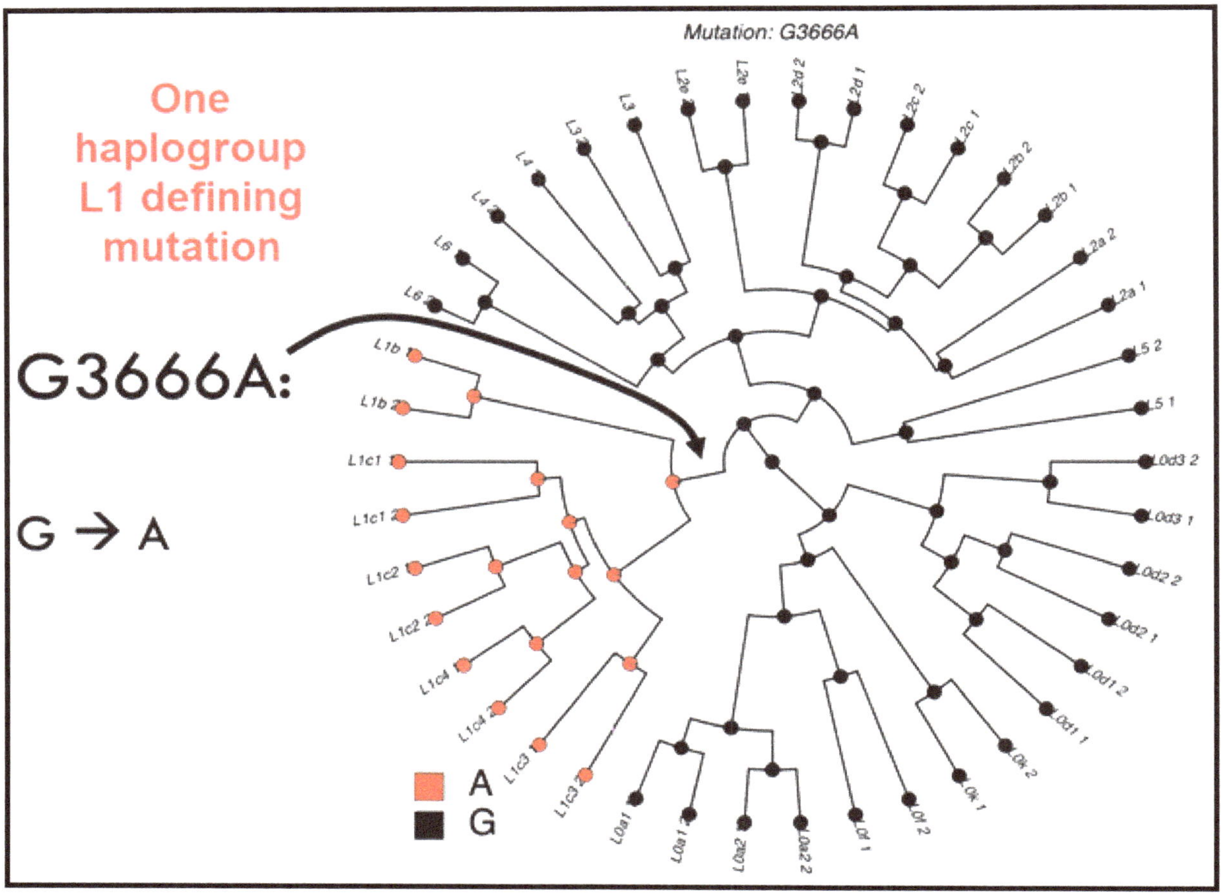

This graphic, courtesy of Dr. Paul Maier, shows the branching tree structure where mutation G3666A occurs in haplogroup L1. The reference or standard G nucleotide became an A. The arrow shows the location where that mutation happened. Every downstream haplogroup also has the A at position 3666 and is colored red in the wheel.

Occasionally, another mutation occurs in the same location. In other words, the A at location 3666 could become T, C, or G. That would be a new mutation at that branch point in the haplogroup, defining a new subgroup.

If the value of that mutation was G, the original reference value, that's considered a reverse mutation.

Reverse Mutations

Reverse mutations essentially stagger forward and backward – the drunken sailor effect.

Reverse mutations occur when a mutation occurs, then, later, reverts to the original value, as shown in this image. Mitochondrial phylogenetic tree spiral graph images are courtesy of Dr. Paul Maier.

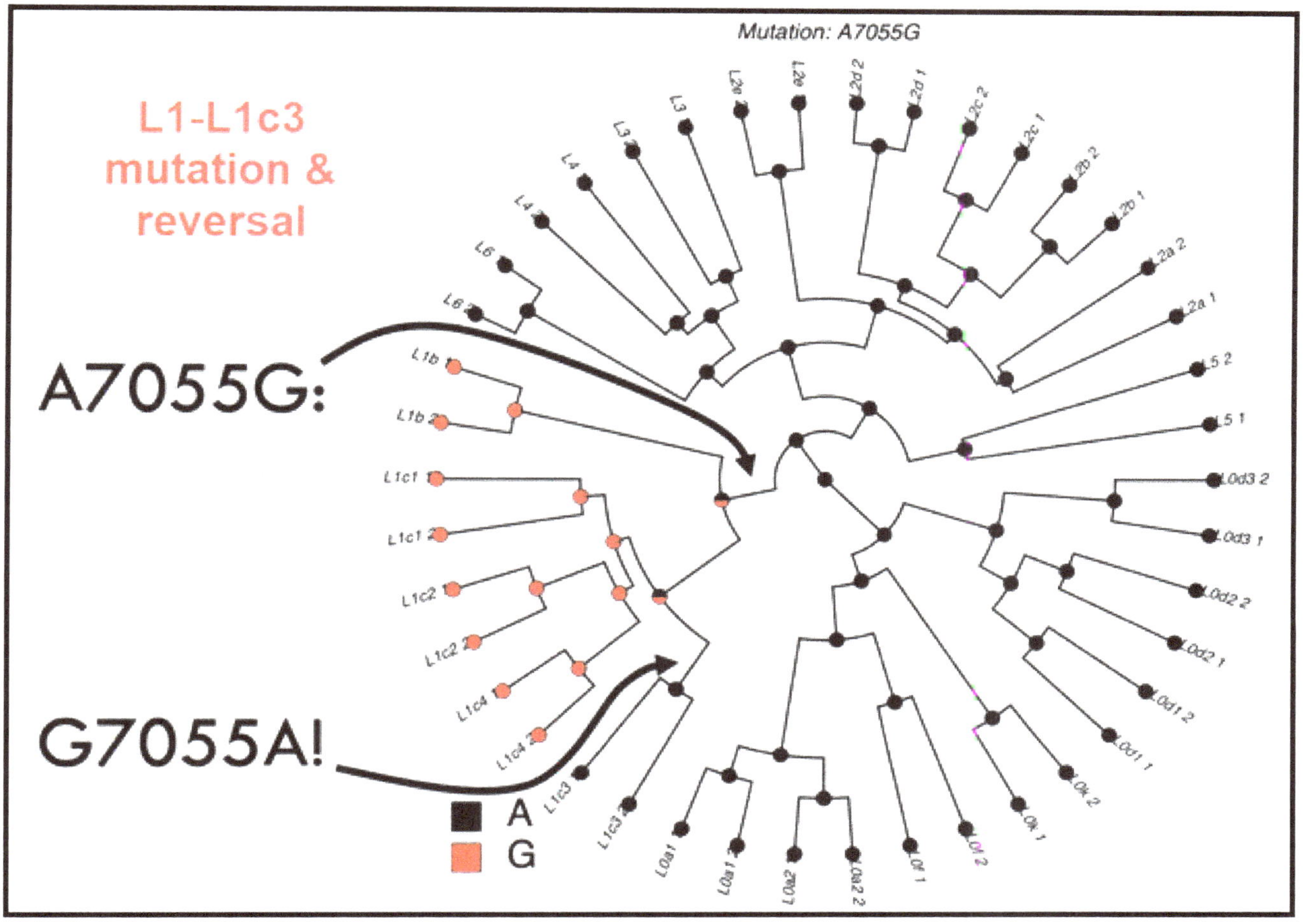

In the notation, G7055A!, the "!" indicates that a back mutation has occurred. Sometimes you see mutations followed by multiple !! which means backward, then forward again, one time for each "!".

Sometimes reversals only occur once, but other times we find several in a branch. How many back-and-forth reversals in a branch are too many when defining haplogroups? Should we include or ignore all of them, some of them, or none of them?

Unstable Mutations

Unstable mutations occur many times in the tree of womankind. For example, mutation C150T is found in 4 different locations in just this small portion of the tree.

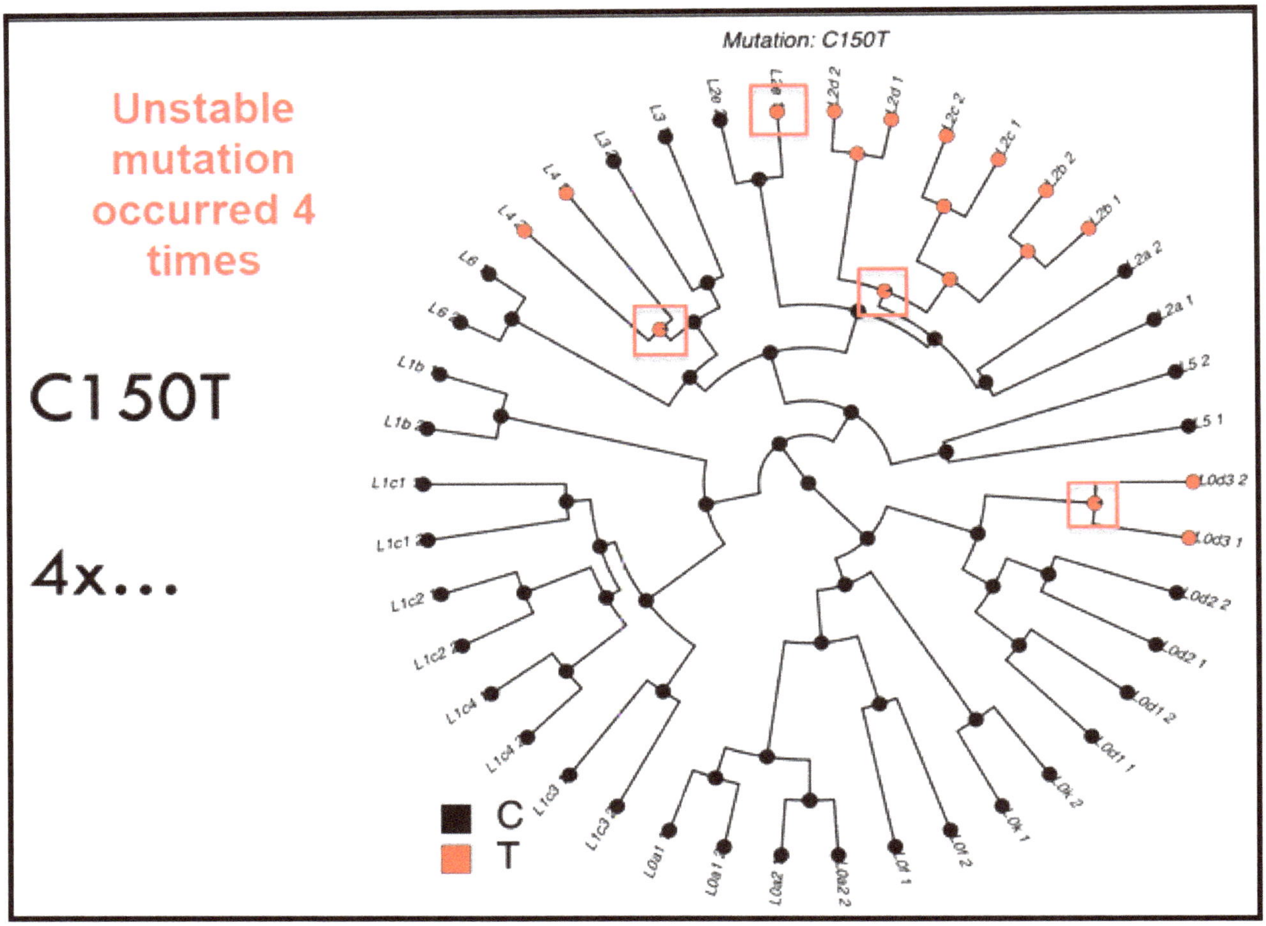

For some reason, this mutation occurs often, in multiple lines. How often is too often?

Should this and similarly unstable mutations be used for haplogroup formation? Are they reliable?

Should this mutation be used for matching?

Another very common but unstable mutation is the insertion, 315.1C.

Heteroplasmies

Heteroplasmies are mutations on steroids, or maybe mutations in progress would be a more apt description.

Heteroplasmies occur when two (or more) different nucleotides are found at the same location in a tester's sample.

Symbol	Meaning	Symbol	Meaning
A	A (Adenine)	T	T (Thymine)
C	C (Cytosine)	G	G (Guanine)
M	A or C	S	C or G
R	A or G	Y	C or T
W	A or T	K	G or T
H	A or C or T	V	A or C or G
D	A or G or T	B	C or G or T
N	G or A or T or C	X	G or A or T or C

If two values are found at the same location greater than 20% of the time, both values are reported. However, instead of combining an A and a C, for example, the circumstance where A and C are both found is reported by the letter M.

So, using our last example of A7055 that has both an A and a C occurring more than 20% of the time, we would find that location noted as A7055M.

Anytime you see the trailing letter value listed as anything other than T, A, C, G, or lowercase "d," you know you are dealing with a heteroplasmy.

Generally, but not always, one of the two values reported is the reference value, and the second is a different value.

Very occasionally, 3 or 4 values are detected above 20%.

Two decades ago, it was thought that heteroplasmies were mutations in progress and, within a generation or two, would resolve one way or the other. We now know that isn't always the case. The work of professional genealogist, Peter Sjölund, on the descendants of Kerstin Nilsdotter, born about 1610, shows a total of 111 DNA transmission events through three of her daughters' lines in a total of 15 living people who all carry the same heteroplasmy.[115]

If heteroplasmies have occurred recently, they may be a cause for non-matching between testers, especially if they occur in the HVR1 or HVR1+2 regions where one mismatch or a genetic distance of 1 causes two people not to match. Heteroplasmies occurring in the coding region are less likely to result in not matching because the matching algorithm allows a genetic distance of 3.

115 https://www.facebook.com/peterDNA/photos/a.381740412304249/1126554791156137/

Transitions Versus Transversions

You may notice that some of your mutations have a capital first letter, but a lowercase second letter, such as T7624a. That means that a transversion[116] has occurred. A transition occurs when a mutation between C and T or A and G takes place. A transversion occurs when any other mutation combination occurs.

Put simply, transitions are more likely to occur than transversions[117].

Mutation	Transition (Capital)	Transversion (Lower case)	More or Less Common
T to C	Yes		More Common
C to T	Yes		More Common
A to G	Yes		More Common
G to A	Yes		More Common
A to t		Yes	Less Common
T to a		Yes	Less Common
G to c		Yes	Less Common
C to g		Yes	Less Common
A to c		Yes	Less Common
C to a		Yes	Less Common
T to g		Yes	Less Common
G to t		Yes	Less Common

Back mutations are less likely to occur when a mutation is a transversion.

In terms of matching and genealogy, the only reason this matters is that you may wonder why one of your mutations ends with a lowercase letter. It's not a typo.

Insertions

Insertions happen when a copy error occurs, and a nucleotide is duplicated and inserted between two other locations.

Remember 315.1C from the Haplotree Branch Definition section? That's an insertion of one copy of C at the location of 315.

116 https://en.wikipedia.org/wiki/Transversion

117 https://www.mun.ca/biology/scarr/Transitions_vs_Transversions.html#:~:text=DNA%20substitution%20mutations%20are%20of,ring%20%26%20two%2Dring%20structures

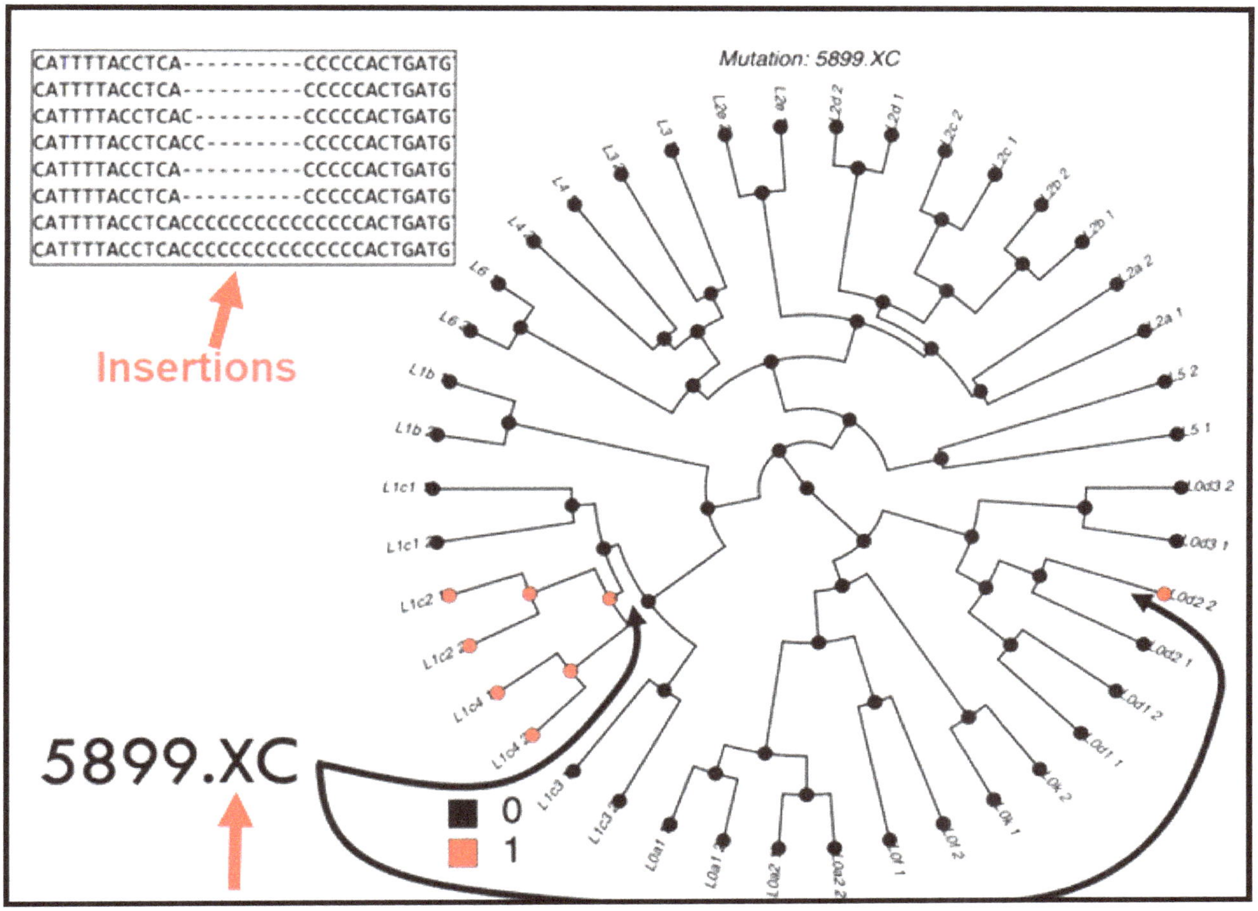

You might see the designation of XC, as in 5899.XC. That means there's an insertion of C after location 5899, but the number of insertions is uncertain. It could be 1, 2, or more Cs in this case, as shown in the box at the top left of this graphic by Dr. Paul Maier.

Deletions

In another graphic by Dr. Maier, we see that deletions are locations where the DNA has disappeared.

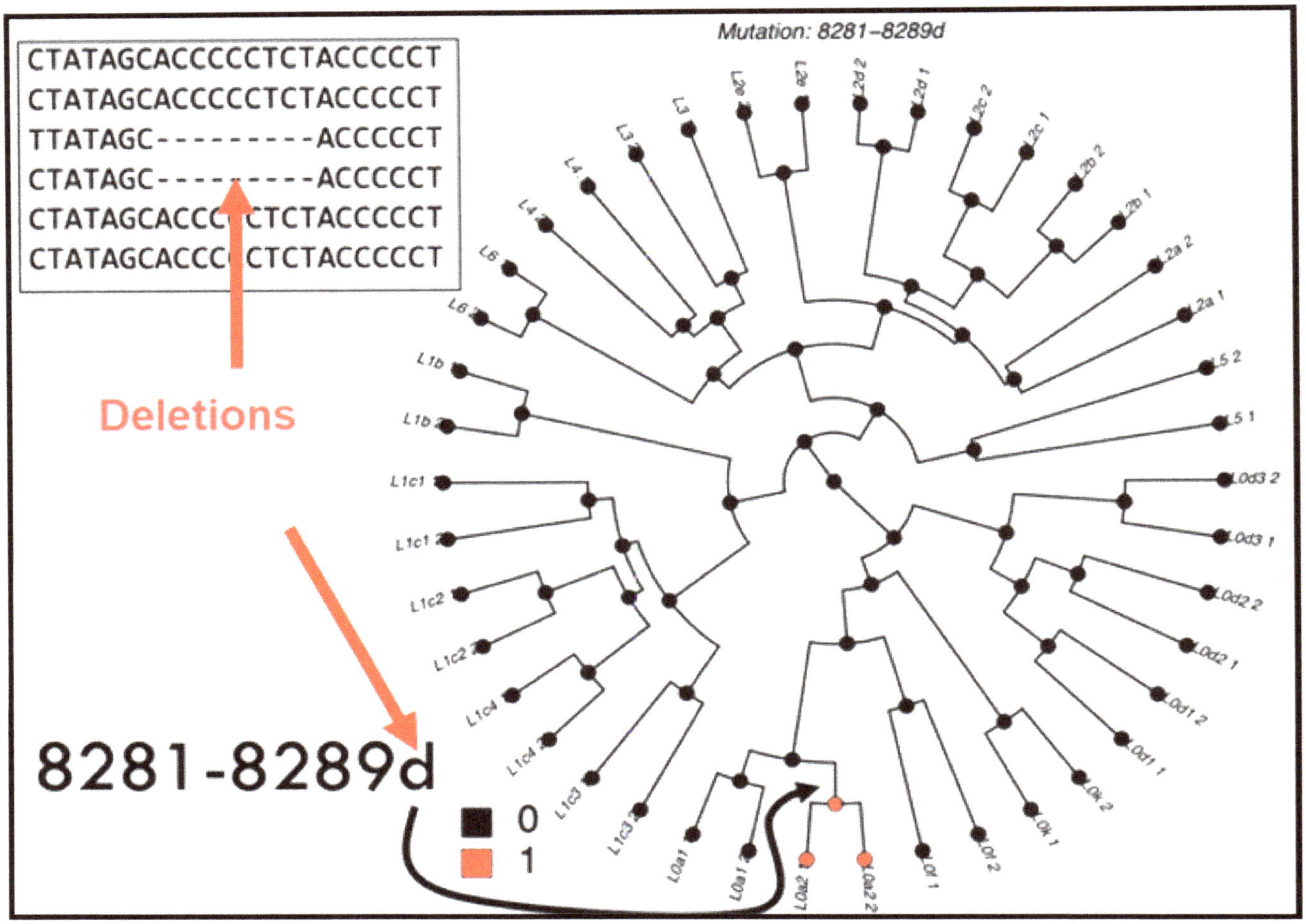

In this case, there's a 9 base-pair deletion from location 8281 through 8289, inclusive.

Mitochondrial DNA Dashboard

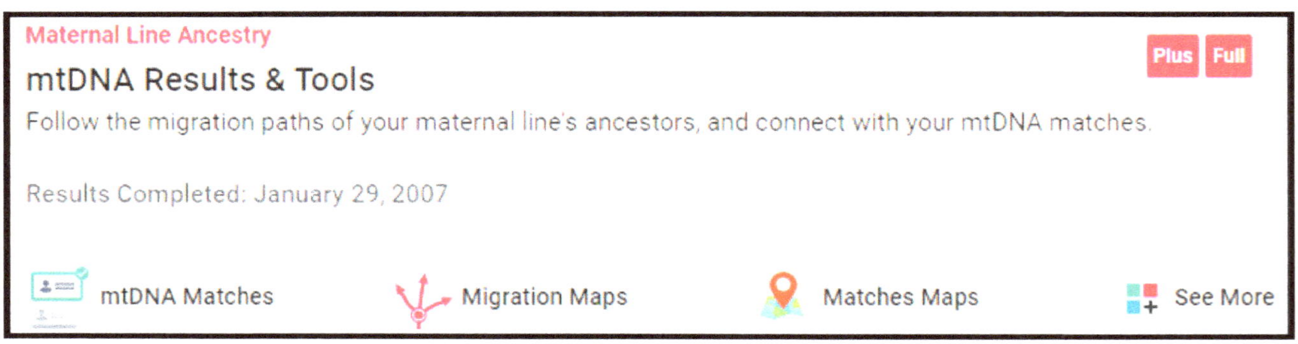

To determine your testing level, check the icon at the upper right-hand side of the mitochondrial DNA section on your personal page.

- If you haven't tested at all, you won't have this section.

- If you only tested at the HVR1 level, years ago, then both the Plus and Full will be greyed out.
- If you have taken the HVR1+HVR2 test(s), Plus will be colored red, but Full will be greyed out.
- If you have taken the mtFull, full sequence test, both Plus and Full will be colored red, as seen, above.

If you haven't taken the full sequence test, please upgrade by clicking on the "Full" button. Your results will help both your research and science by building the tree of womankind.

Mutations

The first thing most people want to see is their matches, but before we review matches, let's look at your actual marker values, which are your mutations.

You'll see those results by clicking on "See More," above, then on "Mutations."

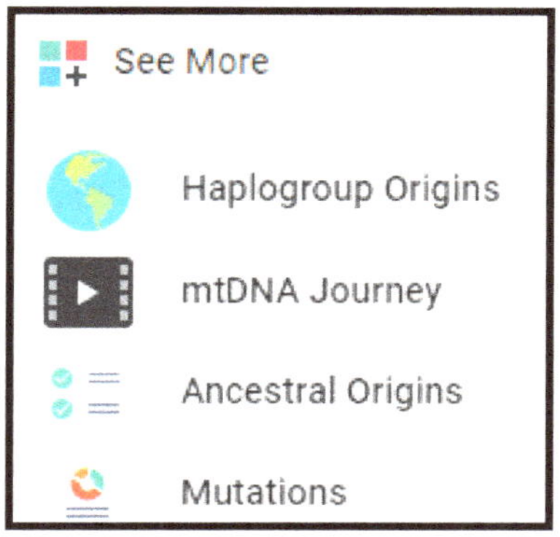

When clicking on the Mutations button, the default display is the RSRS values.

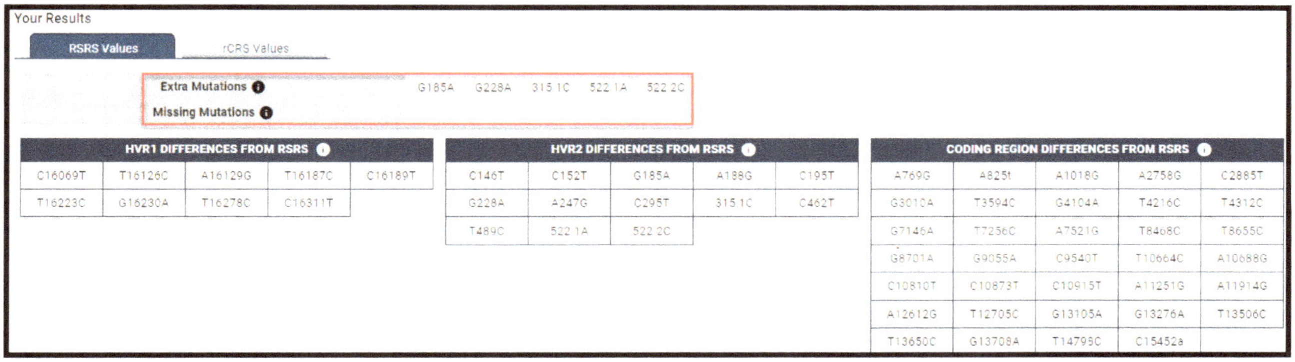

Your Results

RSRS Values | rCRS Values

Extra Mutations: G185A G228A 315.1C 522.1A 522.2C

Missing Mutations

HVR1 DIFFERENCES FROM RSRS				
C16069T	T16126C	A16129G	T16187C	C16189T
T16223C	G16230A	T16278C	C16311T	

HVR2 DIFFERENCES FROM RSRS				
C146T	C152T	G185A	A188G	C195T
G228A	A247G	C295T	315.1C	C462T
T489C	522.1A	522.2C		

CODING REGION DIFFERENCES FROM RSRS				
A769G	A825t	A1018G	A2758G	C2885T
G3010A	T3594C	G4104A	T4216C	T4312C
G7146A	T7256C	A7521G	T8468C	T8655C
G8701A	G9055A	C9540T	T10664C	A10688G
C10810T	C10873T	C10915T	A11251G	A11914G
A12612G	T12705C	G13105A	G13276A	T13506C
T13650C	G13708A	T14798C	C15452a	

The mutations, or "differences from RSRS," listed in the HVR1, HVR2, and Coding Regions, are the cumulative mutations that define your haplogroup. In this case, the tester is haplogroup J1c2f, so you're seeing all of the accumulated mutations from Mitochondrial Eve through when haplogroup J1c2f was defined.

Extra Mutations	G185A	G228A	315.1C	522.1A	522.2C
Missing Mutations					

The Extra and Missing Mutations, at the top, show mutations that this tester has or doesn't have as compared to their haplogroup definition. These mutations may be haplogroup-defining in the future, but currently are not.

Extra Mutations are mutations this tester has that have not been used to define this haplogroup, and Missing Mutations are expected haplogroup-defining mutations that were not found. For example, if a back mutation has occurred and is not already used to define an existing haplogroup, it would be listed in Missing Mutations.

Based on the discussions in the Mutations section, we can discern the following information about this tester who has:

- An insertion mutation at location 315.1C, which is one of the unstable regions and is not counted in either haplogroup definition or matching.
- Two insertions at location 522. The first mutation is an insertion of an A, and the second mutation is the insertion of a C.
- Mutations at locations G185A and G228A have no special significance other than their relevance when matching.
- There are no deletions, missing, or reverse mutations.

The extra mutations for this tester all fall in HVR2.

Scanning the rest of this tester's mutations, I notice that they have transversions at locations A825t and C15452a. Because these are not shown in the Extra Mutations section, we know that both of these are haplogroup-defining someplace in the mitochondrial DNA tree.

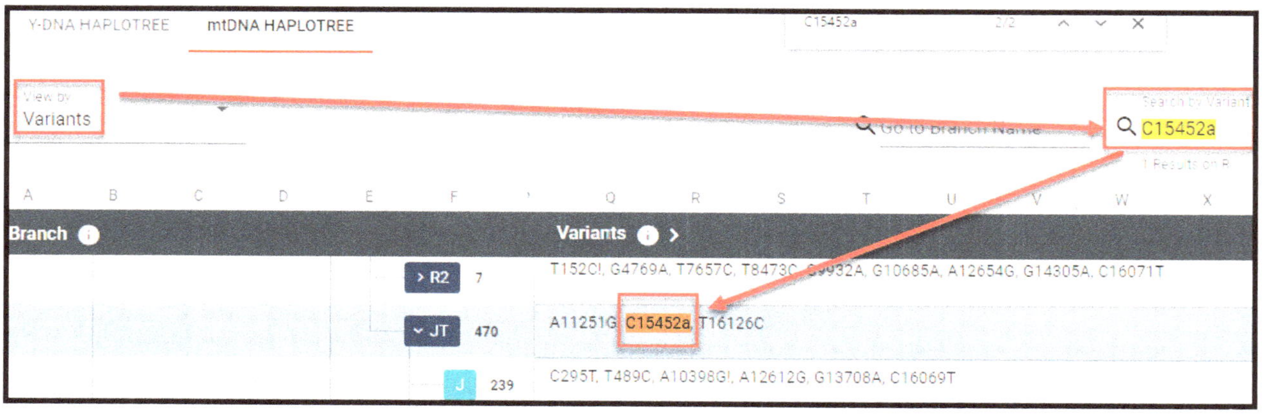

To confirm or locate the haplogroup defined by any mutation, you can go to the Public Tree at Family-TreeDNA[118], and execute the following steps:

- Select "View by Variants" at upper left.
- Search by Variants, at the upper right, and enter the name of the variant, meaning mutation, you wish to view.
- If the variant is present (make sure there's not a space in front of or behind the entry), text will appear below the search blank, such as "1 Result on R," meaning haplogroup R.
- Click the letter R in the haplogroup bar, just below the search box..
- The branch where the variant appears will be grey.
- I do a Browser search (Control+F on your keyboard) to find the mutation quickly on the resulting tree.
- View the haplogroup at left. In this case, C15452a is a haplogroup-defining mutation for haplogroup JT, the parent haplogroup of J.

Now, we're ready to look at mitochondrial DNA matches.

Matches

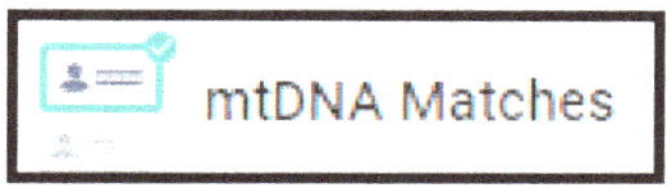

On your Matches page, the display defaults to people who match you on your highest-level test and in the entire database. You can select other match criteria, including testing levels and various projects that you've joined.

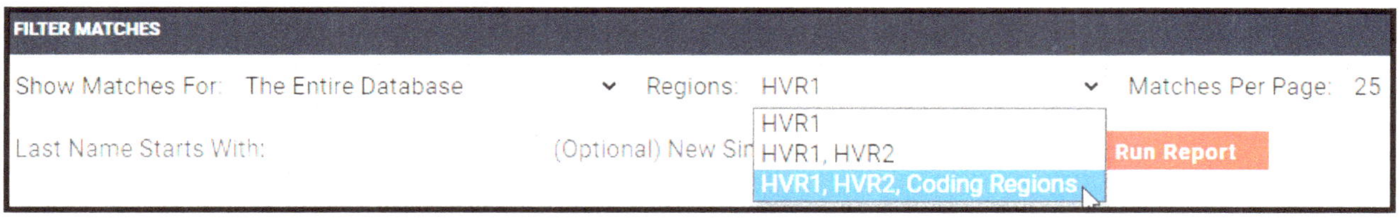

In this case, our tester took the mtFull full sequence test, so those results, noted as "HVR1, HVR2, Coding Region," will be displayed first. However, do NOT neglect to view the HVR1 and the HVR1+HVR2 match results because someone may have tested only to one of those levels years ago and entered ancestral information or included a tree that is critical to your research.

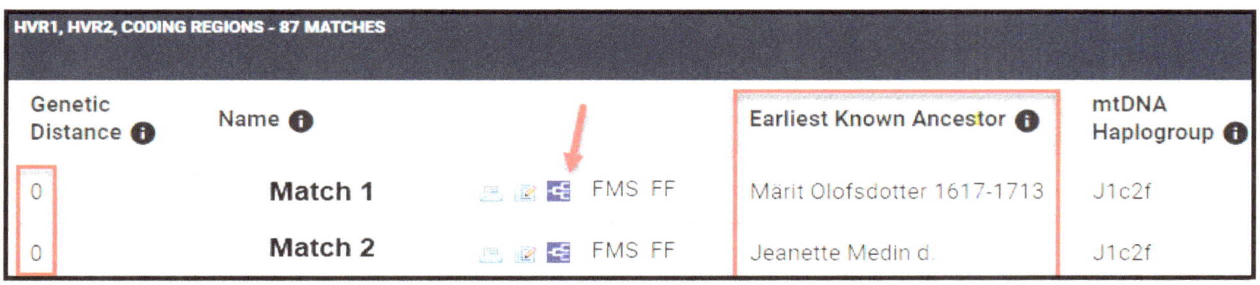

118 https://www.familytreedna.com/public/mt-dna-haplotree/L

When viewing the full sequence level matches, you will only see people who match you at that level and are members of your haplogroup. For HVR1 or HVR1+HVR2 matches, you'll see them as matches if they are members of your haplogroup or an upstream haplogroup such as J1c.

Haplogroups of testers at the HVR1 and HVR1+HVR2 levels cannot be determined at the resolution of full-sequence testers, so you will only receive a high-level or intermediate-level haplogroup assignment, depending on where haplogroup-defining mutations fall in the mitochondrial sequence.

You will also be able to see if your matches have taken a Family Finder test. If so, you may want to check your Family Finder match list or use Advanced Matching to see who matches you on both tests.

Eventually, when possible, the mitochondrial DNA haplogroups will be extracted and provided for Family Finder customers. Some autosomal DNA files uploaded from other vendors either include minimal mitochondrial haplogroup SNP locations, or none at all, so some people may not receive a mitochondrial haplogroup from an uploaded file.

The genetic distance (GD) of the full sequence matches in the above illustration is 0, which means you and that tester match exactly. These matches have all of the extra and/or missing mutations that you have, so eventually, these mutations, together, may form a new downstream haplogroup.

The Earliest Known Ancestor (EKA) is an important clue, both genealogically and further back in time to discern the origins of your mitochondrial family. If you notice a male EKA for a mitochondrial DNA test, the tester was confused or misunderstood the directions. The earliest mitochondrial ancestor must be a woman – your mother's direct line matrilineal ancestor as far back as you know.

Be sure to check your matches' trees by clicking on the pedigree icon. Many times, the trees have more or even different information than the EKA. Leave no stone unturned.

TIP: It's important to remember that the EKA information is NOT extracted from trees, so be sure to check both.

The instructions and steps for entering your Earliest Known Ancestor and their geographic location on a map are found under the Y-DNA Matches Map section in this book. Be sure to enter this information for your direct matrilineal line[119] mitochondrial ancestor, too.

119 Matrilineal line is your mother's mother's mother following all women up your tree as far as you can.

Techniques for Making Matches More Useful

Now's a good time to discuss techniques to make matching more useful. You'll want to gather as much information about your matches as possible, including by clicking on the match name which displays their profile card.

I wrote detailed step-by-step instructions about what to do, and how, in the article "*Mitochondrial DNA: Part 4 – Techniques for Doubling Your Useful Matches*."[120] While I penned this article specifically about mitochondrial DNA matches, it's every bit as relevant and useful for Y-DNA too.

I recommend starting a spreadsheet with the information that can be gathered and gleaned when you first test, or now. Build on it as you go.

Please note that you can also use Genetic Affairs AutoTree Clustering[121] and select either Y-DNA or mtDNA to begin the ancestor matching and tree construction with either of those types of tests.

Matches Maps

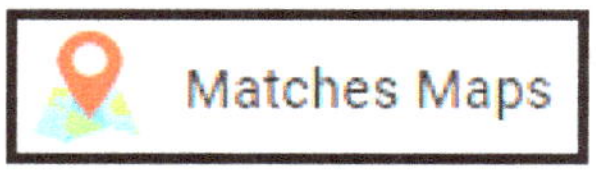

The Matches Maps display the EKA locations entered by your matches for their ancestors.

Some of these ancestors will be found in the region of the world where your ancestor is from, but other locations probably reach back before the adoption of surnames. You may have a surprise waiting. I certainly did.

120 https://dna-explained.com/2019/07/03/mitochondrial-dna-part-4-techniques-for-doubling-your-useful-matches/

121 https://dna-explained.com/2019/12/02/genetic-affairs-reconstructs-trees-from-genetic-clusters-even-without-your-tree-or-common-ancestors/

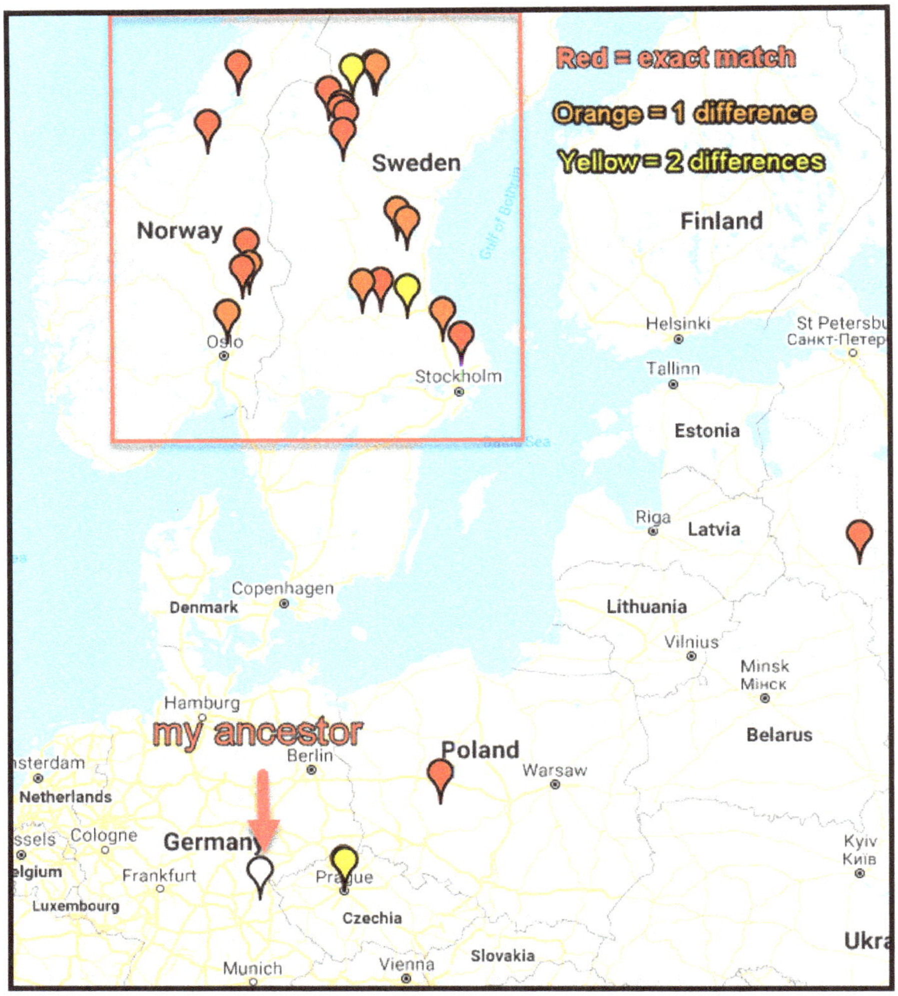

My white pin on this map is near the bottom, with the red arrow by the "y" in Germany.

- Exact matches are red pins
- Genetic distance of 1 is orange
- Genetic distance of 2 is yellow

In general, red pins are more relevant and more closely related to you than orange or yellow pins unless something unusual is involved, such as heteroplasmies[122] which might preclude matching or cause someone who would otherwise be a close match to appear as a more distant match.

In my case, my earliest known ancestor was found in Germany in 1621, but most of my exact matches, except for two, are found in either Sweden or Norway, conveying the message that her ancestors were found in Scandinavia. The question, of course, is when, how, and why did her maternal ancestor arrive in Germany? Evaluating the history of the region provided critical clues.

122 https://dna-explained.com/2021/06/10/what-is-a-heteroplasmy-and-why-do-i-care/

Migration Maps

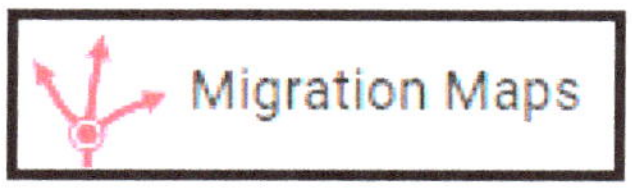

The mitochondrial DNA Migration Map displays the path out of Africa from about 140,000-150,000 years ago until your base-level haplogroup was formed.

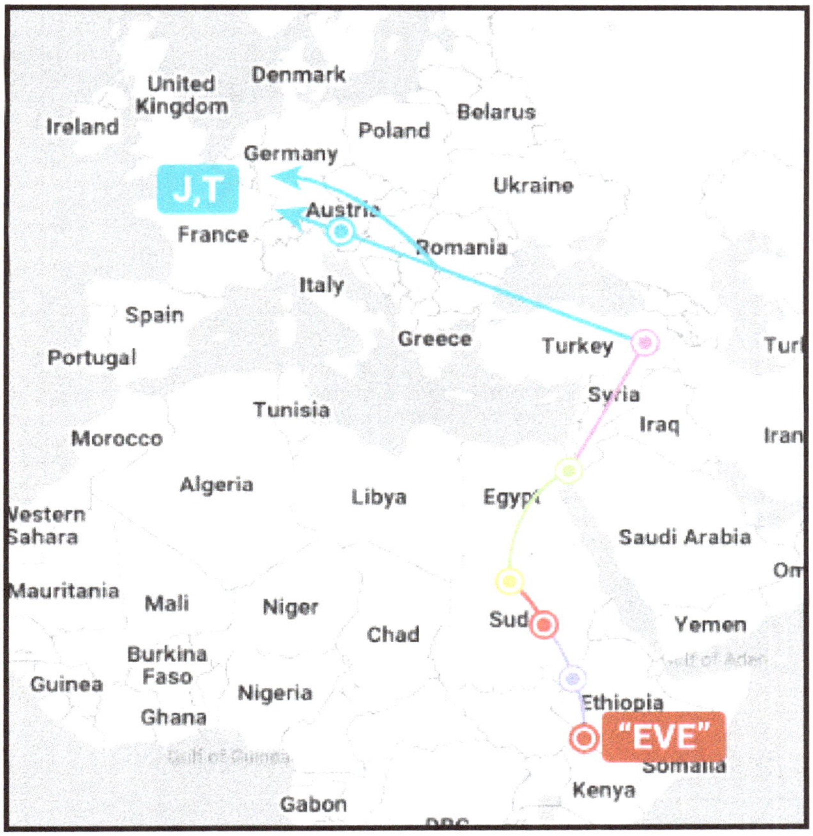

Haplogroup Origins

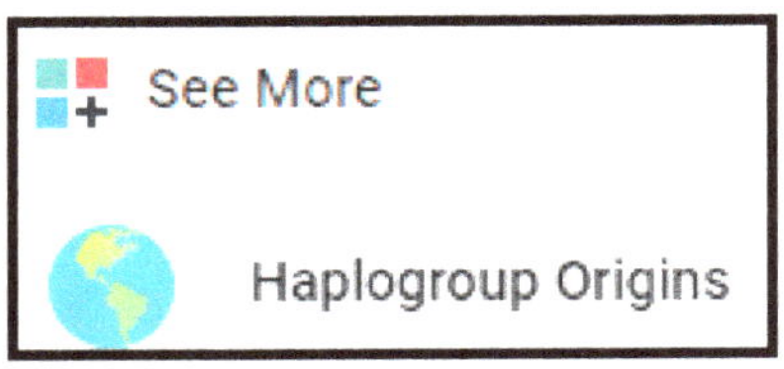

Under "See More," Haplogroup Origins shows the locations of the Earliest Known Ancestors of people who share your haplogroup. Some origins may be very vanilla in nature, but others may be quite useful.

This person matches several people with the same haplogroup, in various locations, whose ancestors were Sephardic or Ashkenazi Jews.

mtDNA - Haplogroup Origins

HVR1

No Matches Found

HVR1 AND HVR2 MATCHES

Haplogroup	Country	Comments
H	Russian Federation	-
H4a1a3a	Morocco	Sephardic
H4a1a3a	Poland	Ashkenazi
H4a1a3a	Russian Federation	Ashkenazi
H4a1a3a	Spain	-

This person discovered that their haplogroup A2f1a indicated a Native American ancestor.[123]

mtDNA - Haplogroup Origins

HVR1 MATCHES

Haplogroup	Country	Match Total
A	Canada	18
A	United States (Native American)	9
A2f1a	Canada	15
A2f1a	Canada (First Nations)	8
A2f1a	France	1
A2f1a	United States (Native American)	3

Be aware of two caveats:

- Some people record oral history which turns out to be incorrect. For example, people often record their mitochondrial EKA as Native American because "someone on mother's side is supposed to be Native American." If the haplogroup is NOT a documented Native American haplogroup and there is a stray Native American designation, be aware that people record what they believe at the time, which is often before testing. Few people think about going back and updating that information later.

123 https://dna-explained.com/2013/09/18/native-american-mitochondrial-haplogroups/

- Incorrect information can work in both directions. In this example, haplogroup A2f1a is confirmed as Native American, but one person entered France, probably because they knew their ancestor was "French-Canadian." I see this same scenario often when people of Mexican, Central, or South American heritage record "Spain," but their ancestor turns out to be Native based on Y-DNA or mitochondrial DNA haplogroups.

Ancestral Origins

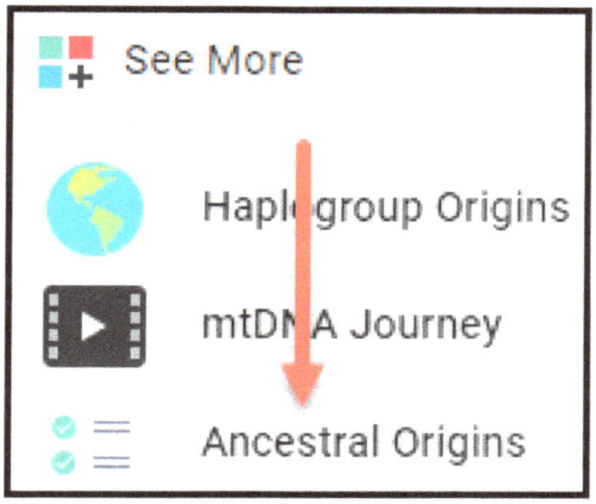

Under "See More," then "Ancestral Origins," you'll find a summary of your matches' EKA locations. Just like with Haplogroup Origins, some are very useful, and others are only mildly interesting.

For example, this individual has four matches, and three of the four indicate Ashkenazi or Sephardic Ancestral Origins.

HVR1, HVR2, AND CODING REGION MATCHES

EXACT MATCH				
Country	Match Total	Country Total	Percentage	Comments
Morocco	1	105	1%	Sephardic (1)
Russian Federation	1	2435	< 0.1 %	Ashkenazi (1)
GENETIC DISTANCE -1				
Country	Match Total	Country Total	Percentage	Comments
Poland	1	3479	< 0.1 %	Ashkenazi (1)
Spain	1	1419	0.1%	

This tester discovered that they have a Native American/First Nations direct maternal ancestor with several Canadian connections.

HVR1, HVR2, AND CODING REGION MATCHES

EXACT MATCH	
Country	Match Total
Canada	8
Canada (First Nations)	14
GENETIC DISTANCE -1	
Country	Match Total
Canada	2
Canada (First Nations)	5
United States (Native American)	2
GENETIC DISTANCE -2	
Country	Match Total
United States (Native American)	1
GENETIC DISTANCE -3	
Country	Match Total
Canada (First Nations)	1

Journey Video

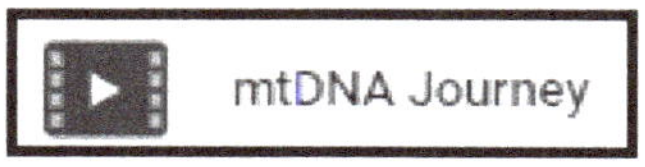

Under "See More," you'll find your mtDNA Journey video, which explains the basics of what your results are telling you.

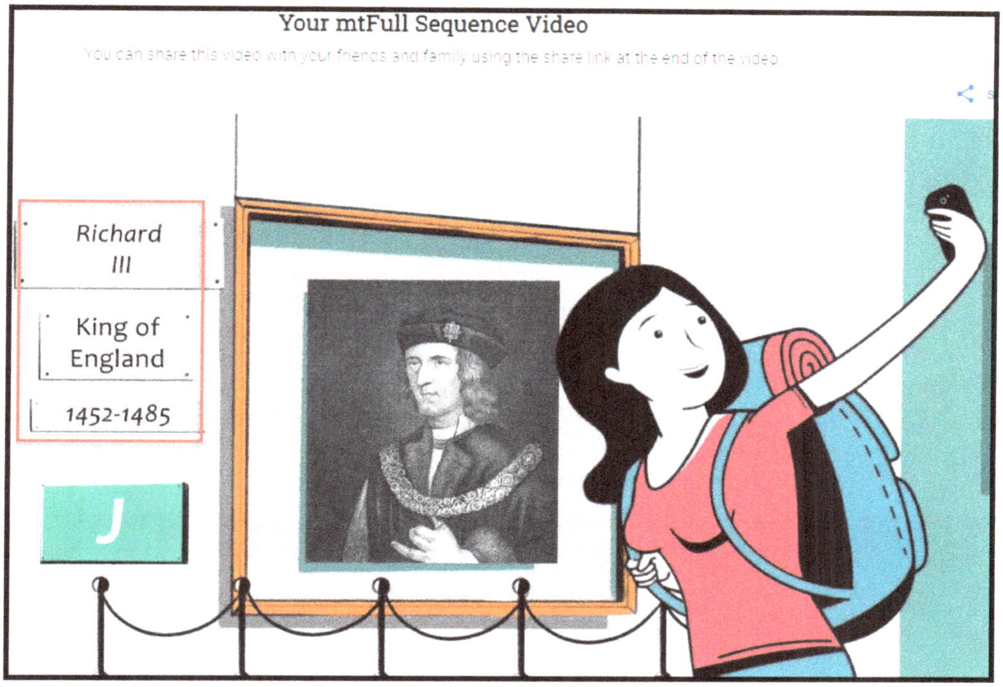
Your mtFull Sequence Video
You can share this video with your friends and family using the share link at the end of the video.
Richard III
King of England
1452-1485
J

My favorite part is discovering which famous person you share an ancestor with at some point in time. The Journey videos would be prime candidates for replacement in the future with a tool similar to the Y-DNA Discover™ Haplogroup Reports,[124] which are updated regularly.

Discover™ Mitochondrial Time Tree

While the mitochondrial version of Discover™ has not been released as of this book's publication, the features will be essentially the same as found in the Y-DNA Discover™ Haplogroup Reports.

These tools provide critical information about the age of the haplogroup, where it is found, and where ancient DNA samples may be found as well. All of this information, cumulatively, is the history of your ancestors.

Steps ↑ ⓘ	Haplogroup ⓘ	Age Estimate ⓘ	Archaeology Era ⓘ	Time Passed ⓘ	Immediate Descendants ⓘ	Tested Modern Descendants
1	J1c2f	500 BCE ⓘ	Metal Ages/ Imperial	6,050 years	44	96

This early, internal R&D version of mitochondrial Discover™ reveals that my haplogroup, J1c2f, was born about the year 500 BCE, so about 2500 years ago. There are 44 descendant branches, and 96 people have tested and been assigned to haplogroup J1c2f. Additional Discover™ information, not included here, shows that the majority of haplogroup J1c2f is found in Sweden, followed by Norway. My ancestor was found in Germany, in 1647, just before the Thirty Years' War, in which the majority of German records

124 https://dna-explained.com/2022/06/30/familytreedna-discover-launches-including-y-dna-haplogroup-ages/

were destroyed, ended. How did my ancestors get to Germany from Scandinavia during that time? Haplogroup age dates provide brackets of time in which to search for relevant historical evidence that is not available any other way.

Advanced Matching for mtDNA

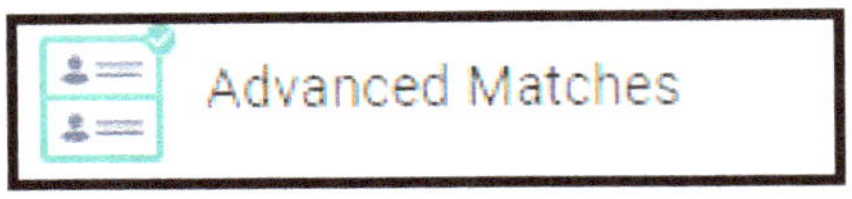

Advanced Matching, found under Additional Tests and Tools, can be quite useful for mitochondrial DNA matches. Advanced Matching provides the ability to compare your mitochondrial matches to determine who is also a Family Finder autosomal test match.

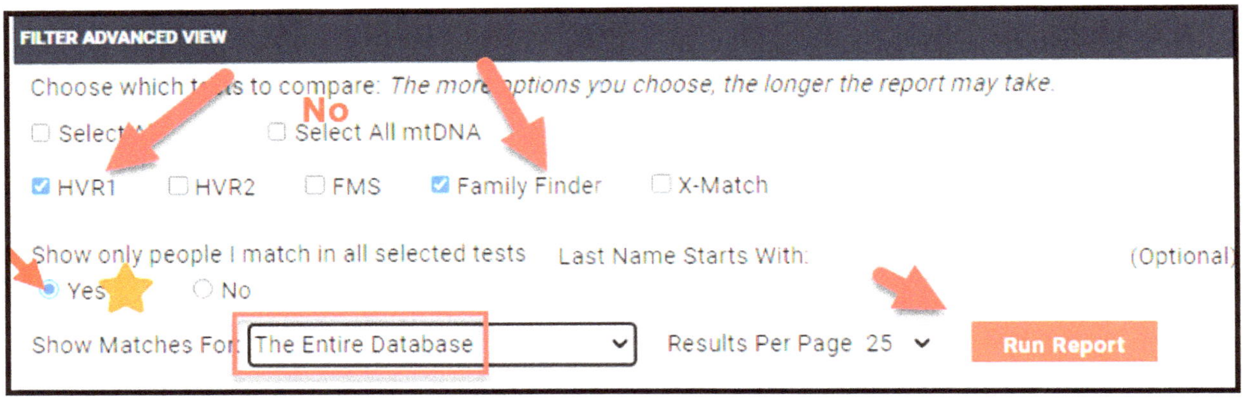

Select Family Finder and **ONE** level of mitochondrial DNA test, **NOT** "All mtDNA" tests. If you select "All," you will have to match the person on all levels of the test. If you have one mismatch in the HVR1 region, you won't match in that region, so you won't show as a match to "all" of the mtDNA criteria.

If you want to know who matches you on the FMS, or full sequence, just select that option. I generally select one mtDNA test level at a time, combined with Family Finder.

Be sure to check yes for "Show only people I match in all selected tests," or you will see your entire match list for all tests, not just the intersection of criteria.

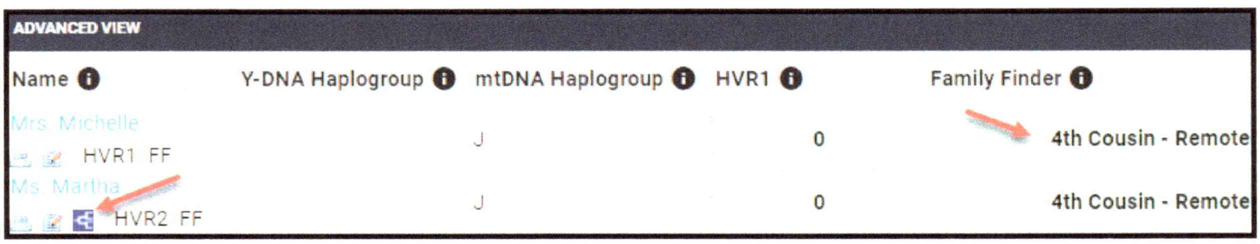

The resulting report, above, shows the people who match the tester at the HVR1 level, regardless of whether they have tested at a higher level, haplogroups where available, their genetic distance at the HVR1 level, and Family Finder estimated relationships.

It's important to note that the Family Finder match may not be due to the mitochondrial line, but a match is a research clue.

Selecting Mitochondrial Projects

We'll review step-by-step procedures for finding and joining projects[125] in the Projects chapter, but mitochondrial DNA testers may benefit by joining the following types of projects:

- Relevant surname projects, if allowed by the volunteer project administrators
- Geographic projects, such as England, France or New Mexico
- Groups such as American Indian or Acadian Amerindian
- Mitochondrial haplogroup projects, such as haplogroup J
- Mitochondrial lineage projects focused on a specific family line

Mitochondrial DNA Case Studies

Mitochondrial DNA can assist genealogists in many ways.

The most immediate benefit of mitochondrial DNA, aside from matching, is determining where your ancestral line originated. You can think of this as ancestor-specific ethnicity.[126]

Case 1 – Mother's Heritage Was a Surprise

Based on who you match, and where your haplogroup is found, you'll know where in the world your ancestor originated. This information sometimes comes gift-wrapped as a surprise. I wrote about that in the article, "*Dorcas Johnson's Mitochondrial DNA Secret Revealed*" [127], as well as my own experience in the article, "*Where Did My Mitochondrial DNA Haplogroup Come From?*"[128]

In both cases, we thought we knew where our matrilineal ancestors were from, and in both cases, we were wrong. We would have NEVER made that discovery without mitochondrial DNA testing. My line was found in Germany, but originated in either Sweden or Norway, either during or before the Thirty Years' War which began in 1618. Dorcas's line was brick-walled in the US but was from either Sweden or Finland instead of being Scots-Irish as told through oral history.

125 https://dna-explained.com/2019/08/14/mitochondrial-dna-part-5-joining-projects/

126 https://dna-explained.com/2021/05/04/want-ancestor-specific-ethnicity-test-mitochondrial-dna/

127 https://dna-explained.com/2022/05/08/dorcas-johnsons-mitochondrial-dna-secret-revealed-52-ancestors-357/

128 https://dna-explained.com/2021/05/01/where-did-my-mitochondrial-dna-haplogroup-come-from/

Case 2 – Found the Sister, Then Found the Parents of Both Sisters

Mitochondrial DNA can break through brick walls when you don't know surnames. That's exactly how we discovered that my ancestor, Phebe, wife of Jotham Brown, was the sister of Lydia Cole and that they were both the daughters of Mary Mercy Kent and John Cole. The article, "*Mitochondrial DNA Bulldozes Brick Wall*"[129] explains exactly how a mitochondrial DNA match led to an unknown sister, then pointed us to a location in colonial New Jersey to search for records. We subsequently located baptism records once we knew where to look.

Case 3 – Lydia Brown is the Mother of Phebe Crumley, not Elizabeth Johnson

Using mitochondrial DNA matching to descendants of multiple daughters, we were able to determine that Lydia Brown,[130] [131] the wife of William Crumley, was indeed the mother of Phebe Crumley,[132] and by proving that relationship, we also proved that this William Crumley (because of course, there's more than one William Crumley) did not marry Elizabeth Johnson after Lydia supposedly died.[133]

Case 3, Part 2 – This William Crumley did NOT Marry Elizabeth Johnson

Based on the fact that the mitochondrial DNA of William Crumley's three daughters, who were born both before and after one William Crumley's marriage to Elizabeth Johnson, match exactly, we can eliminate this William as a candidate for that marriage. A different William Crumley, probably his father,[134] married Elizabeth Johnson. Based on mitochondrial DNA, we know that William Crumley's first (and apparently, only) wife, Lydia Brown,[135] was the mother of my ancestor, Phebe Crumley, along with her older and younger sisters.

Using mitochondrial DNA, we:

- Proved Phebe Crumley was Lydia Brown's daughter
- Proved Phebe matched her two sisters, one born before and one born after her mother, Lydia, was believed to have died based on a marriage record for William Crumley marrying Elizabeth Johnson prior to Phebe's birth.
- Found Lydia Brown's sister and parents

---

129 https://dna-explained.com/2019/01/10/mitochondrial-dna-bulldozes-brick-wall/

130 https://dna-explained.com/2018/11/24/lydia-browns-3-daughters-or-were-they-mitochondrial-and-autosomal-dna-to-the-rescue-52-ancestors-218/

131 https://dna-explained.com/2015/06/28/lydia-brown-c1790-18401850-buried-or-attending-a-wedding-52-ancestors-78/

132 https://dna-explained.com/2020/12/19/phebe-crumleys-mother-really-is-lydia-brown-c1781-c1830-52-ancestors-318/

133 https://dna-explained.com/2015/11/22/phebe-c1747-c1803-is-jotham-browns-wife-zopher-johnsons-daughter-52-ancestors-99/

134 https://dna-explained.com/2019/06/29/county-formation-petitions-resolve-long-standing-mystery-which-william-crumley-got-married-52-ancestors-244/

135 https://dna-explained.com/2020/12/19/phebe-crumleys-mother-really-is-lydia-brown-c1781-c1830-52-ancestors-318/

- Proved a total of 5 relationships - Phebe and her older sister to her mother Lydia, then Lydia to her sister, which led to their parents
- Disproved the marriage of Phebe's father William Crumley to Elizabeth Johnson
- Clarified that William Crumley's father, also named William, was the most likely candidate to marry Elizabeth Johnson.

Case 4 – Direct Matrilineal Ancestor is Native American

Many people have both discovered and confirmed that their mitochondrial ancestor was Native American. Many had no idea before they tested. That's exactly what happened to my cousin, who discovered her haplogroup was A2f1a, clearly Native American.

TIP: I've also used mitochondrial DNA to prove an ancestral line was Native when there were absolutely no records, not even the woman's name.

Of course, a mitochondrial DNA test can also put those rumors to rest and disprove Native ancestry in your direct matrilineal line. Wouldn't it be nice to know for sure? I wrote about that in the article, "*Native American: Is She or Isn't She?*"[136]

Here's the bottom line. Everyone can test their own mitochondrial DNA. You don't know what you don't know, and you're never going to know if you don't test.

136 https://dna-explained.com/2022/11/09/native-american-is-she-or-isnt-she/

Chapter 5

AUTOSOMAL DNA – THE FAMILY FINDER TEST

The heart of genetic genealogy is DNA matching, and the most common type of test taken by consumers is the autosomal test. At FamilyTreeDNA, the autosomal test is called the Family Finder test.

How greatly you benefit from an autosomal test, whether you test directly with FamilyTreeDNA or upload your raw DNA results file[137] from another vendor, has a lot to do with your goals and how much effort you're willing to invest in your results.

That's not a lot different from the rest of genealogy.

While Y-DNA focuses on the direct paternal line for males and mitochondrial DNA focuses on the direct matrilineal line for everyone, autosomal DNA provides matching to people based on all of your genealogical lines.

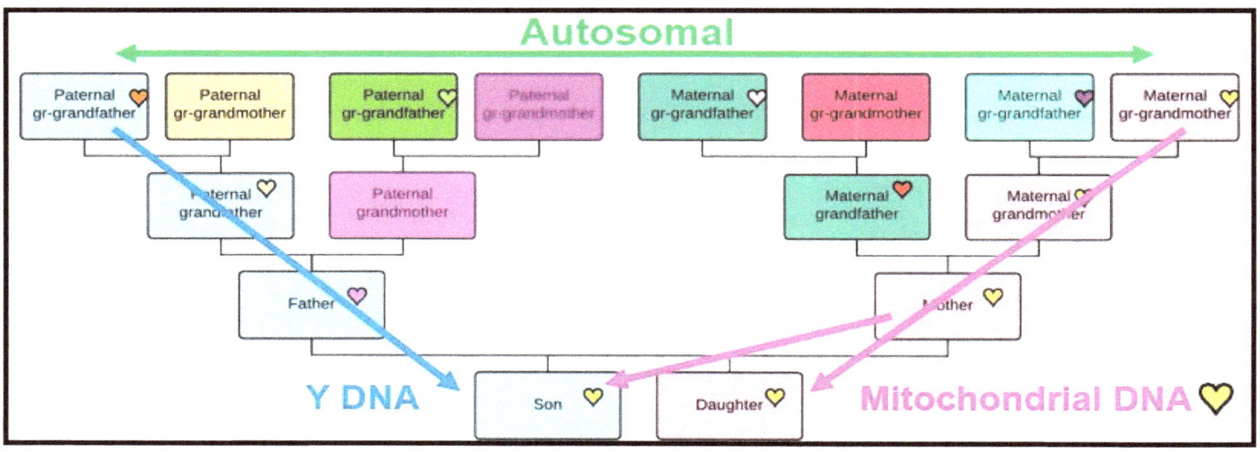

The good news is that you'll probably have more matches because you will match cousins from a wide variety of ancestors.

The bad news is that autosomal DNA is divided in half in each generation, so, over time, less and less of any specific ancestor's DNA will be passed to descendants. You need to figure out your common genealogy line for each match – unlike Y-DNA and mitochondrial DNA, where you know exactly which line those matches pertain to.

137 https://dna-explained.com/2018/08/28/family-tree-dna-step-by-step-guide-how-to-upload-download-dna-files/

Autosomal Testing Goals

Autosomal testing goals might include:

- Finding cousins through DNA testing
- Collaborating with newly discovered cousins
- Confirming your ancestors
- Discovering your ancestors
- Breaking through brick walls by using DNA
- Identifying unknown parents, grandparents, or siblings[138]
- Discovering your population breakdown, meaning ethnicity
- Accumulating evidence to prove or disprove family oral history
- Identifying pieces (segments) of your DNA that descend from specific ancestors

FamilyTreeDNA makes autosomal testing easy because they:

- Accept uploads from other major vendors if you have already tested elsewhere.
- Divide your matches maternally and paternally if you upload or create a tree and link known matches.

Uploads

In the article, *DNA File Upload-Download and Transfer Instructions to and from DNA Testing Companies,*[139] I provide detailed step-by-step instructions for how to download your raw DNA data file from each of the vendors, and how to upload to FamilyTreeDNA, MyHeritage, and GEDmatch, the major vendors who accept uploads.[140]

FamilyTreeDNA accepts uploads[141] from the three other major vendors:

- Ancestry – All versions except their Health/NGS
- MyHeritage – Tests taken at MyHeritage after May 7, 2019.
- 23andMe – V3 and higher, which are tests taken in December 2010 and later[142]

---

138 https://dna-explained.com/in-search-of-unknown-family/

139 https://dna-explained.com/2019/11/04/dna-file-upload-download-and-transfer-instructions-to-and-from-dna-testing-companies/

140 https://dna-explained.com/2019/11/04/dna-file-upload-download-and-transfer-instructions-to-and-from-dna-testing-companies/

141 https://help.familytreedna.com/hc/en-us/articles/4402392808463-Autosomal-DNA-Transfers-Guide

142 This feature is currently paused because 23andMe is not currently not allowing customers to download their raw DNA data file, and because FamilyTreeDNA has paused 23andMe DNA file uploads in response to the 23andMe data exposure incident.

Matches, shared matches, the Matrix, and parental side matching are always free, but advanced features can be unlocked for only $19.

Feature	Included with Free Upload	Requires $19 Unlock
Matching	Full match list	
	Parental side matching aka bucketing	
	Shared matching	
	Matrix – reports if your matches also match each other	
Chromosome Browser		Compares your DNA with your matches on your chromosomes[143]
myOrigins (ethnicity)		Percentages and locations
Chromosome Painter		Paints your ethnicity segments on your chromosomes
ancientOrigins		Archaeological digs provide category percentages
Y-DNA and mitochondrial DNA[144] haplogroups, when available		MyHeritage files yield the same haplogroup resolution as FamilyTreeDNA files, but files from other vendors may not[145]

TIP: If you upload your DNA file from another DNA testing company, be aware that you're uploading your raw DNA file, just the sequences of your DNA – not your matches from that site.

If you upload a file instead of taking a test directly at FamilyTreeDNA, after uploading, they process your DNA file and display your matches in the FamilyTreeDNA database.

FamilyTreeDNA has a full generation of testers that the other vendors don't have, so it's important to test or encourage all of your known relatives[146] to upload too.

143 https://dna-explained.com/2022/12/13/concepts-your-matches-on-the-same-segment-are-not-necessarily-related-to-each-other/

144 Mitochondrial DNA haplogroups are not yet available from Family Finder tests and uploads, but will be after the Y-DNA haplogroups are fully rolled out, and after the new mitochondrial tree is introduced.

145 Both MyHeritage and Vitagene are processed in the Gene by Gene lab, along with the Family Finder tests. Those vendor files are considered vendor-to-vendor imports, contain the same SNPs as the Family Finder test, and produce the same haplogroup results as a Family Finder test. Tests from other vendors do not contain exactly the same Y or mtDNA SNPs, but the customer will receive the best haplogroup possible from the file provided. Haplogroup results from Ancestry and 23andMe are not shared with your matches, but haplogroups from the other files are. https://dna-explained.com/2023/11/30/familytreedna-provides-y-dna-haplogroups-from-family-finder-autosomal-tests/

146 https://dna-explained.com/2016/10/19/concepts-why-dna-testing-the-oldest-family-members-is-critically-important/

FamilyTreeDNA's first customers tested in 2000 and many have since purchased the Family Finder test – or their families upgraded their kit after they passed away.

- If you have already taken a Y-DNA or mitochondrial DNA test at FamilyTreeDNA, upload your autosomal DNA file to the same account so you can utilize the combined test types available in the advanced matching tool.
- If you upload an autosomal file from another vendor and want to add a Y-DNA or mitochondrial DNA test, order that test from your existing FamilyTreeDNA account. Don't worry, FamilyTreeDNA will mail you a swab kit.

Autosomal Test Features

Genealogists take the Family Finder test for two primary reasons:

- Matching – matches with other testers that lead to the identification of common ancestors
- myOrigins – population-based ethnicity results

Let's look at the features and tools by category, beginning with matching.

Family Finder Dashboard

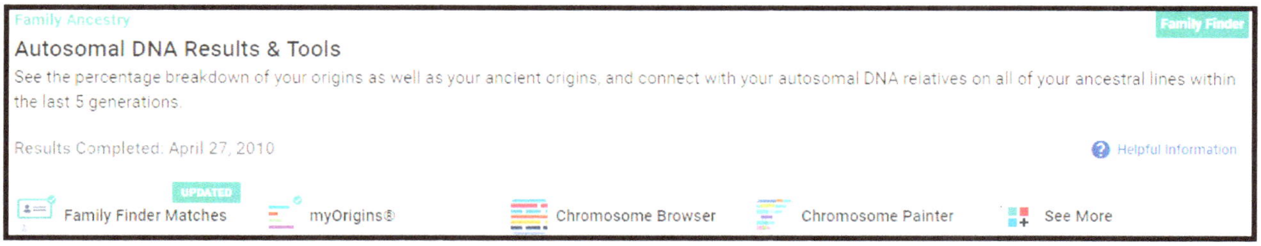

Under the "See More" button:

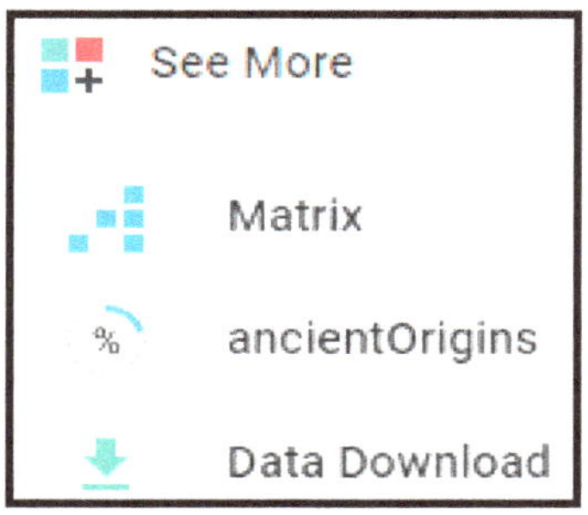

Let's review each feature.

Family Finder Matches

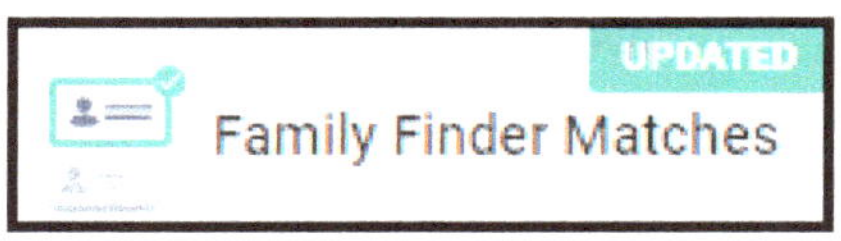

FamilyTreeDNA provides a list of people whose DNA matches yours:[147]

- On at least one 7 centimorgan[148] (cM) segment, or larger, although 6 cM matching segments are shown if your match also has a 7 cM minimum segment match.
- After factoring in quality assurance calculations and adjusting for endogamy. If your family history includes endogamy, your total cM is likely to be significantly higher than an equivalent non-endogamous match.[149]
- Assigned (when possible) to either paternal, maternal, or both parental sides if you create or upload a tree and link known relatives.

FamilyTreeDNA includes X chromosome matching, which is omitted by some other vendors.[150]

The goal is to provide you with identical by descent (IBD) matches[151] that can be attributed to a common ancestor in a genealogical timeframe.

After matching, FamilyTreeDNA:

- Estimates relationship ranges based on both total centimorgans[152] (cMs) shared, and longest segment shared, which is a more accurate predictor in endogamous populations. Closer relationship predictions tend to be more accurate than more distant relationships, in part, because the same amount of shared DNA can be found in multiple levels of distant relationships.[153] I utilize DNAPainter's Shared cM Project tool[154] to visualize relationships and to view contributed relationship calculations.[155]
- Compares matches to tree-linked relatives (when you link matches to their profile card in your tree) to assign additional matches maternally or paternally based on shared segments.

147 https://blog.familytreedna.com/wp-content/uploads/2021/08/Family_Finder_Matching_WhitePaper.pdf

148 A centimorgan, also written centiMorgan, is a standard unit of recombination used to measure genetic distance. The amount of matching DNA with another person is expressed as the number of centimorgans, abbreviated as cM or cMs.

149 https://dna-explained.com/2022/08/11/dna-in-search-ofsigns-of-endogamy/

150 https://dna-explained.com/2018/02/07/who-tests-the-x-chromosome/

151 https://dna-explained.com/2016/03/10/concepts-identical-bydescent-state-population-and-chance/

152 https://dna-explained.com/2022/12/13/concepts-your-matches-on-the-same-segment-are-not-necessarily-related-to-each-other/

153 https://help.familytreedna.com/hc/en-us/articles/4476783220495-Family-Finder-Relationship-Ranges-#how-accurate-are-family-finder-s-relationship-ranges--0-0

154 https://dna-explained.com/2019/10/14/dnapainter-instructions-and-resources/

155 https://dnapainter.com/tools/sharedcmv4 - Please note that the DNAPainter Shared cM Tool provides charts and is calculated based on the community contributed data from all vendors submitted to Blaine Bettinger for the Shared cM Project.

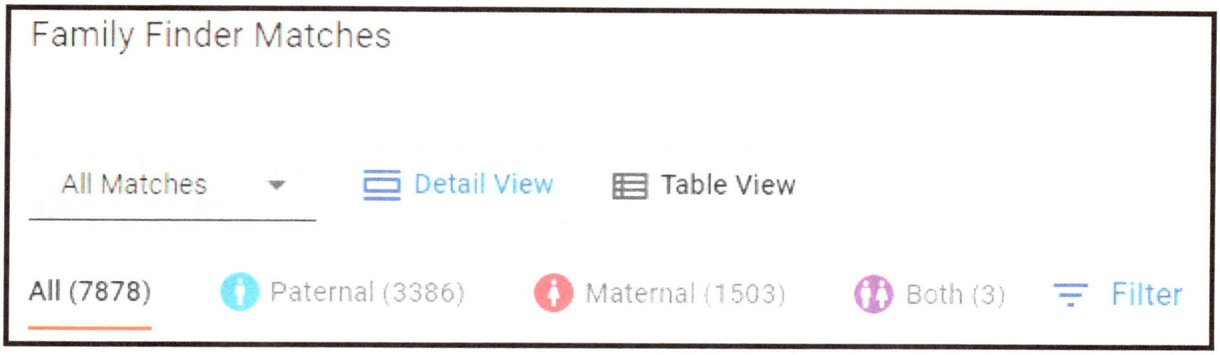

I'm using my own results for these examples.

I have 7878 total matches, of which 3386 are paternal, 1503 are maternal, and 3 people match me on both sides. Matching on both sides is expected for full siblings, sibling's children and their descendants, and your children and their descendants.

People with significant endogamy[156] or whose parents are related to each other will also have matches to both sides.

You will notice that the sum of Paternal, Maternal, and Both is less than the All category. The difference is 2986 matches that cannot be assigned to either a maternal or paternal category.

This is normal and can be a result of a few different factors:

- Both of your parents haven't tested, so not all of your DNA can be compared to a parent for matching. For complete matching, you need all 23 of your chromosomes to be fully covered by matches attributable to one side or the other.
- Neither of your parents has tested, so your match assignments are predicated upon other known, linked family members. Therefore, probably not all of your DNA is assigned to parental sides. This is one reason we encourage everyone to test as many of your closest upstream relatives as possible if both of your parents can't test.
- More people on one side of your family have tested than the other.
- Roughly 20%, and possibly more, of your matches will be a function of identical-by-chance, meaning that you match that person because either your DNA or their DNA just happened to match the other person as a result of chance recombination.

4cM	4cM
Mom	Dad
You	
Your Match	

156 https://dna-explained.com/2022/08/11/dna-in-search-ofsigns-of-endogamy/

Here's an example. Let's say your Mom contributes 4 cMs of pink DNA, and your Dad contributes 4 cMs of adjoining tan DNA. In you, this equals 8 contiguous cMs of DNA.

Now, let's say that you match someone on that 8 cM segment of DNA.

That 8 cMs of your DNA does not descend from one ancestor or one parent. That 8 cMs is divided between two sources – your mother and your father. Therefore, your match cannot match you due to ONE common ancestor. They match you because you inherited smaller matching DNA segments from both of your parents, side by side, by chance – which just happened to match someone else over the 7 cM matching threshold when combined.

This scenario could be reversed, where you inherit 8 cMs from one parent, but your match inherited their 8 cMs by chance from their two parents. Therefore, your match will also match your parent, but the match is still identical by chance, on their side.

I explained and provided many examples in the article "*Concepts – Identical by...Descent, State, Population and Chance.*"[157]

How Are Your Matches Divided into Parental Buckets?

FamilyTreeDNA utilizes your tree[158] combined with matches that you can identify in order to compare matching segments with other people in order to assign them to a particular maternal or paternal side.

Let's use an example.

Let's say that both of your parents have also taken a DNA test, and their results are available at FamilyTreeDNA, along with yours.

You either create a tree at FamilyTreeDNA or upload a GEDCOM file from another source, such as your personal genealogy software on your computer. Common programs are RootsMagic, Family Tree Maker, or Legacy Family Tree software. You can also download your tree from Ancestry if you have one there, or simply link to your existing tree at MyHeritage.[159] FamilyTreeDNA has announced tree-integration with MyHeritage, which is expected in 2024.[160]

The goal is to attach people on your match list to their profile card on your tree. That's how you tell FamilyTreeDNA which side of your family your matches are on, which, in turn, is how they identify other matches as maternal, paternal or both.

Clearly, the best matches to link are both parents, plus grandparents, of course. 100% of your DNA came from your two parents, combined, so if both of your parents have tested, all of your valid matches can be assigned to one side or the other.

157 https://dna-explained.com/2016/03/10/concepts-identical-bydescent-state-population-and-chance/

158 In 2024, FamilyTreeDNA will partner with MyHeritage to utilize their family trees. The functionality of the Family TreeDNA products is expected to remain the same.

159 https://dna-explained.com/2020/06/30/download-your-ancestry-tree-and-upload-it-elsewhere-for-added-benefit/

160 https://dna-explained.com/2023/12/11/familytreedna-2023-update-past-present-and-future/

Unfortunately, testing parents isn't always possible, so testing close relatives provides portions of the same DNA that you inherited from your parents. Connecting those people, such as aunts, uncles, cousins, and grandparents, to their profile card on the proper side of your tree triggers in-common-matching. People who match both you and your relative on a common segment will be assigned to the maternal, paternal, or both buckets.[161]

For example, let's say your mother hasn't tested, but her sister has and appears on your match list. You connect your aunt to her profile card on your tree.

Next, Jane Doe matches both you AND your aunt on a specific common segment or segments. Jane is then assigned to your maternal bucket because she triangulates with you and your aunt on at least one segment.

Uploading or Creating Your Tree and Linking

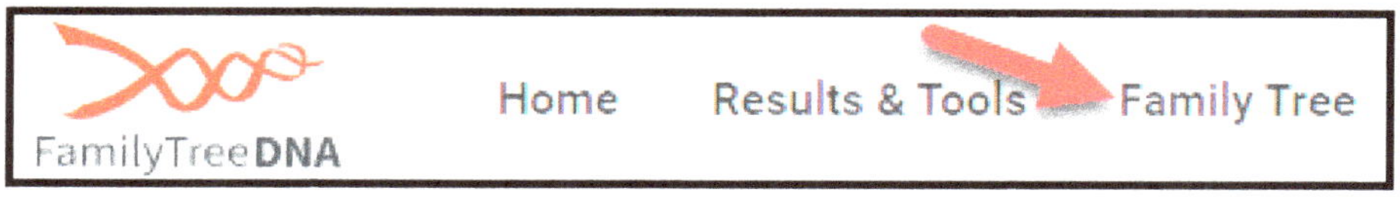

Click on either Family Tree at the top of your page, or Family Tree under Additional Tests and Tools.

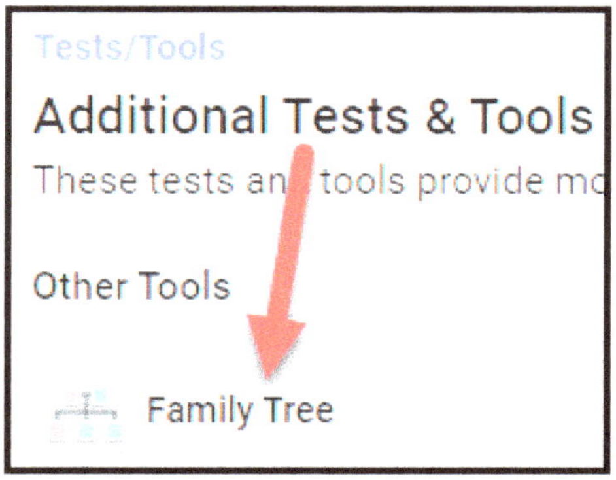

After uploading or creating your family tree, you'll view your tree when you click on either of those links.

Your matches in the order of highest to lowest amount of shared DNA will be shown, at left.

161 https://dna-explained.com/2019/11/06/triangulation-in-action-at-family-tree-dna/

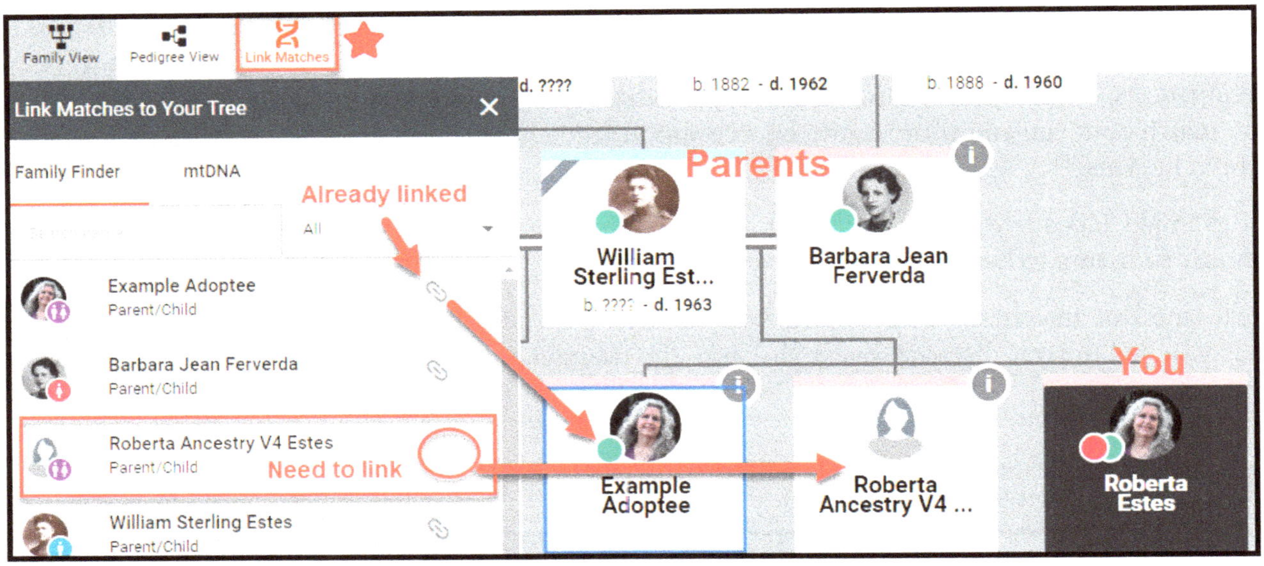

In this example, I, the tester, am the dark profile card in the bottom right corner. I've uploaded two more of my own DNA files (from other vendors) in order to have two "siblings" to show for examples. I don't recommend uploading multiple autosomal tests for the same person, but I broke that guideline here in order to have examples for this book and my blog articles.

The goal is to link your identified matches with their profile card in your tree. People you've already linked are shown with a little link to the right of their name in the list, plus a green dot on their profile. Unlinked people have no link beside their name and no green dot on their profile.

The first test is named "Example Adoptee," and I previously linked that match. The second test, which is not linked, is named Roberta Ancestry V4.

It's very easy to link.

Be sure the profile card is created for the person in the tree that you wish to link your match to.

If a profile card doesn't exist for the person you want to link, you'll need to create a card by confirming that the intermediate people exist in the tree path between you and the person you want to link, then add any missing branches/people to the tree.

In this case, I'm going to link Roberta Ancestry V4 Estes as a full sibling to myself, so I would begin with either my mother or father and add "Roberta Ancestry V4" as their child.

Create Profile Card

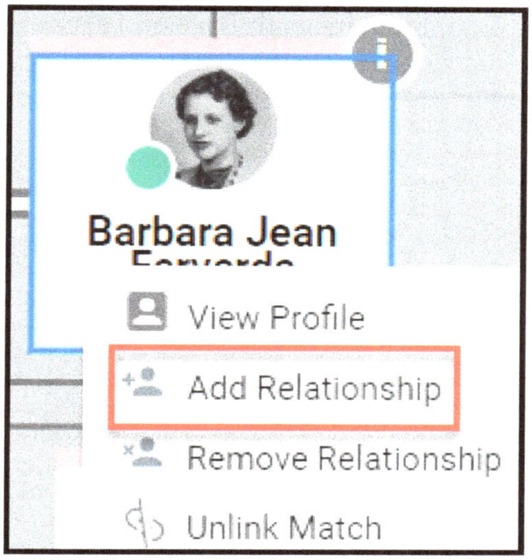

To create a new profile card in your tree, click on one of the relevant parents and select "Add Relationship."

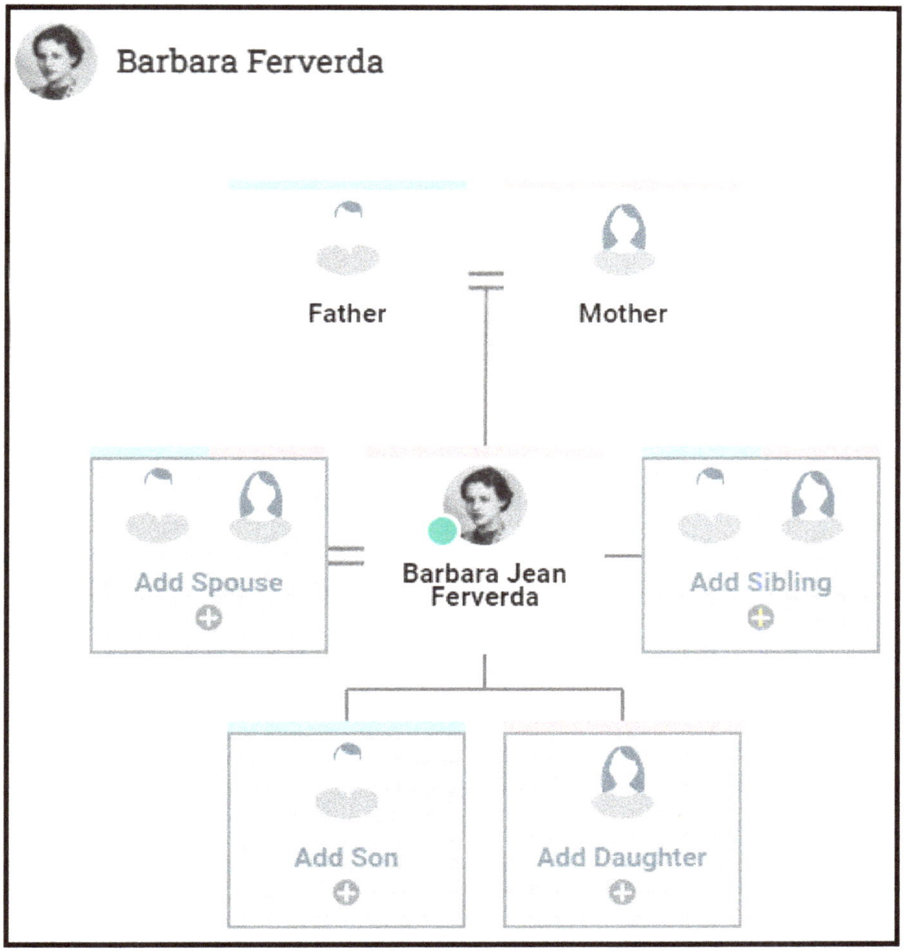

Then click on the type of relationship you want to add.

In this case, I would click on "Add Daughter" beneath Barbara Ferverda.

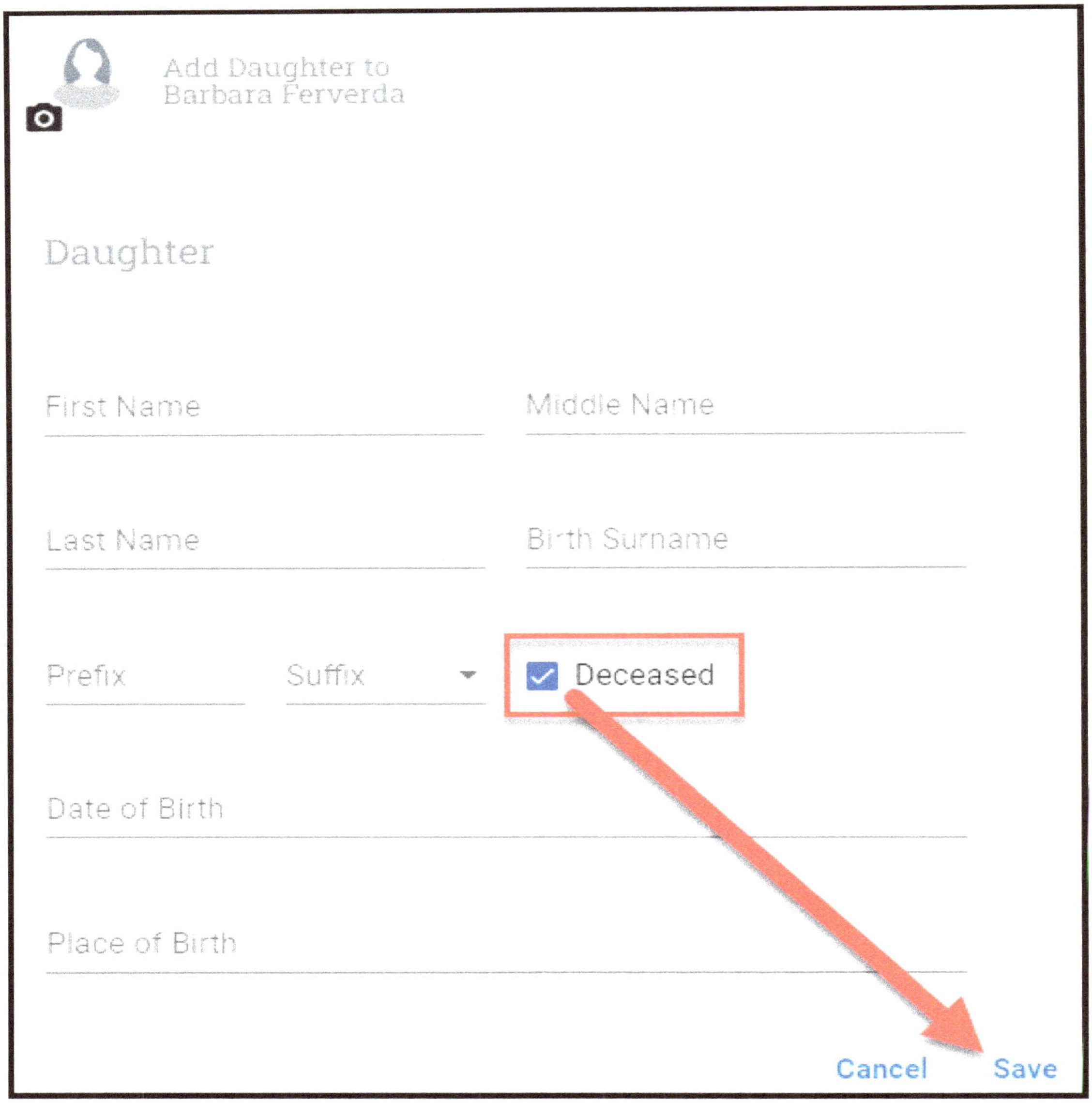

Please note that when entering profile card information, you **MUST** click the "Deceased" box if you want your matches to be able to view that profile card.

While it's common practice not to display living people, you surely DO want your matches to be able to see the identity of your deceased great-grandparents, for example. That's the entire point of matching and identifying your common ancestor.

I strongly recommend including birth and death years, if known, and a location, which can be an important match hint.

TIP: Be sure to click "Save" when finished.

After creating the profile card for your match who took the test, you'll just drag and drop the match, at left, onto their profile card.

Don't worry if you make a mistake. It's easy to unlink, (and relink,) by clicking on the profile card.

Remember, the more people you can link in their proper place in your tree, the more of your unknown matches can be automatically bucketed.

Maternal and Paternal Matching, aka Bucketing

FamilyTreeDNA uses the information you've provided about how you're related to people to bucket that person, and others, to specific sides of your tree.

Let's look at some match examples to explain. Let's say that your mother hasn't tested, but you match your maternal aunt, maternal uncle, and your maternal 1st cousin through a different aunt. All three people, and you, are descendants of your maternal grandparents through different children.

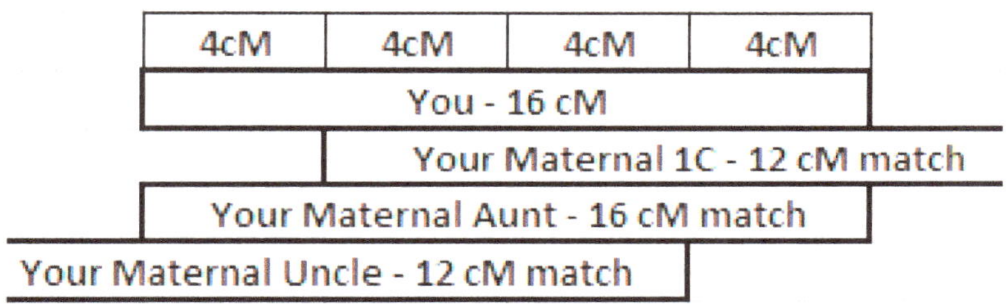

Let's also say that the maternal aunt that you linked in your tree matches you exactly on a 16 cM segment. This tells FamilyTreeDNA that people who match you and this aunt on that same segment(s) should also be assigned to the maternal side of your tree.

Therefore, the FamilyTreeDNA system determines who matches you maternally based on the 16 cM match to your aunt, as follows:

- People who match both you and your linked maternal aunt
- On all or a portion of the same segment(s) over the match threshold of a minimum of 7 cMs.[162]

You can see in our example that your maternal first cousin (1C) matches both you and your maternal aunt on 12 cMs of this segment.

You can see that your maternal uncle matches both you and his sister, your maternal aunt, on 12 cMs of this segment, but not exactly the same 12 cMs as your aunt and first cousin.

162 https://blog.familytreedna.com/wp-content/uploads/2021/08/Family_Finder_Matching_WhitePaper.pdf

Everyone matches each other on the middle 8 cMs.

Therefore, all three of these matches will be assigned to your maternal bucket because you linked your aunt to her profile card. So will anyone else who matches you and your aunt on at least 7 contiguous cMs of those same segments.

Every match that you can assign to a place in your tree should be linked to that individual's profile card. In other words, now you need to link both your maternal uncle and your maternal 1C so that people matching all of those matching segments can be bucketed as well.

The only possible exception is if both of your parents have tested at or uploaded to FamilyTreeDNA because all of your legitimate matches will match both you and one of your parents on at least one segment – so you don't necessarily need to link everyone, although I often do anyway.

Some people may match you and both parents and will be placed in the "Both" bucket.

People who don't match you and either of your parents will remain unassigned. If both parents have tested and you've linked them as your parents in your tree, this means that unassigned matches are identical by chance.

If both of your parents have NOT tested, meaning that Family Matching is being performed based on other linked known relatives, your unassigned matches MAY be unassigned because there simply isn't a linked relative who matches you and that person on the same segment.

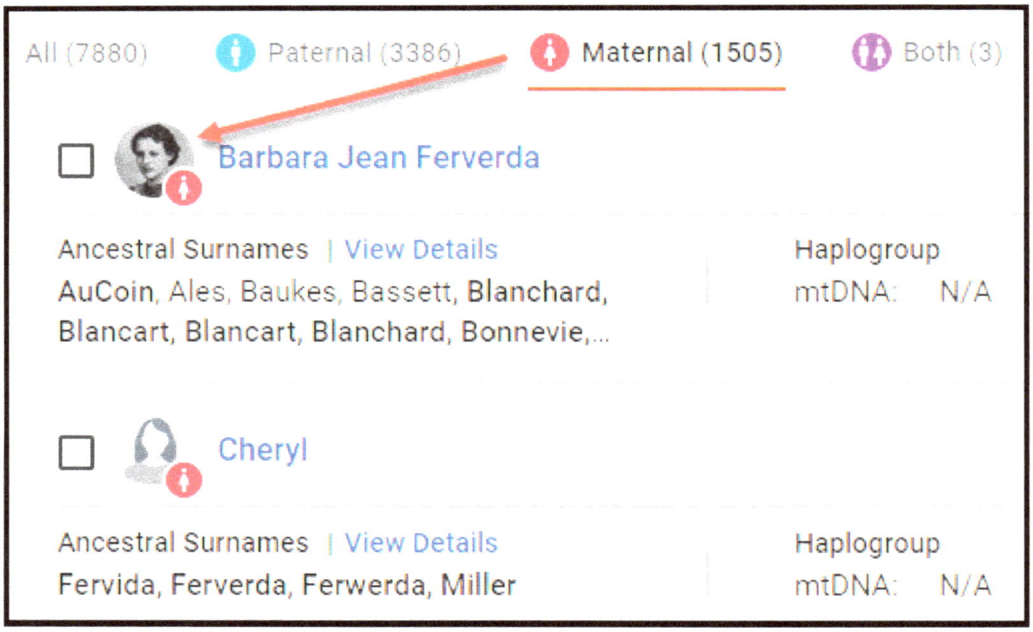

By clicking on the Maternal icon at the top, only maternal matches are displayed, meaning both the people I've linked and the balance of the people that have been assigned maternally by FamilyTreeDNA based on who I've linked.

Triangulation

Triangulation is a technique used to verify segments that descend from a specific ancestor. Triangulated segments[163] confirm descent from that ancestor.[164]

Triangulation attributed to a specific ancestor occurs when:

- At least three (not closely related) people match[165]
- On the same reasonably sized segment, generally 7 cMs or larger
- The people who match can be confirmed to be descended from a common ancestor, ancestral couple, or line

Maternal or paternal bucketing can occur:

- When known relatives are linked to their profile card on the tester's tree AND
- By triangulation, when a match matches the tester and the tester's linked relative on the same segment

I have written articles about triangulation,[166] both general concepts[167] and triangulation techniques specifically at FamilyTreeDNA.[168]

TIP: Please note that every segment has its own individual history.

This means that you may match one person on two (or more) different segments that descend from two completely unrelated lines, especially when the families live or originate in the same geography.

I've discovered some matches with whom I share ancestors from both my mother's and father's lines, even though that's very unlikely given their different ancestry. Yet, it happened. One of my mother's German ancestors' descendants migrated to Tennessee, where my father's family lived, and the rest is history.

163 https://dna-explained.com/2019/10/18/hit-a-genetic-genealogy-home-run-using-your-double-sided-two-faced-chromosomes-while-avoiding-imposters/

164 https://dna-explained.com/2020/12/16/triangulation-resources-in-one-place/

165 https://dna-explained.com/2021/04/18/a-triangulation-checklist-born-from-the-question-why-not-use-close-relatives-for-triangulation/

166 https://dna-explained.com/2020/12/16/triangulation-resources-in-one-place/

167 https://dna-explained.com/2019/10/18/hit-a-genetic-genealogy-home-run-using-your-double-sided-two-faced-chromosomes-while-avoiding-imposters/

168 https://dna-explained.com/2019/11/06/triangulation-in-action-at-family-tree-dna/

Family Finder Filter

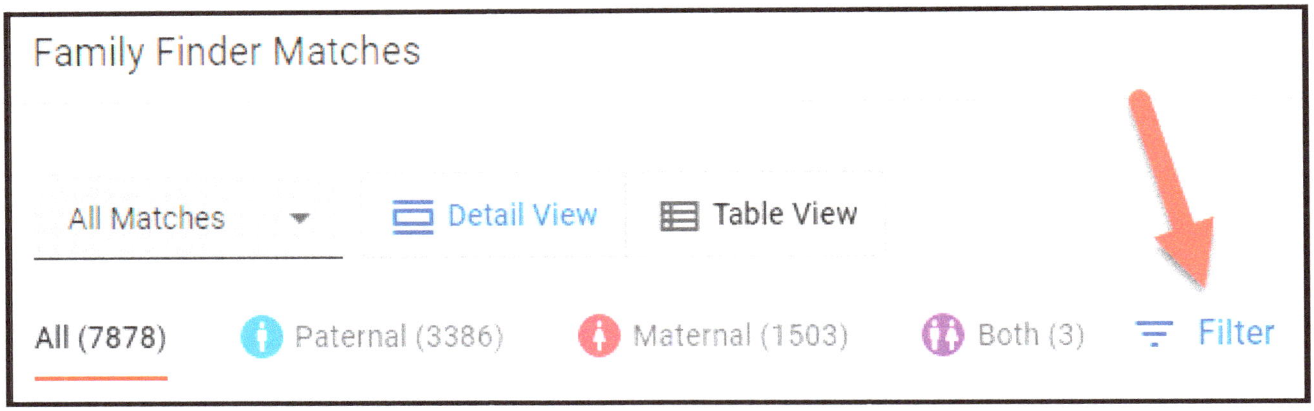

The Family Finder filter option allows users to apply filters in order to view only specific groups of matches.

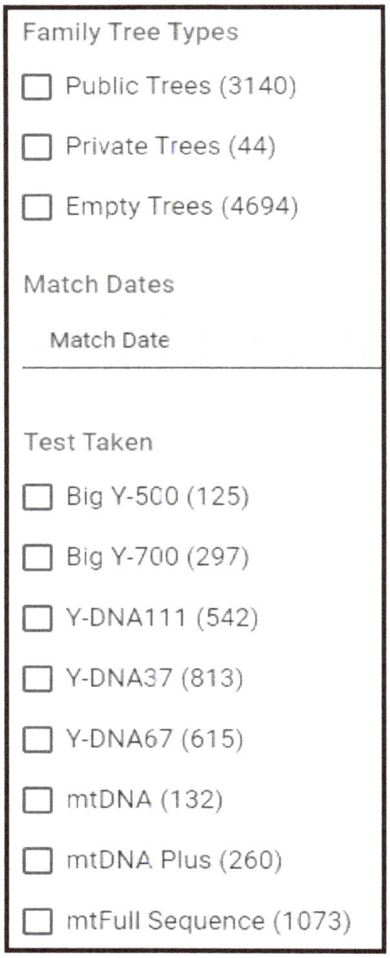

Multiple options can be selected.

Family Finder Sort and Export

At the upper right of your match list, you'll see the sort options, plus an export function.

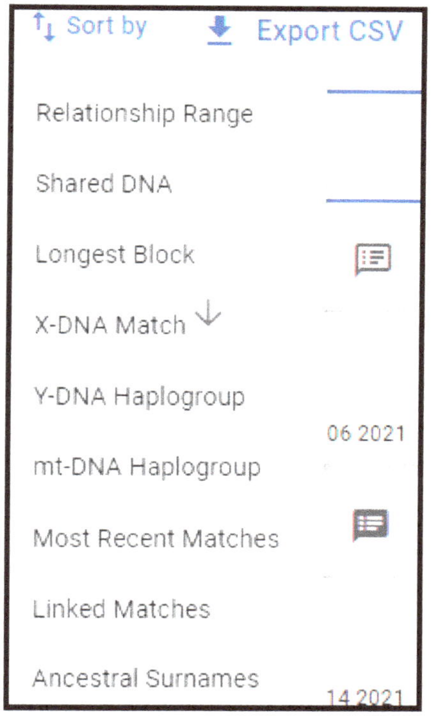

To the right of the Sort is the Export CSV link, which gives you the option of downloading all of your matches, or only matches currently selected using a filter.[169]

Family Finder Match Export File

This export is a .csv file of information about your matches.[170] This is not the Chromosome Browser Results centimorgan segment matches which are provided in a separate export file, found on the Chromosome Browser.

This Match file includes the following columns:

- Full Name
- First Name
- Middle Name
- Last Name
- Match Date
- Relationship Range

169 https://dna-explained.com/2023/12/21/whats-changed-autosomal-dna-vendor-feature-changes-since-the-23andme-data-compromise/

170 This has been paused as a result of the 23andMe data compromise, but will hopefully be restored in early 2024.

- Shared DNA cM total amount
- Longest Block of matching DNA
- Linked Relationship based on how this person is linked to your tree
- Ancestral surnames
- Y-DNA Haplogroup
- mtDNA Haplogroup
- Notes
- Matching Bucket
- X-Match – either the number of cMs or "no match"

I find this file most useful to download at the same time as I download the companion Chromosome Browser Results centimorgan segment file so they are in sync.

This file provides the ability to perform the following features:

- By viewing the Linked Relationship column, it's easy to sort and see at a glance all of the people who I've linked to profile cards in my tree. This makes it easy to discern who else I can link.
- Spreadsheet search for any word, which is particularly useful for surnames.
- It's easy to filter for the matching bucket (maternal, paternal, both) which I use to combine with the companion Chromosome Browser Results segment spreadsheet found on the Chromosome Browser.
- Provides me with the ability to sort by X match.
- For me, viewing matches in a spreadsheet format is easier and allows me to scan and work without needing to click through and do searches. When I find something interesting, I use the Family Finder Matches page to search for shared "in-common" matches and utilize tools like the chromosome browser.
- I record notes in a specific format in the system. I use the notes field to record when I painted this match at DNAPainter, so I can quickly see which matches I've painted along with the identified common ancestor, and which ones I have not. All matches where I've identified the common ancestor have DNAPainter as the first word in the note.

Displays

Family Finder matches are displayed in two formats – the default Detail View and a second, more compact, Table View.

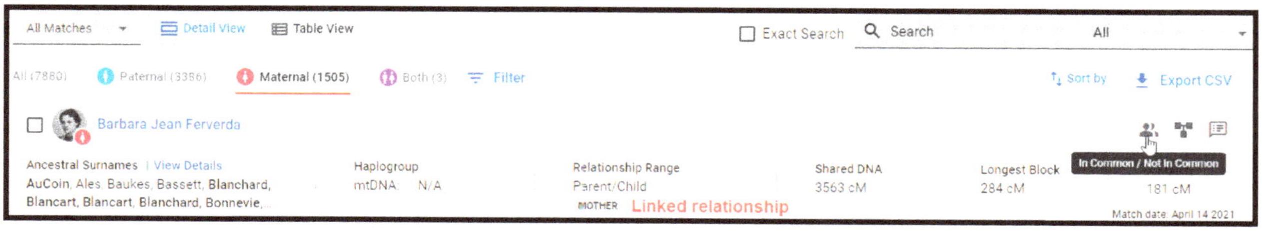

There's a lot of information to be gleaned from match information.

- Your match's name is displayed, along with a profile picture if they have uploaded one.
- If they are bucketed, there's a little pink female, blue male, or purple "both" icon beside their profile picture.
- Beneath their name is a list of ancestral surnames, if they have provided that information. Ancestral surnames are extracted from trees during upload, but that has not always been the case. Initially, no surnames were extracted. Then, at one point, ALL surnames were extracted, not just those on your direct ancestral lines, so if a match uploaded during that period, some ancestral surnames may not be directly relevant to them. Also, additions or modifications to the tree are not reflected in the surname list, so always check both resources.
- Their Y-DNA and mitochondrial DNA haplogroups are displayed if they have taken those tests, or if they have been assigned as a result of the Family Finder test.[171]
- The predicted relationship range is provided. For more distant relationships, several possible relationships will be included. I utilize the Shared cM Project tool at DNAPainter to visualize the various potential relationships.[172]
- If you have linked this match on your tree, the linked relationship is shown.
- The total amount of shared DNA is displayed, along with the longest block of shared DNA.
- The final column is the amount of X chromosomal DNA that you share with this match. X-DNA has a unique inheritance path, which we will discuss in the X-DNA chapter.

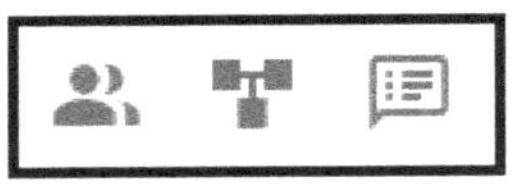

At the far right side of each match, you'll see three icons.

- The first icon that looks like 2 people is the shared DNA or "in common with/not in common with" icon.
- The second icon, the one of a pedigree, indicates, if dark blue, that your match has a family tree that you can view. If it's not dark blue, your match has no tree.
- Clicking on the third icon provides the ability to make notes.

The primary difference between the Detail and the Table View is that in the Table View, no photo is displayed, and the display is more compact.

---

171 Mid-level haplogroups are assigned and displayed to your autosomal matches for Y-DNA from Family Finder tests performed at FamilyTreeDNA and uploaded from MyHeritage. Mitochondrial haplogroups will be added after the Y-DNA haplogroups are complete and after the updated mitochondrial tree has been published. Haplogroups from uploaded files from other vendors will be provided when possible, at the level possible based on the file received, but will not be displayed to matches.

172 https://dnapainter.com/tools/sharedcmv4

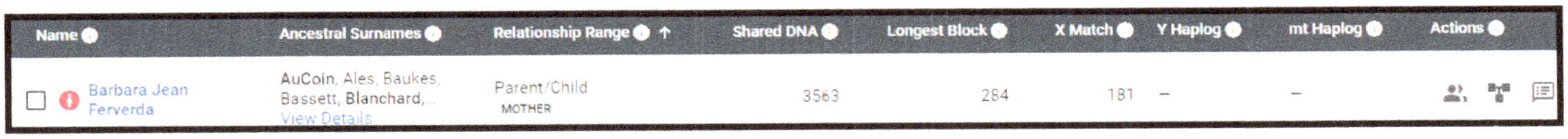

On both views, Ancestral Surnames are displayed.

Bolded names indicate surnames found in both your Ancestral Surname list and your matches' Ancestral Surname list.

Clicking on View Details under Ancestral Surnames provides two lists.

The first is a list of all Matched Surnames in common, along with a location if provided.

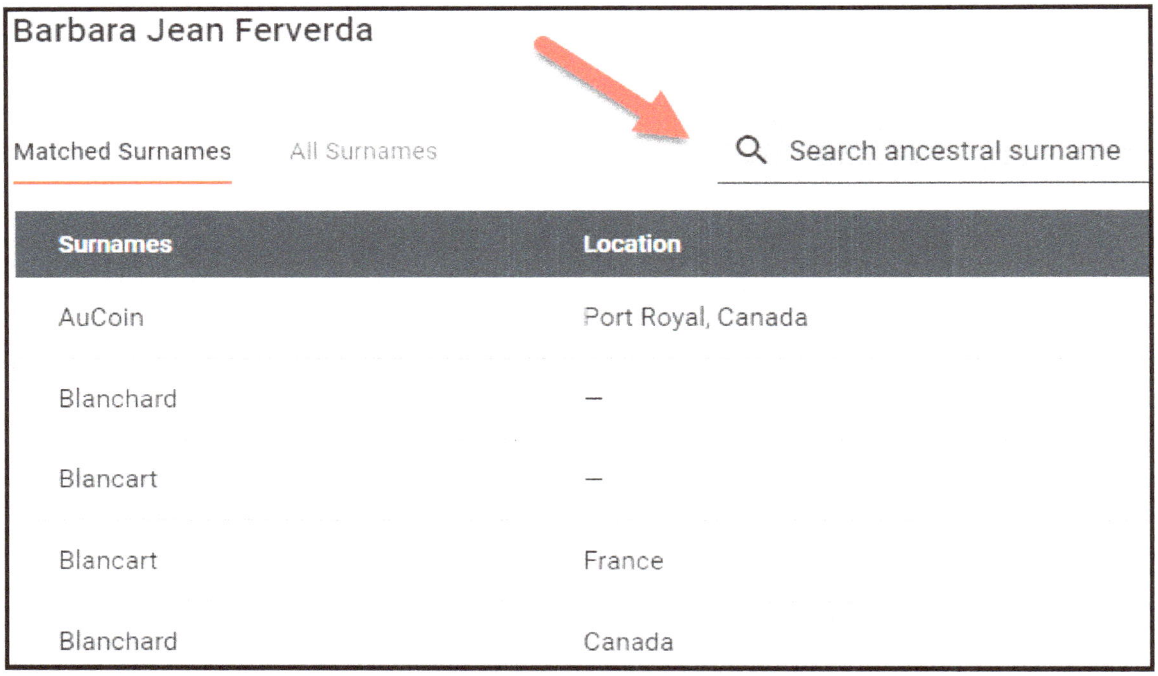

You can also search for a specific surname.

The second list, "All Surnames," means both matching and non-matching surnames.

In Common With, or Not

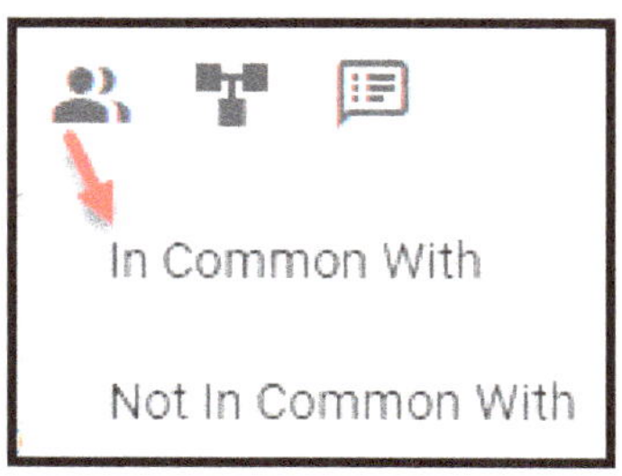

The "In Common With" icon provides the ability to search for people who match you "in common with" or "not in common with" another match.

Selecting the "In Common With" option provides a list of people who match you and your selected match, both. I've selected Cheryl, my mother's first cousin, for this example.

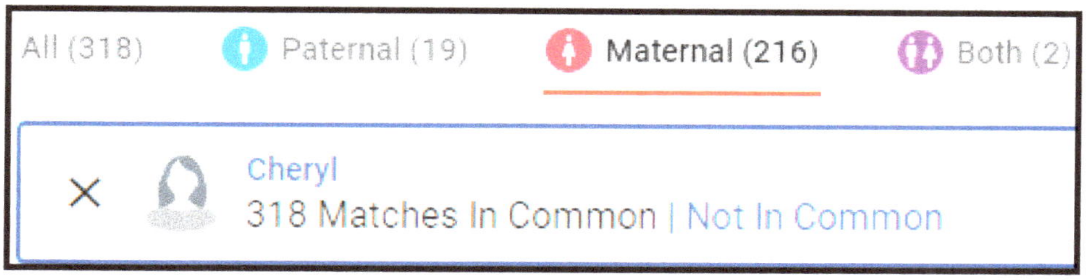

The numbers displayed above the match when "In Common With" is selected indicate how many people in total and in my buckets match me and my selected match, Cheryl.

TIP: Remember, this is always from the perspective of the person who tested, not their match. In other words, I match Cheryl on a total of 318 matches, 19 on MY father's side, (not her father's side), 216 on MY mother's side, (not her mother's side), and 2 through both of MY parents.

I'm related to Cheryl through my mother's side, evidenced by the 216 shared maternal matches plus our proven genealogy. Where did those 19 very unexpected paternal matches (from my perspective) come from? They could be by chance, of course, but as it turns out, they aren't.

My mother's father and Cheryl's father were siblings, but one of Cheryl's maternal ancestors married someone who is from the area where my father's ancestors lived. Hence, 19 of Cheryl's matches also are bucketed matches to me on <u>my</u> paternal side.

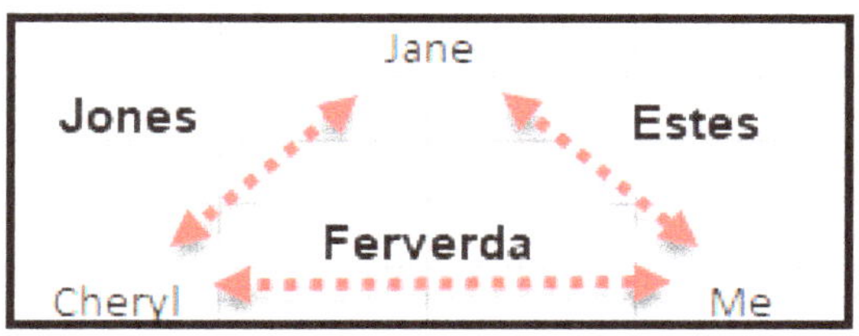

I match Jane, one of those matches, on my paternal Estes line, and Cheryl matches Jane on a Jones line that I thought was unrelated to me. Those 19 paternal matches in common are a result of Cheryl's Jones connection.

We tracked the ancestors of our common Jones match back to the geographic region where my father's ancestors lived.

- The moral of this story is that you can never assume, in either direction.
- Shared matches are clues, but do not necessarily mean common shared DNA segments, nor shared ancestors between all 3 people.
- Shared or "in common" matches alone are hints and can be deceiving. You and another match could both match a third person on different segments, through two completely different ancestors.
- Bucketed matches, assigned maternally, paternally, or both, require at least one common segment between all three people, which assures a triangulated segment. You, the bucketed match, and someone that you've linked in your tree share a common segment and a common ancestor, presuming the match is not identical by chance.
- When common matches are involved, triangulation is critically important.

Profile Card

Clicking on your match's profile card displays additional information, including their email address and both their paternal and maternal Earliest Known Ancestors, haplogroup, and Ancestral Surnames. If they have not created or uploaded a tree, this is another avenue to obtain at least some information.

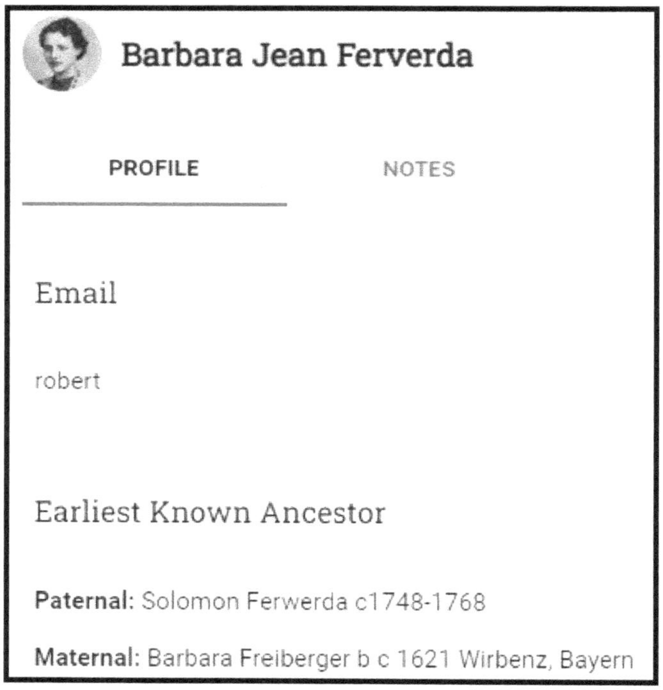

Match Search

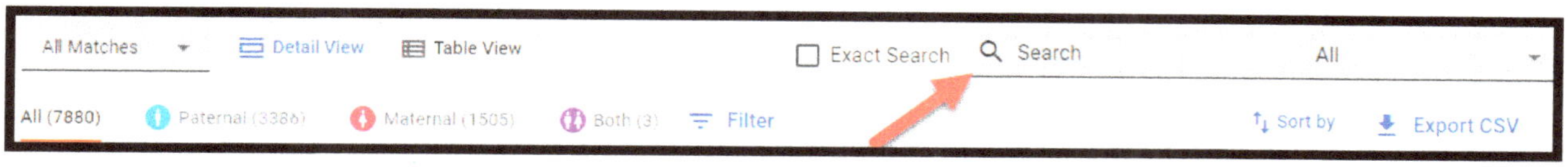

At the top of your match page, you can search for matches by specific criteria.

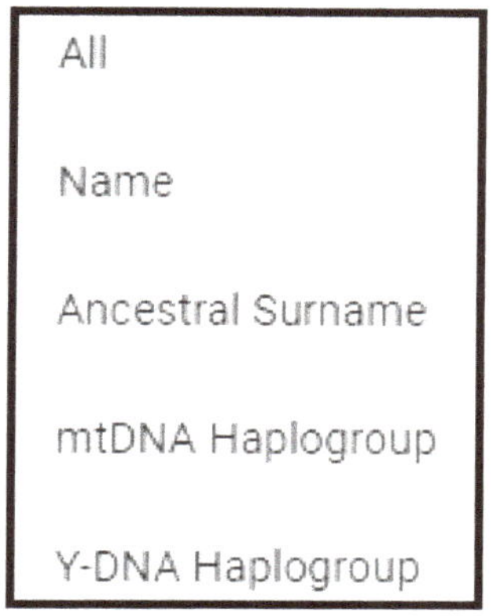

Showing "All" matches is the default, but you can select other options.

- I can enter just the name Estes to see everyone who shows Estes as any part of their name, or in their Ancestral Surnames.
- By selecting "Name" from the dropdown list, only those people where Estes appears as any part of their name will be displayed.
- By selecting Ancestral Surname, only people who have included Estes in their Ancestral Surname list will be displayed, not people with Estes as part of their name. This does not search their tree.

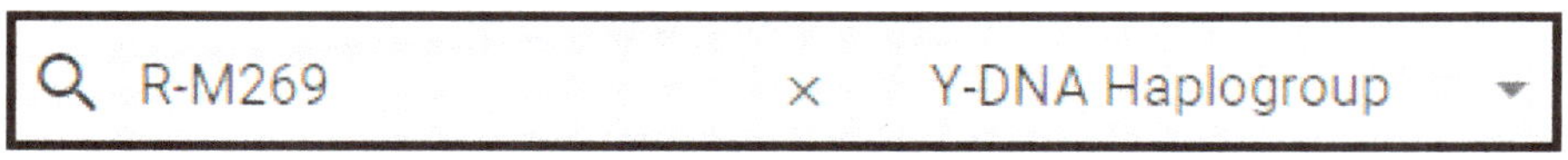

- The haplogroup search facilitates searching for matches with a specific haplogroup.
- For mitochondrial haplogroups, entering a partial haplogroup, like J1c, for example, results in displaying everyone who has J1c as any part of their haplogroup name. However, checking the Exact Search box limits matching to only what has been entered in the search box.

Feel free to experiment with combinations of filters, sort order, shared matches, and search criteria.

TIP: Don't forget to clear your filters at the top of the Filter dropdown page if you'd like to start fresh. Otherwise, you may still be filtering and not realize it.

Chromosome Browser

A chromosome browser is a canvas that uses your 22 chromosomes as the background upon which to compare and display matching DNA segments of your matches with your DNA.[173]

You can compare up to 7 individuals at a time whose matching DNA segments to you will show on individual copies of your chromosomes.

You can access the Chromosome Browser in one of two ways.

On your Family Finder match page, you can select several matches from either your list of all matches, or your paternal, maternal, or both buckets. I've selected my maternal bucket.

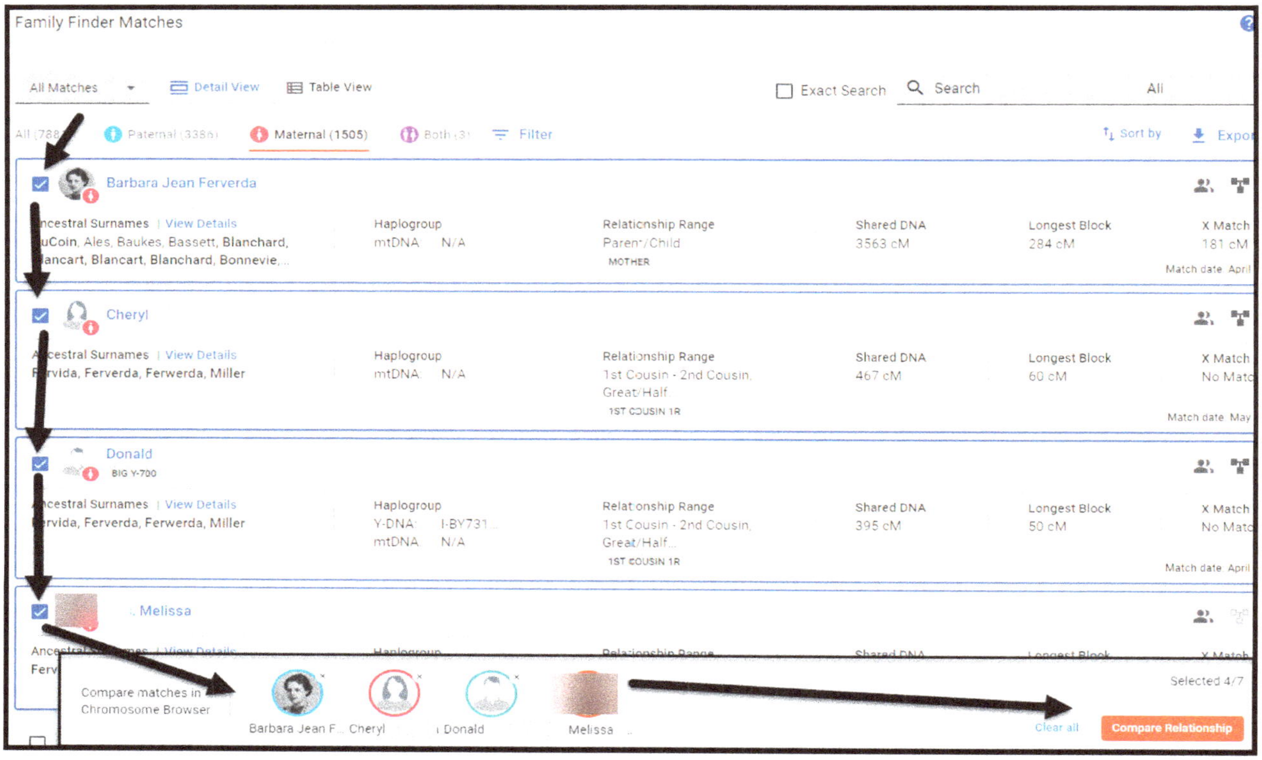

Check the little box to the left of your match's name, and a maximum of seven people will be added to a selection box at the bottom of the page. When finished selecting, click "Compare Relationship."

The second way to access the Chromosome Browser is on the Autosomal DNA Results and Tools section of your personal page.

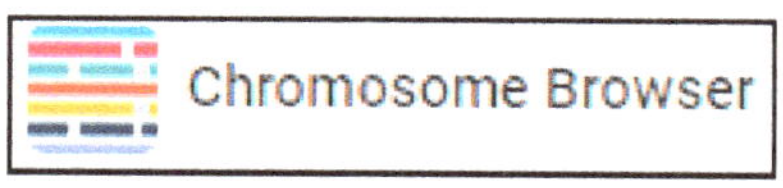

If you click on the Chromosome Browser button, you will see your DNA matches displayed in a slightly different format.

173 https://dna-explained.com/2022/12/13/concepts-your-matches-on-the-same-segment-are-not-necessarily-related-to-each-other/

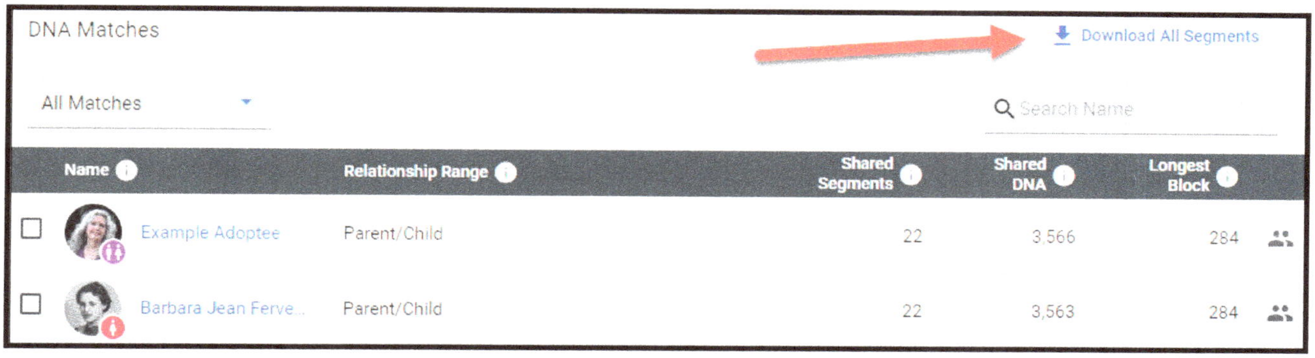

Note, at the upper right, the "Download All Segments" icon. This allows you to download a .csv file that contains the centimorgan matching segment information for ALL of your matches in the Chromosome Browser Results file.[174] We don't need that right now, but you will want to know where it is and how to find it.

Tip: You can use the dropdown box, above the match names, to filter matches, and you can search just like on the other match page.

I'm selecting my maternal matches in the dropdown box. This is important, because all of the matches that will be displayed for match selection will be assigned to my mother's side. This means that if I match any of these people on the same DNA segment, we know that segment descends from my mother's ancestors.

This means that these matches are both:

- Phased, meaning assigned maternally or paternally
- Triangulated[175], meaning those that match me on the same segment MUST descend from the same ancestral line.

TIP: Phased matches means that those matches are from the side of one of your parents.

Please note that if you do NOT select either the maternal or paternal bucket, people from both sides can match you on the same segment, which is neither phased nor triangulated. In other words, those matches on the same segment could be due to a maternal ancestor, a paternal ancestor, or a match by chance. Only selecting bucketed matches will resolve that issue and display only maternal or paternal matches.

174 This feature has been paused temporarily following the 23andMe data exposure.

175 https://dna-explained.com/2017/05/16/concepts-why-genetic-genealogy-and-triangulation/

You can see the maternal icon, beside the profile photos, below.

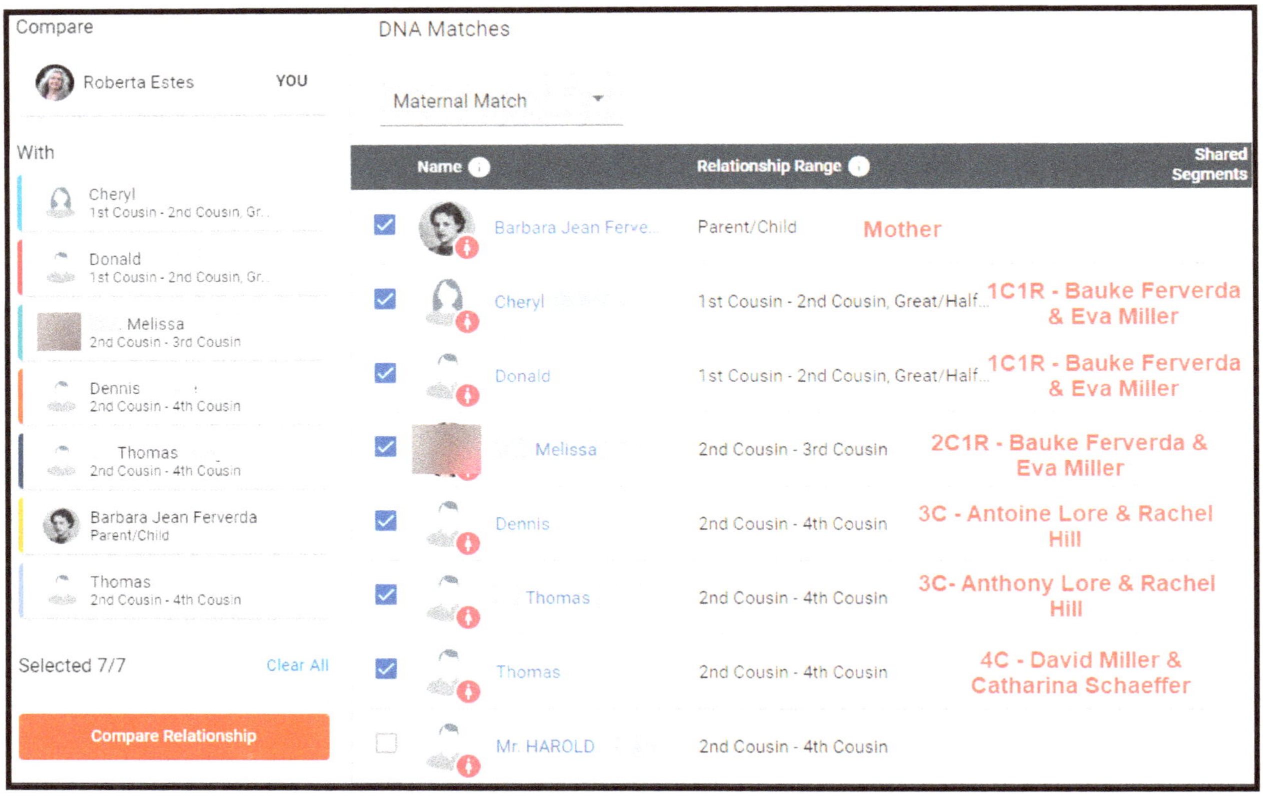

Select the matches whose DNA you want to compare on your chromosomes. I have noted, at right, my actual relationship to each of the selected matches and through which ancestor.

I added my mother to this list only to illustrate that I match my mother on every chromosome.

Therefore, all of these people, if they descend from my mother's ancestors, will match me and my mother, both.

After making your selection, click on "Compare Relationship."

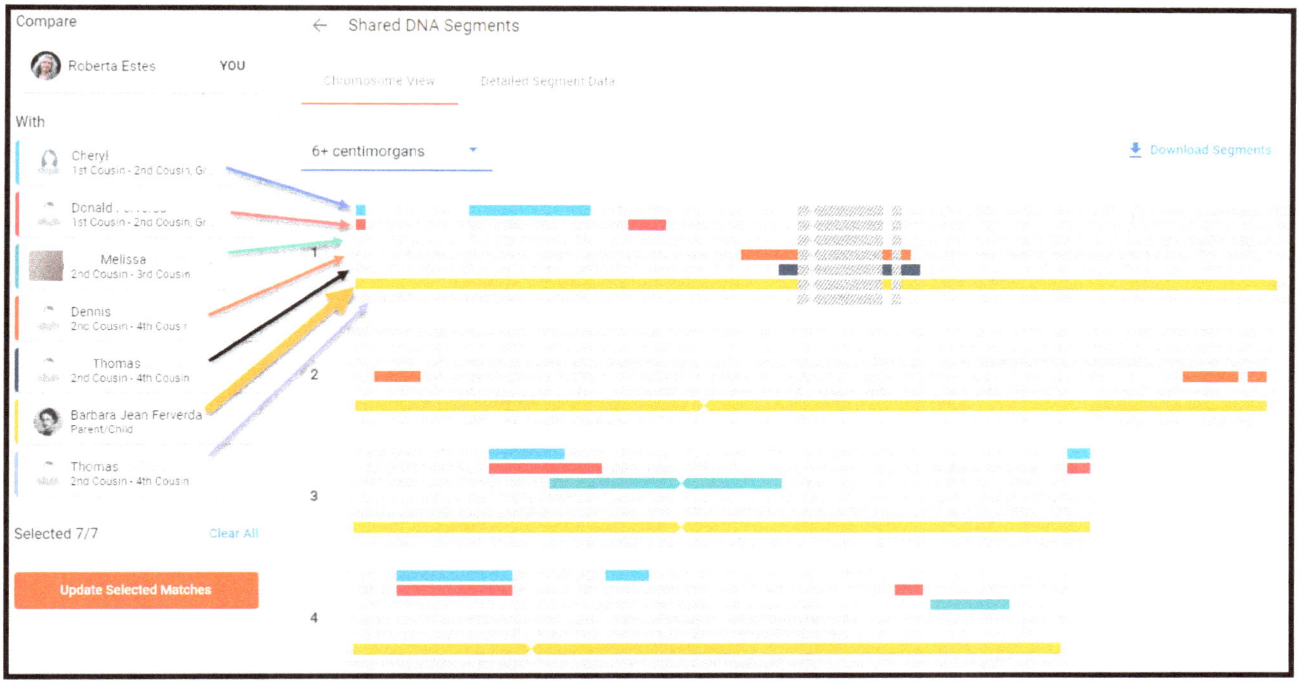

On your Chromosome Browser page, all 23 chromosomes, including the X chromosome, will be displayed, but for brevity, I'm showing only 4 chromosomes here.

The background light grey bands of each chromosome are "me."

The area where every person matches me on that chromosome is shown on their own band of my chromosome. All 7 people are stacked up for each chromosome so I can see them side by side.

Viewing Chromosome 1, at the top, we see that Cheryl's match to me is shown first in band 1. On a color image, her matching DNA to me is blue. Her band of my chromosome shows the segment or segments where she matches me on Chromosome 1.

Other matches are stacked below in their own band of my Chromosome 1.

Her brother, Donald's match to me is shown on band 2.

Melissa's match to me is shown on band 3. It's empty because Melissa does not match me on Chromosomes 1 or 2, but she does on Chromosomes 3 and 4.

Other matches have their own bands as well, with results colored to match their profile tab, at left. I've drawn arrows for each one.

Note my mother's, Barbara Jean Ferverda's larger (yellow) arrow in band 6. I match her on every segment of every chromosome. I received half of Mother's DNA, meaning some portion of her mother or father's segments at every location, so I will match her across every chromosome.

We don't know whether I received her mother's DNA or her father's DNA at any specific location. We need to determine which based on who else we both match at that location.

Based on the common ancestors of my matches, I know immediately that the segments of DNA where my mother and I match Cheryl, Donald, Melissa, and Thomas K. are from my mother's paternal line, and that the DNA where Mother and I match Dennis and Thomas M. (bands 4 and 5) are from my mother's maternal line.

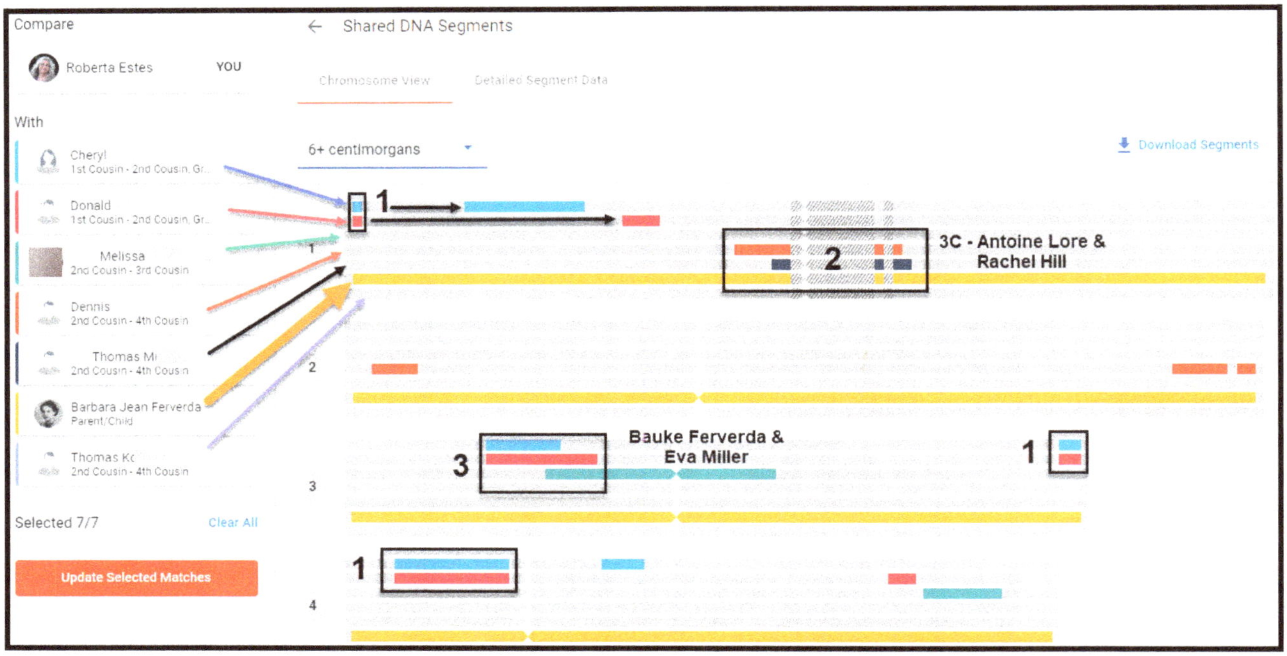

I've numbered and boxed the areas we'll discuss.

#1 – Cheryl and Donald are full siblings. I've included both of them to illustrate why it's important to test siblings. In three locations that are labeled "1," they both match me and mother on the same segments. We all inherited those segments of DNA from our common ancestors, Bauke Ferverda and Eva Miller. However, in other locations, as you can see on Chromosome 1 to the right of the "1" black box, Cheryl and Donald inherited different segments of DNA from their parents. Mother and I match Cheryl on one segment of DNA that Donald doesn't share, and vice versa.

Everyone who matches me, Mother, and Donald or Cheryl on those segments will have received those segments from our common known ancestor, through a common ancestor upstream who contributed them to all of us.

Given that each person triangulates for all matches involved on a specific segment, chances of false positive, invalid, or identical by chance matches are minimal, especially with larger segments over 10 cMs or so.

#2 – On Chromosome 1, further to the right, we see that Mother and I match both Dennis and Thomas M., who are both my third cousins, and both descend from Antoine Lore & Rachel Hill. Notice that this match spans the centromere[176] of the chromosome (hashed markings and white diamond) or the waist of the chromosome, where matching is not performed because of quality issues within that region, regardless of the vendor. However, due to the matching portions on both sides of the centromere, it's still counted as a valid, contiguous match.

#3 – Example three shows three cousins who don't match me on exactly the same segment, but do match on overlapping segments of DNA. In this case, Cheryl and Donald match each other on a significant portion of that segment, where they both match me. So do Donald and Melissa, but Melissa and Cheryl only overlap on a small portion. While they all match me, and by inference, mother, they don't all match each other on this entire segment.[177]

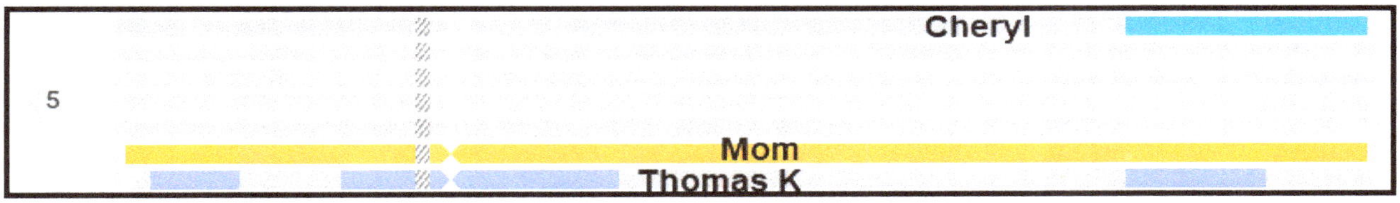

Thomas K. only matches me and Mother on Chromosome 5, but on three separate segments that, together, comprise over 70 cMs of shared DNA. He also matches Cheryl on the third segment on Chromosome 5, but Cheryl's match to me extends beyond that of Thomas's.

Our shared ancestors with Thomas K. descend through Evaline Louise Miller (1857-1939),[178] through her father, John David Miller (1812-1902),[179] and through his parents David Miller (1781-1851)[180] and Catharina Schaeffer (c1781-1826)[181].

Therefore, we know these shared segments descended from David Miller and Catharina Schaeffer to Mother and then to me. I love knowing which of my ancestors contributed my DNA segments.

176 https://help.familytreedna.com/hc/en-us/articles/4418230173967-Glossary-Terms-#c-0-2

177 As the Ferverda DNA Project administrator, I have access to the match lists of project members.

178 https://dna-explained.com/2019/06/22/evaline-louise-miller-ferverdas-will-estate-and-legacy-52-ancestors-243/

179 https://dna-explained.com/2016/07/04/john-david-miller-1812-1902-never-in-his-wildest-dreams-52-ancestors-125/

180 https://dna-explained.com/2016/07/17/david-miller-1781-1851-tamed-3-frontiers-52-ancestors-126/

181 https://dna-explained.com/2016/07/24/catharina-schaeffer-c1775-c1826-and-the-invisible-hand-of-providence-52-ancestors-127/

Segment Data

To view the actual segment data for these matches, click on Detailed Segment Data at the top of the Chromosome Browser display. You will view the segment match information for the individuals that you've selected.

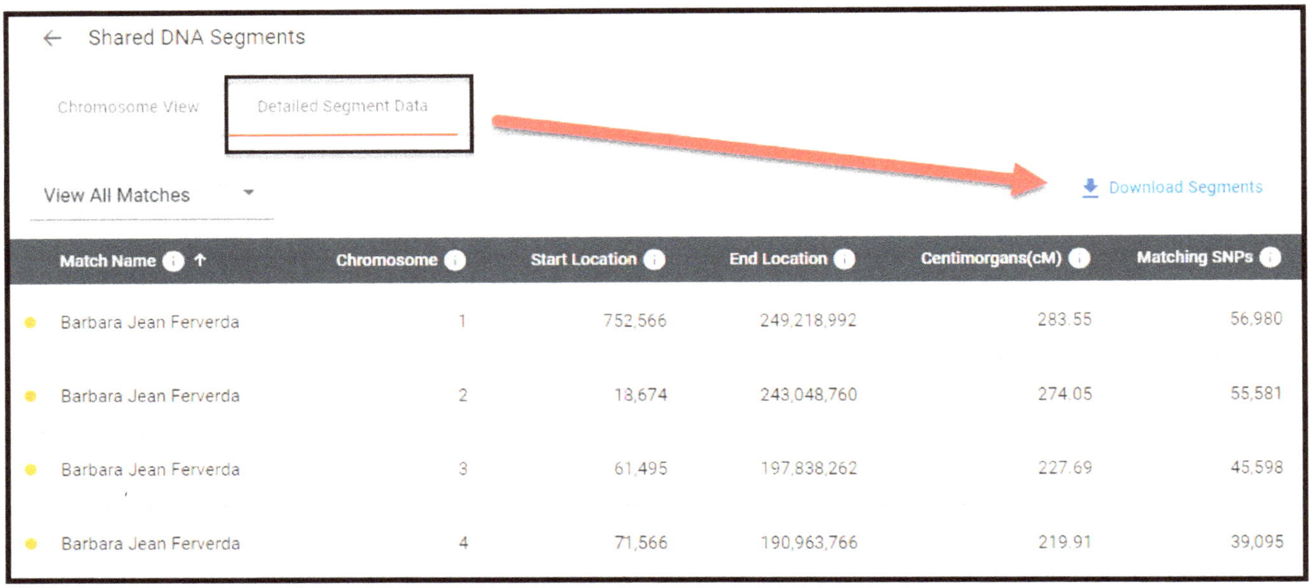

Match Name	Chromosome	Start Location	End Location	Centimorgans(cM)	Matching SNPs
Barbara Jean Ferverda	1	752,566	249,218,992	283.55	56,980
Barbara Jean Ferverda	2	18,674	243,048,760	274.05	55,581
Barbara Jean Ferverda	3	61,495	197,838,262	227.69	45,598
Barbara Jean Ferverda	4	71,566	190,963,766	219.91	39,095

My match with my mother is shown first. We match on the full length of all chromosomes, or the portion that is used for matching. Often, both tips of the chromosomes, known as the telomeres, are omitted, as evidenced by the start location being something larger than position 1.

To download just the matching segments of people you've selected to compare, not your entire match list, click on "Download Segments."[182]

TIP: To remember which Chromosome Browser results segment download is which, if it doesn't say "all," you're not downloading all, just the matches selected for display. All segments are downloaded[183] only prior to selecting individuals to display in the Chromosome Browser.

Parental Segments Versus Unassigned Segments

In the example I'm using, we know that all of the matches have been assigned to my maternal side using triangulation because I selected the maternal bucket.

182 This feature has been paused due to the 23andMe compromise.

183 Please note that the download for all segments and match information was paused as a result of the 23andMe data exposure, which you can read about here: https://dna-explained.com/2023/12/07/23andme-concludes-their-investigation-6-9-million-customers-data-exposed/

Therefore, we know that anyone who matches me and my mother on the same segment is related through an ancestor on my mother's side. Based on who else matches on that same segment, and which of our ancestors that person descends from, we can assign that segment to a specific ancestor or ancestral couple.

However, in the situation where you don't know which side people are assigned to, meaning whether they match you through your mother or father's side, you have no assurance that two people matching you on the same segment are from the same side of your family.

Remember, you have two copies of each chromosome, one from your mother and one from your father. I wrote about this in "*Concepts: Your Matches on the Same Segment are NOT Necessarily Related to Each Other*."[184]

Here's the best example I can possibly show you.

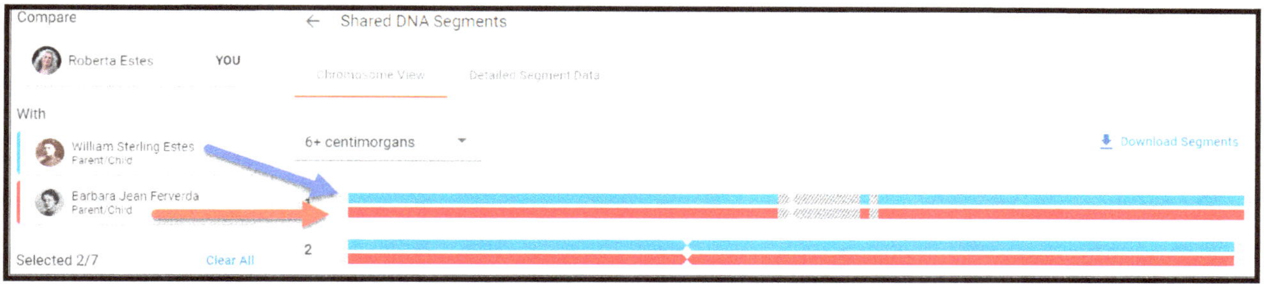

I've selected my father and my mother and **compared them to my chromosomes**. I match both of them on the entire length of every chromosome, of course, but that does not mean they match each other. They don't.

Remember, the chromosome browser is ALWAYS from the perspective of the tester.

Now, let's say I'm an adoptee and don't have a DNA test for either parent nor do I know how I'm related to any of my matches.

Here are 7 people who match me at the beginning of Chromosome 1. You've already met Cheryl.

Are these people related to me on my mother's side, or my father's side, or are they identical by chance?[185]

184 https://dna-explained.com/2022/12/13/concepts-your-matches-on-the-same-segment-are-not-necessarily-related-to-each-other/

185 https://dna-explained.com/2016/03/10/concepts-identical-bydescent-state-population-and-chance/

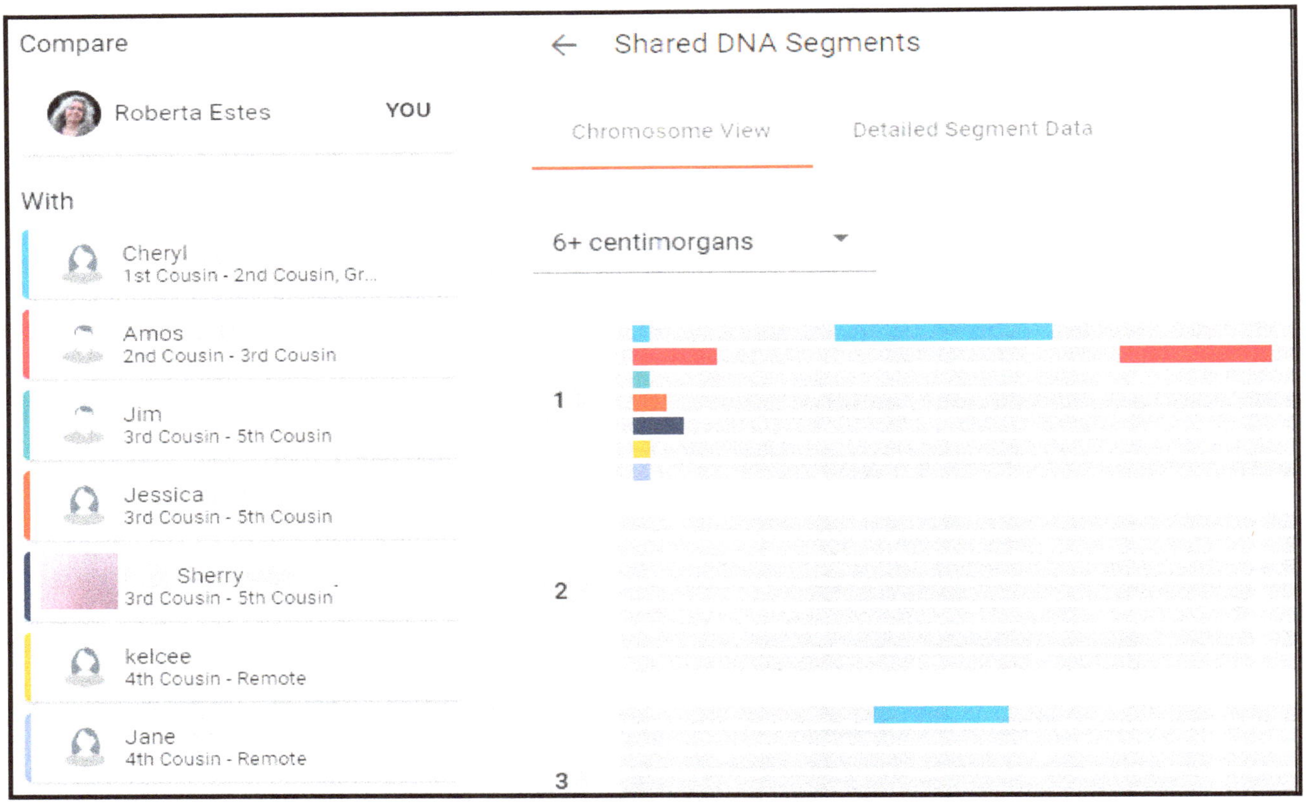

In this example, no one is bucketed or assigned paternally or maternally, so these matches could be from either side, or neither side, meaning they are identical by chance.

There's no way to tell without additional information.

The best way is bucketing, but that's not always possible.

Identifying common ancestors is useful too, but remember that every segment has its own history. Just because you share a specific common ancestor with a match doesn't necessarily mean that ALL of your common segments are from that same ancestor, or that all matching segments are valid matches.

TIP: Identical start and end segment locations do NOT indicate a common ancestor. That's a common fallacy.

Notice that all of these matches begin at the same location, and several have the same end segment too.

Care to guess whether these segment matches are maternal or paternal?

In display order, these segments are attributed as follows:

- Cheryl – assigned and confirmed maternal side
- Amos – assigned and confirmed paternal side
- Jim – assigned and confirmed maternal

- Jessica – assigned and confirmed paternal
- Sherry – assigned and confirmed paternal
- Kelcee – not bucketed and does not match either parent, identical by chance
- Jane – not bucketed and does not match either parent, identical by chance

Do Your Matches Match Each Other?

It would be very helpful to be able to see if my matches on Chromosome 1 also match each other, given that one of the fundamental requirements of triangulation is that you match both people on the same segment, and they also match each other.

FamilyTreeDNA provides a Matrix tool where you can view up to 10 people at once to see if they also match each other.

Matching each other in the Matrix:

- Does NOT mean they match each other on the **same segment** as they match you.
- Does NOT mean that their match with each other is due to the **same ancestor** as their match with you.

We will talk about using the Matrix in the Matrix section.

Identifying Segment Matches

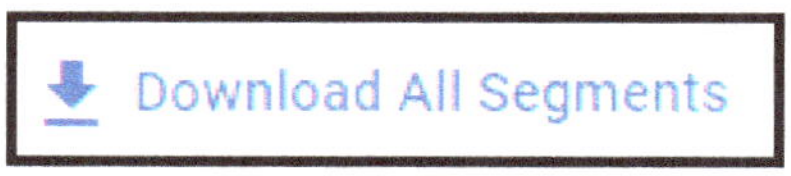

To find the list of all of your matches that match you on some portion of the same segment, click on "Download All Segments"[186] on the Chromosome Browser. This produces a .csv file of all matching segments on every chromosome for every match in the Chromosome Browser Results file.

Once downloaded, I utilize spreadsheet filters and sort, in order:

1. Chromosome end location smallest to largest
2. Chromosome start location smallest to largest
3. Chromosome number smallest to largest

You will then have the list of your matches, sorted by chromosome order. Each chromosome will begin with the smallest match locations, so you'll see matches on the leftmost side of each chromosome first.

186 Please note that "Download All Segments" has been paused in the aftermath of the 23andMe data exposure as other vendors evaluate their security strategies and make changes.

The segments probably won't all match exactly, but groups of matches will overlap, shifting right, little by little, as shown in the example above.

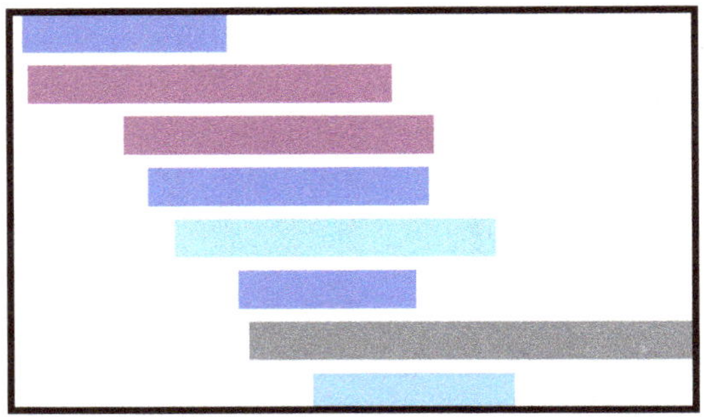

Identical by Descent and Identical by Chance

Be aware, and this concept is **fundamentally important**, that you will have three types of matches for each segment:[187]

1. A group of people who will match you (and your mother if she has tested) on your mother's side. These people are identical by descent, or IBD, meaning you share a common ancestor on your maternal side. This assumes you match one of your matches' parents on this segment too. Both people in a match pair need to evaluate each match to ensure they are IBD.
2. A group of people who will match you (and your father if he has tested) on your father's side. These people are identical by descent, or IBD, assuming you match one of your matches' parents on this segment too.
3. A group of people who will match you, but are actually identical by chance (IBC) because a piece of your mom's DNA and a piece of your dad's DNA just happened to combine in you to match them. Conversely, a piece of their mom's and dad's DNA just happened to combine to match you (and your parent.)

All of these people technically match you, but the question is why.

- A legitimate match, meaning that you match someone because you both inherited that same piece of DNA from a common ancestor, is considered to be identical by descent, or IBD.
- A false positive match is when you match someone, but only because random recombination on either their side or yours caused the match. Those matches are identical by chance, or IBC.

Of course, the only way to tell if you match someone genealogically is to identify a common ancestor, and then determine if you and they also match other people who descend from that common ancestor on that same segment.

187 https://dna-explained.com/2016/03/10/concepts-identical-bydescent-state-population-and-chance/

The best way to eliminate someone from being identical by chance, at least on your side, in the first generation, is to determine whether they match one of your parents. Of course, the same goes for them. If you're lucky and you match their parent, and they match your parent, you've confirmed IBD for at least one generation in each direction.

Next, you'll want to see if they also match other known relatives on that same side of your tree.

That's where the Matrix tool enters the picture. But first, you'll want to prepare your spreadsheet if you have bucketed matches, or know which side, maternal or paternal, some of your matches are from.

Prepare the Spreadsheet

In this example, I only want to work with the first matching segments on Chromosome 1 using the entire Chromosome Browser Results[188] segment file, meaning all of my matches and all of their matching segments to me.

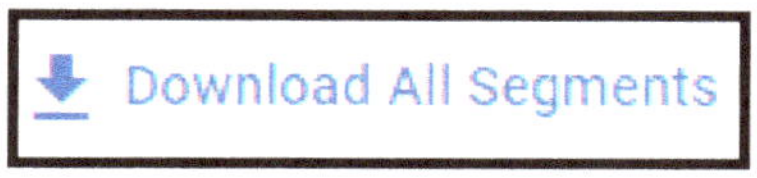

As a reminder, you download the "All Segments" file from the Chromosome Browser, without having selected people to compare. Otherwise, only the people selected to compare will be downloaded.

This file is titled, "Chromosome Browser Results."

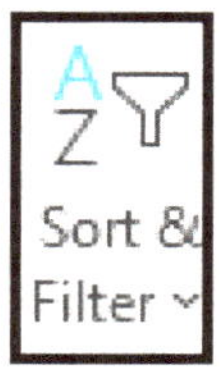

You can use a spreadsheet sort, but I've had issues in the past with not all columns sorting correctly, so I would strongly recommend using the filter option by adding filters to the spreadsheet header row.

188 This download file has been paused as a result of the 23andMe incident. Until this functionality is restored, you can create your own spreadsheet to achieve the same thing and revisit this section after the download ability has been resumed. The concepts are pertinent, regardless of the download ability.

Match Name	Chr	Start Location	End Location	Centimorgans	Matching SNPs	Bucketed
James	1	725266	4744206	9.803617	1614	mother
Cheryl	1	725266	5764879	13.141793	2168	mother
Cody	1	725266	5777457	13.166938	2151	mother
Sherry	1	725266	10713765	21.004978	4053	father
William Sterling Estes	1	725266	249222527	284.03668	82095	**father**
Donald	1	725266	5764879	12.653017	1582	mother
Jim	1	725266	5922308	13.553952	1663	mother
Jessica	1	725266	7537500	15.894821	2141	father
Amos	1	725266	15050177	29.553602	4096	father
Barbara Jean Ferverda	1	725266	249218992	283.5479	56980	**mother**

I downloaded the entire Chromosome Browser Results spreadsheet and filtered/sorted the spreadsheet as described above so that all of my matches on Chromosome 1 begin with those who match me on the smallest-numbered start location, or the furthest left portion of the chromosome.

My matches are bucketed, so I colored my matches above accordingly to reflect which parent they match.

- My maternally bucketed match rows, including my mother, James, Cheryl, Cody, Donald, and Jim, are colored red, which show up as dark grey.
- My paternally bucketed matches, including my father, Sherry, Jessica, and Amos, are colored light blue, which show up as lighter grey

You have two options available for color-coding your matches to identify which people on the spreadsheet are assigned maternally, paternally, or both.

Option 1: Manually color code your spreadsheet rows

If you're only dealing with a few rows, or if you're not terribly comfortable with manipulating spreadsheets, you may just want to manually color a portion of your spreadsheet.

In the example above, I can do that easily by checking a match on the match list or the spreadsheet to determine how they are bucketed.

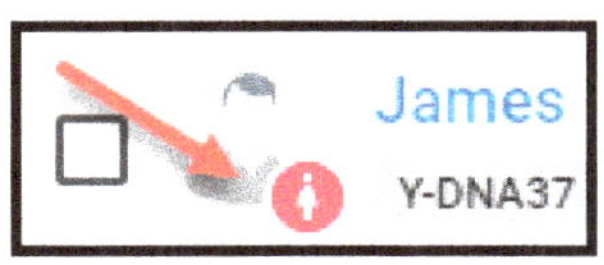

You can see that the first match, James, is maternally bucketed, and I've colored his row red.

If your parent has tested, even if you haven't uploaded a GEDCOM file or created a tree for bucketing, you can see if James matches you in common with one of your parents by using the "In Common With" filter. Color appropriately.

The second and easiest method of determining how people are bucketed is by downloading[189] your Family Finder Matches Spreadsheet, shown in Option 2, below, and viewing the Matching Bucket column. Of course, this presumes that you have bucketed matches.

Option 2: Combine your Chromosome Browser Results Spreadsheet with your Match Spreadsheet data.

Creating a combined spreadsheet is by far the easiest option.

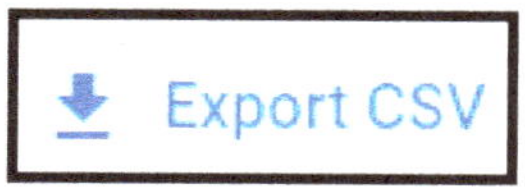

By clicking on the Export CSV link[190], at right on your Family Finder Matches page, above your first match, you will download a Family Finder Matches spreadsheet that includes information about your matches, but not segment information which is found in the Chromosome Browser Results "All Segment" file, above.

The reason that there are two spreadsheets is that you may match one person on several segments, but you only need their information once. You also need to know if they are bucketed, and to which side. That information is found in this match spreadsheet, not the segment spreadsheet.

In this example, I've removed surnames, but each individual will be listed by their entire name in the Match Name column in the Chromosome Browser Results Segment Spreadsheet, above, and the Full Name column in the Family Finder Matches spreadsheet, below.

Full Name	Matching Bucket
Barbara Jean Ferverda	Maternal
Jessica	Paternal
Donald	Maternal
Cody	Maternal
Jim	Maternal
William Sterling Estes	Paternal
Sherry	Paternal
Amos	Paternal
James	Maternal
Cheryl	Maternal

189 Downloading your matches spreadsheet is one of the features paused in the aftermath of the 23andMe data exposure.

190 This download file capability has also been suspended.

I removed the other columns on the Match Spreadsheet, above, leaving only the Full Name and the Matching Bucket. Your matches aren't in the same order between the two spreadsheets, which doesn't matter.

Full Name	Matching Bucket
Barbara Jean Ferverda	**Maternal**
James	Maternal
Cheryl	Maternal
Donald	Maternal
Cody	Maternal
Jim	Maternal
William Sterling Estes	**Paternal**
Sherry	Paternal
Jessica	Paternal
Amos	Paternal

Filter/Sort the "Matching Bucket" column, then color with the legend you want to represent each side. I selected red (maternal) and blue (paternal.)

Match Name	Matching Bucket	Chr	Start Location	End Location	Centimorgans	Matching SNPs	Bucketed
James		1	725266	4744206	9.803617	1614	mother
Cheryl		1	725266	5764879	13.141793	2168	mother
Cody		1	725266	5777457	13.166938	2151	mother
Sherry		1	725266	10713765	21.004978	4053	father
William Sterling Estes		**1**	**725266**	**249222527**	**284.03668**	**82095**	**father**
Donald		1	725266	5764879	12.653017	1582	mother
Jim		1	725266	5922308	13.553952	1663	mother
Jessica		1	725266	7537500	15.894821	2141	father
Amos		1	725266	15050177	29.553602	4096	father
Barbara Jean Ferverda		**1**	**725266**	**249218992**	**283.5479**	**56980**	**mother**

On your Segment Spreadsheet, above, which won't be colored yet, insert a column to the right of the Match Name column and title it, Matching Bucket.

Match Name	Matching Bucket	Ch	Start Locatic	End Locati	Centimorgai	Matching SNP	Bucketed
Amos		1	725266	15050177	29.553602	4096	father
Amos	Paternal						
Barbara Jean Ferverda		**1**	**725266**	**249218992**	**283.5479**	**56980**	**mother**
Barbara Jean Ferverda	Maternal						
Cheryl		1	725266	5764879	13.141793	2168	mother
Cheryl	Maternal						
Cody		1	725266	5777457	13.166938	2151	mother
Cody	Maternal						
Donald		1	725266	5764879	12.653017	1582	mother
Donald	Maternal						
James		1	725266	4744206	9.803617	1614	mother
James	Maternal						
Jessica		1	725266	7537500	15.894821	2141	father
Jessica	Paternal						
Jim		1	725266	5922308	13.553952	1663	mother
Jim	Maternal						
Sherry		1	725266	10713765	21.004978	4053	father
Sherry	Paternal						
William Sterling Estes		**1**	**725266**	**249222527**	**284.03668**	**82095**	**father**
William Sterling Estes	Paternal						

Copy the colored Full Name column contents and the Matching Bucket contents from the Family Finder Matches Spreadsheet and paste them into the first two columns in the Chromosome Browser Results Spreadsheet as illustrated above, **BELOW the existing rows of data. Do not overwrite existing rows of data**.

Your Chromosome Browser Results spreadsheet is already sorted by chromosome size.

Next, filter/sort by Match Name.

Match Name	Matching Bucket	Chr	Start Location	End Location	Centimorgans	Matching SNPs	Bucketed
James		1	725266	4744206	9.803617	1614	mother
Cheryl		1	725266	5764879	13.141793	2168	mother
Cody		1	725266	5777457	13.166938	2151	mother
Sherry		1	725266	10713765	21.004978	4053	father
William Sterling Estes		**1**	**725266**	**249222527**	**284.03668**	**82095**	**father**
Donald		1	725266	5764879	12.653017	1582	mother
Jim		1	725266	5922308	13.553952	1663	mother
Jessica		1	725266	7537500	15.894821	2141	father
Amos		1	725266	15050177	29.553602	4096	father
Barbara Jean Ferverda		**1**	**725266**	**249218992**	**283.5479**	**56980**	**mother**
Barbara Jean Ferverda	Maternal						
Cheryl	Maternal						
Donald	Maternal						
Cody	Maternal						
Jim	Maternal						
William Sterling Estes	Paternal						
Sherry	Paternal						
Jessica	Paternal						
Amos	Paternal						

The results for your entire spreadsheet will be that you can see which matches are bucketed, and which are not.

- Each of these individuals is assigned either maternally or paternally.
- The segment row for that person has no color, but the match spreadsheet row for that person has the color and also which bucket.
- If they are not bucketed, there will be no color beside their name on the matches spreadsheet.

While all rows aren't colored, because they are sorted by name, you can easily see that Amos is paternal, Barbara Jean Ferverda is maternal, and so forth. You don't have to color the rows, but I find it much easier to discern which matches aren't bucketed at all with a visual clue.

TIP: If you have NOT tested both parents, you CANNOT assume that unbucketed matches are identical by chance.

TIP: If you have tested ONLY one parent, you can't assume that matches which aren't assigned to that parent belong to the other parent. You can expect that an average of 15-20% of your matches, and possibly more, will be identical by chance.

Now, let's see if your matches also match each other.

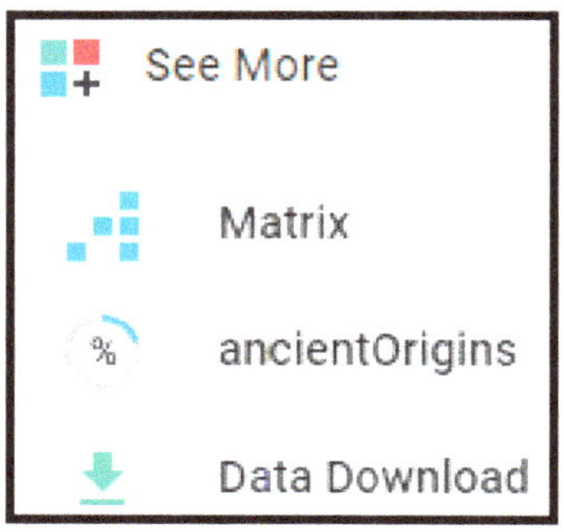

Matrix

The Matrix tool is available under the "See More" tab.

The goal of the Matrix is to determine whether your matches also match each other. I utilize this tool in addition to bucketing or the spreadsheet colorization technique discussed above. This is particularly useful when both parents have not tested, so you don't have complete bucketing.

TIP: Matching on the Matrix does not mean you match on a common segment, only that your matches match each other, or don't.

In the Matrix, scroll, then click to select up to 10 people you wish to compare and "Add" each one. Their name will then appear in the comparison box, at right.

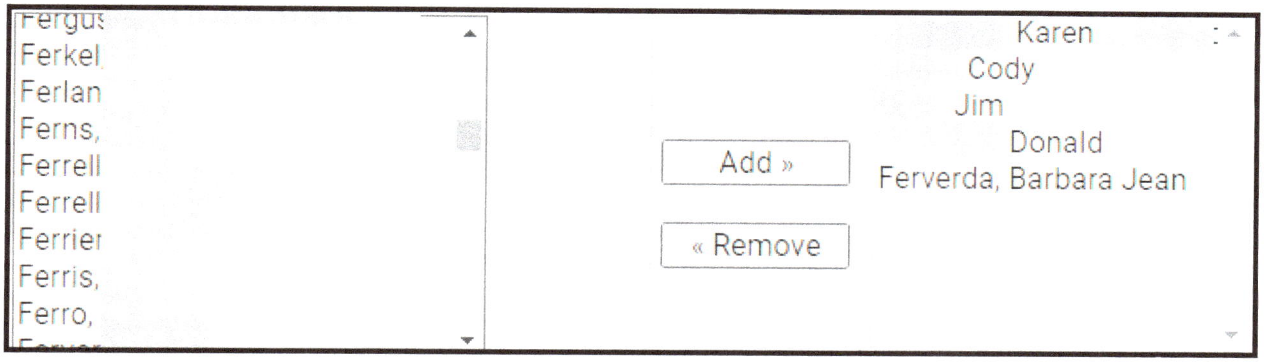

I've selected only my mother and the matches that are bucketed to her on the first segment of Chromosome 1.

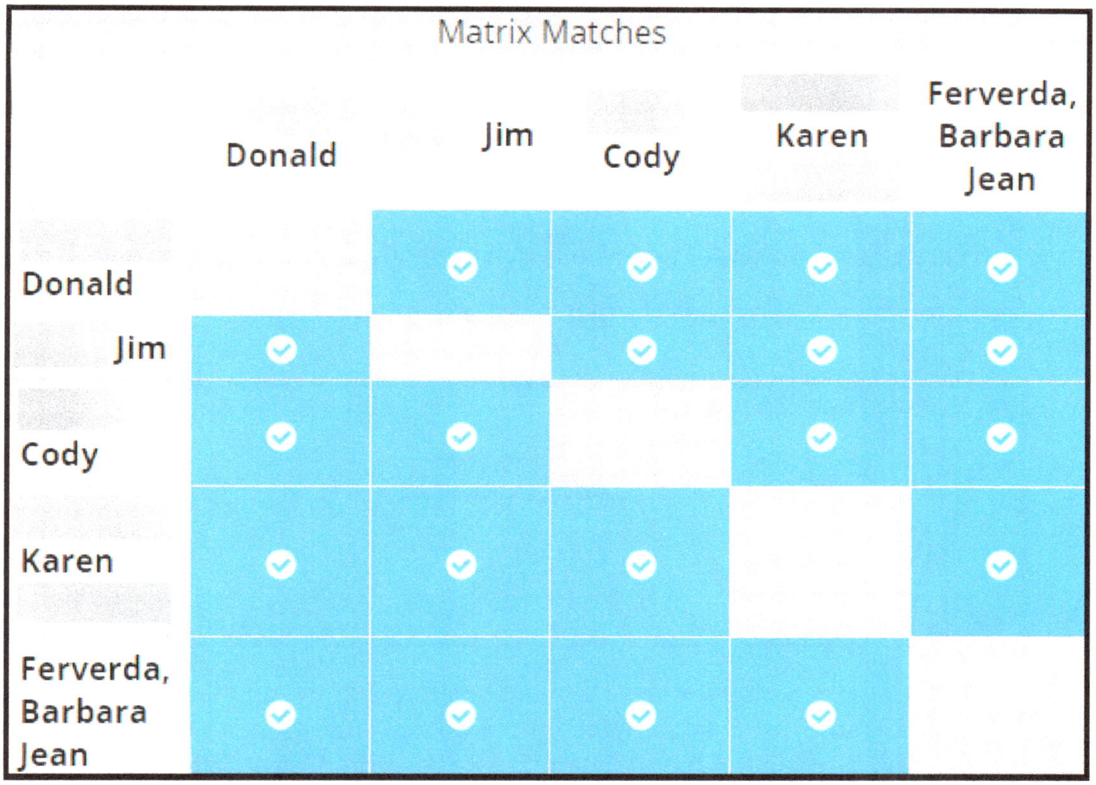

All of these matches also match each other. That's exactly what I expected since we already knew that they match on the same segment, and they are bucketed to my maternal side.

TIP: If we don't know how people are bucketed, we could enter up to 10 people who match me on that segment to see if they also match each other.

Without bucketing, there would be a group from my maternal side, a group from my paternal side, and possibly people that don't match either group.

I selected a group of people known to all have a match to me on the same region of Chromosome 1. However, I could have selected people at random without regard to match location.

When people match, it does NOT mean they necessarily match on the same or a common segment, nor does it mean they match each other because of the same ancestor(s) whose segment(s) they share with you.

People who do not match either the maternal or paternal group are the people who either:

- Are identical by chance, or
- Don't share quite enough DNA to be a match with the other person on that segment. Segments sometimes don't align exactly, which is why you see different start and end locations.
- If I had not selected a group of people known to match on the same segment of the same chromosome, a third reason for someone not matching either my paternal or maternal group is that they simply don't happen to match any of the people I've selected.

When you're not working with known segment locations, you may want to see which members of a group of people match each other to see if they are from the same line.

Let's say I have 4 people bucketed to my mother's side, but none of them match me on the same segment.

Of those four people, we have two sets of two who match each other, too. What can this tell me?

Let's look at a pedigree chart. George and Harriett had a son, John, who married Barbara, the daughter of Elijah and Mary.

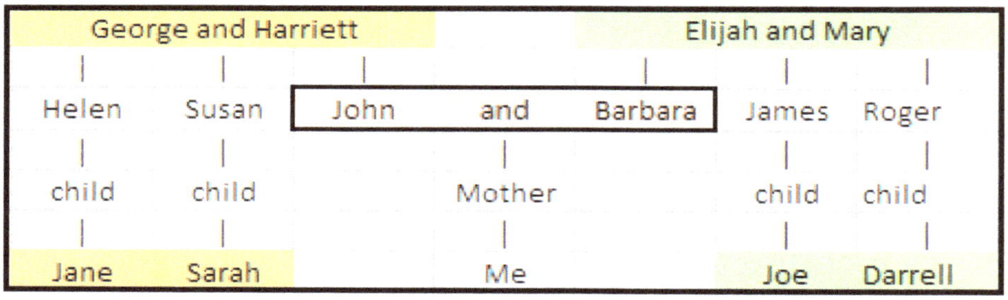

Mother and I both match Jane, Sarah, Joe and Darrell. Therefore, I know that this match is maternal for me. However, the Matrix shows us that Sarah and Jane, who descend through other children of George and Harriett, match each other, but not Joe and Darrell, who descend through different children of Elijah and Mary and also match each other.

If my mother and I share common segments with either Jane and/or Sarah, we can attribute those segments to George and Harriett through my mother's father, John.

If we share common segments with Joe and/or Darrell, those segments can be attributed to Elijah and Mary through my mother's mother, Barbara.

TIP: Your matches may match each other because they share an entirely different ancestor than the one you share with them. For example, Joe and Sarah could potentially match each other through ancestors of their "other parent."

Chapter 6

X CHROMOSOME - UNIQUE INHERITANCE PATH

You inherit two copies of each of Chromosomes 1-22, one copy of each chromosome from each of your parents.

That's why DNA matching works and each match is either designated as "maternal" or "paternal," depending on how your match is related to you. Each valid match will be related either maternally, paternally, or sometimes, both.

Your 23rd chromosome is your sex-determination chromosome and is inherited differently.

You still inherit one copy of Chromosome 23 from each parent, which may contain two X chromosomes (females) or an X and Y chromosome (males.)

- Males inherit a Y chromosome from their father, which is what makes males male.
- Males inherit an X chromosome from only their mother.
- Females inherit an X chromosome from both parents, which is what makes them female.

Chromosome 23	Father Contributes	Mother Contributes
Male Child	Y chromosome	X chromosome
Female Child	X chromosome	X chromosome

Because males don't inherit an X chromosome from their father, X chromosome matching has a unique and specific pattern of descent which allows testers to immediately eliminate some common ancestors.[191]

- Males can only have legitimate X matches on their mother's side of their tree because they only inherit an X chromosome from their mother.
- Females, on the other hand, have matches on both sides of their tree because they inherit an X chromosome from both their mother and father. Their father only has one X chromosome to contribute, so the daughter receives her paternal grandmother's X chromosome intact.
- Both males and females inherit their mother's X chromosome just like any of the other 22 autosomes, meaning it is comprised of the X chromosome of both her mother and father.

191 https://dna-explained.com/2012/09/27/x-marks-the-spot/

This unique X chromosome inheritance path provides us with a fourth very useful type of DNA for genealogy. X-matching is included with your Family Finder test.

The X chromosome, even though it is autosomal in nature, meaning it recombines and divides, is really its own distinct tool that is not equivalent to autosomal matching in the way we're accustomed. We need to learn about the message it's delivering and how to interpret X matches.

FamilyTreeDNA is currently the only vendor[192] that utilizes X chromosome matching, which is another good reason to encourage your matches at other vendors to upload their results to FamilyTreeDNA for free matching.

TIP: The X chromosome is not the same as mitochondrial DNA, but people often confuse the two.[193]

My X Chromosome Family Tree

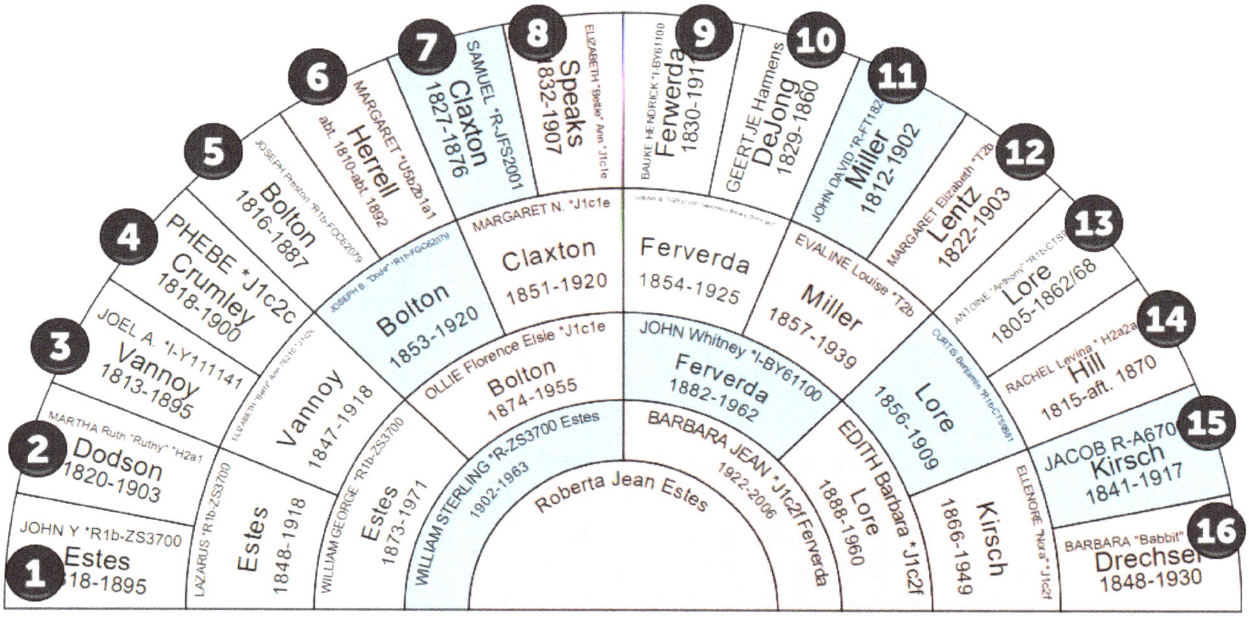

Roberta's 4-Generation X-Chromosome Fan Chart

This fan chart[194] of my family tree colorizes the X chromosome inheritance path. In this chart, males are colored blue and females pink, but the salient point is that I can inherit some portion of (or all of) a copy of my X chromosome from the colorized ancestors, and only those ancestors.

Because males don't inherit an X chromosome from their fathers, they CANNOT inherit any portion of an X chromosome from their fathers' ancestors.

Looking at my chart, you see that, as a female, I inherited an X chromosome from both of my parents, but my father only inherited an X chromosome from his mother.

192 23andMe provided X-DNA segment information prior to their data exposure.

193 https://dna-explained.com/2017/07/26/x-matching-and-mitochondrial-dna-is-not-the-same-thing/

194 https://dna-explained.com/2017/02/07/using-x-and-mitochondrial-dna-charts-by-charting-companion/

Men don't inherit an X chromosome from their fathers. Therefore, I didn't inherit an X chromosome from any of the people whose positions in the chart don't have any color.

X matching for females eliminates 50%, or 8 of 16 4th-generation matches shown on previous page.

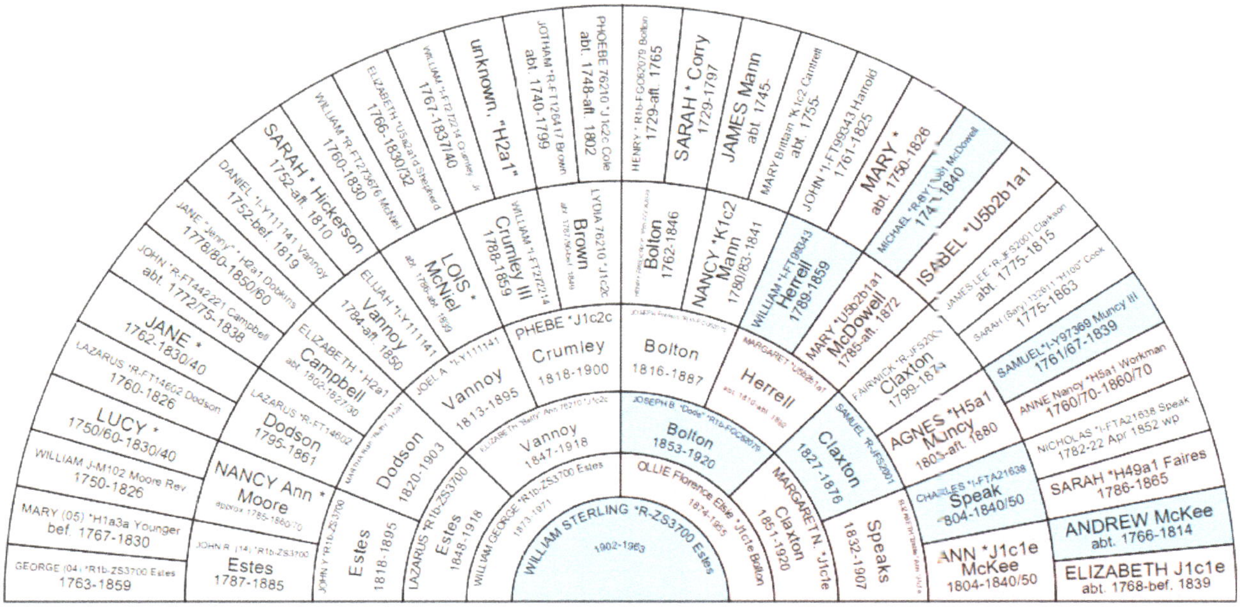

Male 5-Generation X-DNA Fan Chart

I know positively that I inherited my paternal grandmother, Ollie Bolton's entire X chromosome, because hers is the only X chromosome my father, as shown in his fan chart above, had to give me.

X matching for males eliminates 75%, or 24 of 32 possible 5th-generation ancestors, displayed above.

Tip: Sometimes, men appear to have X matches on their father's side, but this is impossible. Those matches must be identical by chance, or somehow related in an unknown way on their mother's side.

On my mother's side, I inherited an X chromosome from my mother, which is some combination of the X chromosomes from her father and mother. It's also possible that I inherited all of my maternal grandmother's or maternal grandfather's X chromosome, meaning they did not recombine during meiosis.

X chromosome matching and analysis is different due to:

- The unique inheritance pattern, meaning fewer recombination events occurred.
- The fact that X-DNA is not inherited from several lines.
- The X chromosome contains fewer SNPs, referred to as SNP density, so less possible locations to match as compared to the other chromosomes.

X-DNA potentially reaches back further in time than autosomal DNA on the other chromosomes at the same generational level, so you may have inherited the DNA of an ancestor on the X chromosome that you did not on other chromosomes. X-DNA represents a golden opportunity to match in a different way.

TIP: You may match someone on both the autosomes and the X chromosome, but each of those segments may have descended from completely different ancestral lines.

X-DNA Chromosome Ancestor Inheritance

X-DNA chromosome matching can't really be equated to matching on the other chromosomes. They are two distinct tools, so the results can't be interpreted identically. I'll explain why, and how X-DNA works before we discuss how to use the X chromosome for genealogy matching.

It's challenging to draw equivalences when comparing X-DNA matching to the other chromosomes due to several variables that make interpretation difficult.

I created the X-DNA Ancestor Inheritance Table, below, to illustrate several points.

Generation	Ancestor Average Chr 1-22	Father's Side X DNA								Mother's Side X DNA								Total
		Estes	Dodson	Vannoy	Crumley	Bolton	Herrell	Claxton	Speaks	Ferwerda	DeJong	Miller	Lentz	Lore	Hill	Kirsch	Drechsel	
		1	2	3	4	5	6	7	8	9	10	11	12	13	14	15	16	
GG-Grandparents	100						100	100	100			100	100		100	100	100	
G-Grandparents	50					Blocked	50	50	50			50	50	Blocked	50	50	50	
Grandparents	25						25	25	25	Blocked	Blocked	25	25		25	25	25	
Parents	12.5	Blocked	Blocked	Blocked	Blocked		12.5	12.5	12.5			12.5	12.5		12.5	12.5	12.5	
Female Tester %	6.25	0	0	0	0	0	6.25	6.25	6.25	0	0	6.25	6.25	0	6.25	6.25	6.25	50
Female Actual %	6.25	0	0	0	0	0	12.5	12.5	12.5	0	0	12.5	12.5	0	12.5	12.5	12.5	100
Male Actual %	6.25	0	0	0	0	0	0	0	0	0	0	20	20	0	20	20	20	100
Non-X Autosome cM	19																	
X Female cM Average	45.25	0	0	0	0	0	45.25	45.25	45.25	0	0	45.25	45.25	0	45.25	45.25	45.25	362
X Male cM Average	36.2	0	0	0	0	0	0	0	0	0	0	36.2	36.2	0	36.2	36.2	36.2	181

X-DNA Ancestor Inheritance Table

- The X-DNA Ancestor Inheritance Table is divided into two "sides," paternal and maternal.
- The first column in the upper section, above the blank dividing row, is the generation.
- The second column, "Ancestor Average Chr 1-22," shows the percent of DNA, on average, that a tester would inherit from their great-great-grandparents, 4 generations back in time, across Chromosomes 1-22. This corresponds to the fan chart, above.

For example, I receive approximately 6.25% of the DNA of any of my great-great-grandparents. Of course, that's assuming that the DNA of our ancestors divides exactly in half in each generation. It doesn't, due to random recombination. Sometimes we receive more or less of the DNA from a specific ancestor. Still, on average,[195] from a 4th-generation ancestor (counting your parents as generation one), you will receive approximately 6.25% of each of their DNA. Your parent would have received about 12.5%.

Clearly, you don't receive an equal amount of each 4th-generation ancestor's DNA on every chromosome, and you may not receive ANY of their DNA on some chromosomes. You inherited approximately 3500 cMs of DNA from each of your parents, for a total of about 7000 cMs between both parents. Dividing each ancestor's DNA in half in every descending generation means, on average, you inherited about 437 cMs of DNA from each of those 16 great-great-grandparents scattered across some combination of your chromosomes.

195 We use averages to set expectations, but all inheritance is subject to random recombination.

However, we know that isn't the case for X-DNA, because you received no X chromosome DNA from several of those ancestors.

Females only inherit X-DNA from 8 of those ancestors, and males only inherit X-DNA from 5 ancestors, as seen on the X-DNA Ancestor Inheritance Table.

The next two sections of the table to the right are further divided into ancestors from the Father's Side and the Mother's Side for a female tester. The chart is the same for a male tester, except males inherit no X-DNA from their father's side, so the "Father's Side X-DNA" can be disregarded for males.

- The surnames in Row 2 reflect the surnames on my fan chart, but regardless of the names, the positions contribute the same average amount of DNA for every female. I receive no X-DNA from the lineage names with red (or grey in black and white) shading.
- Row 3, below the surnames, correlates to the position number in my family tree fan chart.
- I've noted any generation in which the X-DNA is blocked, meaning that person does not pass the X chromosome on.
- In the column titled Estes, position #1, you can see that X-DNA is blocked for a female tester in her father's generation, meaning my father's father did not contribute an X chromosome to my father, so he can't pass it on to me.
- The first four lineage positions, Estes, Dodson, Vannoy, and Crumley, are blocked because my father did not inherit an X chromosome from his father, so he cannot pass any part of an X chromosome from those ancestors on to me.
- Reading further across the chart, we see in the Bolton column, line #5 is blocked because we have two men in consecutive descending generations, so the second person, marked blocked, did not receive and, therefore, cannot pass his father's X chromosome on to descendants. Male to male is always an X block.
- However, the next three lineages, Herrell, Claxton, and Speaks, positions #6-8, descend through my father's mother just like any other autosome.
- You can see the same percentage, 6.25%, in each generation as the autosomal Ancestor Average percent in the second column. That's accurate for autosomal DNA in those generations on Chromosomes 1-22, but not for X-DNA, so we'll need to adjust these appropriately.
- Of course, if the tester is a male, he inherits no X-DNA on his father's side of this chart, so the appropriate adjustment for a male would be zero for his father's X-DNA.
- Moving to the mother's side, male and female testers both receive X-DNA from the same lines. Three lineages, #9, 10, and 13, are blocked by male-to-male (father-to-son) inheritance, so there is no X to pass on to the next generation from that ancestral line.

The final column, "Total," shows the total percentage of DNA descended from the lines in which X-DNA is contributed. You can see that for me, in the "Female Tester %" row, the total percent is 50, but I clearly have 100% of an X chromosome from my father and mother. The inheritance from those ancestors would be 50% if the X were a normally inherited chromosome, but it isn't. The X chromosome has that special inheritance pattern, so I receive a higher percentage of X-DNA from each contributing ancestor.

I inherit a higher percentage of X-DNA from those ancestors because I inherit no DNA from other ancestors. The total for autosomal and X-DNA must be 100%, regardless of which ancestor is contributing.

The next section, below the blank row, shows the actual female and male average percentages that are contributed by each of these lineages.

Calculating X Chromosome Percentages and Centimorgans

How do we calculate the number of expected cMs for the X chromosome?

- On the other autosomes, at 4 generations, Chromosomes 1-22, each of 16 ancestors contribute an average of 6.25%.
- Looking at the "Female Actual %" row, we see that on the X chromosome, a female tester's ancestors contribute twice that amount, 12.5%, because the X chromosome can only be inherited from a maximum of 8 ancestors, not 16.
- Viewing the "Male Actual %" row, we see that on the X chromosome, a male tester's ancestors contribute an average of 20% each, because his X chromosome is only inherited from 5 ancestors, not 16.

Regardless of which ancestor contributes exactly which percent, the total has to be 100% of the size of the X chromosome, and the DNA cannot come from any of the lineages that are blocked.

To understand how the expected number of cMs is calculated in the non-X autosome row, we need to understand the size of our chromosomes.

Each chromosome is a different length, so the total number of both cMs and SNPs on each chromosome is different. Please note that the X chromosome is about the same size in terms of total cMs as Chromosome 10, but the SNP density is a lot smaller, about half the size, so there are fewer SNPs to match along the length of the chromosome.

You might hear that an X match needs to be "larger" than a match on the other chromosomes to be considered genealogically equivalent. This stems from the SNP density of the X chromosome. Normally, 7 cMs of DNA is the generally accepted threshold where approximately 50% of your matches will be valid, identical by descent, and the rest will be invalid, meaning identical by chance. Because the SNP density of the X chromosome is less than the SNP density of the other chromosomes, the rule of thumb is that you need twice as many X-matching SNPs to be equivalent to compensate for the lower density. While SNP density is certainly a consideration, a 15 cM requirement for X-DNA matching is certainly not carved in stone.

There's yin and yang to everything!

Keep the X-matching cM threshold in mind, but also keep in mind that the X-DNA match you're seeing is potentially coming from further back in time and may be extraordinarily enlightening.

Chromosome	Total cM	SNPs	SNP Density Per cM
1	284	56980	200.95
2	274	55581	202.81
3	228	45598	200.27
4	220	39095	177.78
5	209	40546	194.04
6	198	46299	233.53
7	190	36731	192.93
8	173	35641	206.58
9	170	31573	186.15
10	182	37634	206.94
11	161	35174	218.75
12	173	34093	197.56
13	130	26902	207.34
14	117	22460	192.35
15	127	20832	163.59
16	130	21776	167.10
17	127	19442	152.70
18	120	20966	174.52
19	106	14439	136.13
20	110	17695	160.56
21	64	9863	154.66
22	71	10059	141.11
X	181	17406	96.17

This chart shows my exact match to my mother from the Family Finder Chromosome Browser Results file on every chromosome. Everyone's cM match amount on a specific chromosome to a parent may vary slightly due to no-reads and scan differences.

The portion of the X chromosome covered for genetic genealogy is approximately[196] 181 cMs in length, times two for both parents (362) for a female.

Given that females inherit from a maximum of 8 X-chromosome ancestors at 4 generations, I would inherit an average of 45.25 cMs from each of those ancestors, subject to random recombination, which means I could (and probably would) receive more X-DNA from some ancestors and less from others.

A male only has one X chromosome, 181 cMs in length, so he will receive an average of 36.2 cMs from each of 5 contributing ancestors, all from his mother's side.

This is easier to visualize in a chart that compares autosomal DNA cMs from Chromosomes 1-22 to X-DNA inheritance at 4 generations.

196 Different vendors and test versions cover slightly different amount of DNA on each chromosome, hence, the word "approximate." A few cMs difference in coverage makes no difference.

	Autosomes	X Female	X Male
Total cM	7000	362	181
Contributing Ancestors	16	8	5
Ancestor Contribution Calculation	7000/16	362/8	181/5
Total cM Divided by contributing ancestors	437.5	45.25	36.2
Individual ancestor total contribution	437.5	45.25	36.2
Autosomes divided by 22 for everage per chromosome	19.88	45.25	36.2
Ancestor Average per Chromosome	19.88	45.25	36.2

- Total cMs - Total number of cMs for all of the autosomes, meaning Chromosomes 1-22, and separately, the X chromosome for males and females.
- Contributing Ancestors - The number of contributing ancestors for autosomes, chromosomes 1-22 is 16 for both males and females.
- The number of contributing ancestors for the X chromosome is 8 for females and 5 for males.
- Ancestor Contribution - Dividing the total cMs of autosomal DNA by 16 ancestors gives us about 437 cMs of DNA that we expect to inherit, on average, and subject to random recombination, from each of those 16 ancestors, excluding the X chromosome.
- For the X chromosome, the total amount of X-DNA inherited by a female is divided by the 8 ancestors she received it from.
- A female has twice the amount of X-DNA as a male, because she has an X chromosome from both parents, while a male has only one copy of the X chromosome.
- For the X chromosome, the total amount of X-DNA inherited by a male, only from his mother, is divided by the 5 ancestors he received it from.
- Each individual ancestor's expected average total contribution of each type of DNA is shown.
- However, X-DNA is only one chromosome, Chromosome 23, and autosomal DNA is scattered across any (or all) of 22 chromosomes.
- To compare apples and apples, one would need to divide the amount of autosomal DNA by the 22 chromosomes to determine the approximate amount of autosomal DNA, per chromosome, that would be equivalent to the amount of X DNA on that chromosome at the same generational level.
- The average total cMs for all of Chromosomes 1-22 together is 437 cMs. However, dividing by 22, the average cMs expected on each individual chromosome if the DNA were equally distributed across all 22 autosomes would be approximately 19.88 cMs.
- The total number of cMs on the X for both parents for females totals 362 and 181 for males.
- The calculated average for the X chromosome is significantly higher than the average for autosomal by chromosome, shown in the bottom row.

However, this isn't how we see matching cMs expressed. Since we don't know which of the 1-22 chromosomes will hold our ancestral DNA, we can only use the total expected or average cMs for all autosomal DNA.

	16 Ancestors - 4 Generations
Total Autosomal cM Average Minus X	437
Individual Chromosome cM Average	19.88
Female X Chromosome Average	45.25
Male X Chromosome Average	36.2

- We see a total of inherited autosomal cMs which spans all 22 autosomes and excludes the X chromosome at FamilyTreeDNA.[197]
- We see a separate X chromosome inheritance amount for only that chromosome.
- The X inheritance amount appears small when contrasted to the total cM match, which includes the DNA across 22 chromosomes.
- We don't realize that at 4 generations, X-DNA inheritance of 45 or 36 cMs is actually functionally better than the 437 cMs autosomal inheritance. Having said that, the fact that there's significantly more autosomal DNA means there's a greater chance that we'll inherit at least some of it.

For clarity, you can see that my shared DNA with my mother, which is my total match amount for chromosomes 1-22, all chromosomes except for the X chromosome, is 3563 cMs. The longest block is 284 cMs, the entire length of Chromosome 1, the longest chromosome, and the X chromosome match is 181 cMs, which is not included in the total of 3563 cMs.

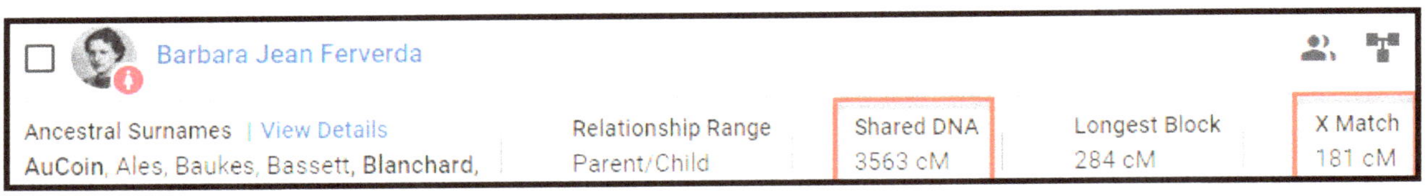
Barbara Jean Ferverda
Ancestral Surnames | View Details
AuCoin, Ales, Baukes, Bassett, Blanchard,
Relationship Range
Parent/Child
Shared DNA
3563 cM
Longest Block
284 cM
X Match
181 cM

It's important to remember when looking at X matching that you're only looking at the amount of DNA on one chromosome. When you're looking at any other matching amount, you're looking at a total match across all 22 chromosomes, which comparatively causes the X-DNA amount to seem small.[198] You're not comparing apples to apples which is why X-DNA needs to be evaluated independently.

197 23andMe includes the amount of matching X-DNA in their total matching cMs.

198 The X is included in the total cM count at 23andMe, but not at FamilyTreeDNA. The X chromosome is not used for matching or included in the match amount at either MyHeritage or Ancestry, but is included in the raw DNA data download files for all four vendors.

TIP: We might inherit a specific amount of DNA from each ancestor, but for DNA matching, the other person must inherit that same segment of DNA over the matching threshold. Normally, people (other than our direct ancestors such as parents) only match on a portion of the DNA inherited from a particular ancestor. Let's say that you and a match both inherited 100 cMs of DNA from a particular ancestor. You may match on the entire 100 cMs, or only on a portion like 10 cMs, for example. It's also possible to not match any DNA at all at the third cousin level, and more distantly. In other words, just because you and another person inherited DNA from the same ancestor doesn't mean you match on that DNA.

Different vendors treat the X chromosome differently, making comparison challenging.

- 23andMe includes not only the X chromosome in their cM total, but doubles the Fully Identical Regions (FIR) when people, such as siblings[199], share the same DNA from both parents.
- Ancestry does not include the X in their cM calculations.
- MyHeritage does not include the X in their cM calculations.
- FamilyTreeDNA shows an X match only when it's accompanied by a match on another chromosome too and does not include the X-matching cMs in the total shared DNA.

X-DNA Summary

Understanding how the X chromosome works helps us understand how to evaluate matches.

Critical takeaway messages for X-DNA analysis:

1. Because there are fewer ancestral lineages contributing to the tester's X chromosome, the percentage of X chromosomal DNA that a tester inherits from the ancestors who contribute to their X chromosome is increased substantially.
2. The increased X-DNA percentage equates to an increased average cM percent contributed from each ancestral lineage, which means it may persist longer without being recombined, reaching further back in time.
3. The X-DNA of the contributing ancestors is more likely to be inherited, because there are fewer other possible contributing ancestors, meaning fewer recombination events or DNA divisions.
4. X matches cannot be compared equally to either percentages or cM amounts on any or all of the other chromosomes because X matching reports only the amount of matching DNA on one single chromosome, while your total cM match amount reports the amount of DNA that matches across all 22 chromosomes.

199 https://dna-explained.com/2022/08/29/dna-in-search-offull-and-half-siblings/

The X chromosome is different and holds clues that the other autosomes can't provide. Don't dismiss X matches even if you can't identify a common ancestor. Given the inheritance path, and the reduced number of divisions, your X-DNA may descend from an ancestor further back in time. I certainly would not disregard X matches, even as low as 7 cMs, without appropriate scrutiny.

X chromosome matching can't really be equated to matching on the other chromosomes. They are two distinct tools, so they can't be interpreted identically.

The X chromosome inheritance pattern means that you're much more likely to carry some amount of a contributing ancestor's X-DNA than on any other chromosome.

- An X-DNA segment may well be "older" because it's not nearly as likely to be divided, given that there are fewer opportunities for recombination.
- When you're tracking your X-DNA back in your tree, whenever you hit a male, you get an automatic "bump" back a generation to his mother. It's like the free bingo X-DNA square!
- With an X-DNA match, you can immediately eliminate many ancestors as your most recent common ancestor (MRCA) for that segment.
- Because X-DNA reaches further back in time, sometimes you match people who descend from common ancestors further back in time as well.

TIP: If you match someone on multiple segments, and one of those matching segments is X-DNA, that segment may have descended from a different ancestor than the segments on Chromosomes 1-22. Always evaluate X-matches carefully.

Sometimes X-DNA is exactly what you need to solve a mystery.

Using X-DNA

Let's say that I have a 30 cM X match with a male.

I know immediately that our most recent common ancestor is on his mother's side.

I know, based on my fan chart, which ancestral lines are eliminated in my tree. I've immediately narrowed the ancestors from 16 to 5 on his side and 16 to 8 on my side.

Two matching males is even easier because you know immediately that the common ancestor must be on both of their mother's sides, with only 5 candidate lines each at the great-great-grandparent generation.

Female-to-female matches are slightly more complex, but there are still 8 immediately eliminated lines each.

In this match with a female second cousin, I was able to identify who she was via our common ancestor based on the X chromosome path. Below, I'm showing the relevant halves of her chart (paternal), and mine (maternal), side by side.

I added blockers on her chart and mine too.

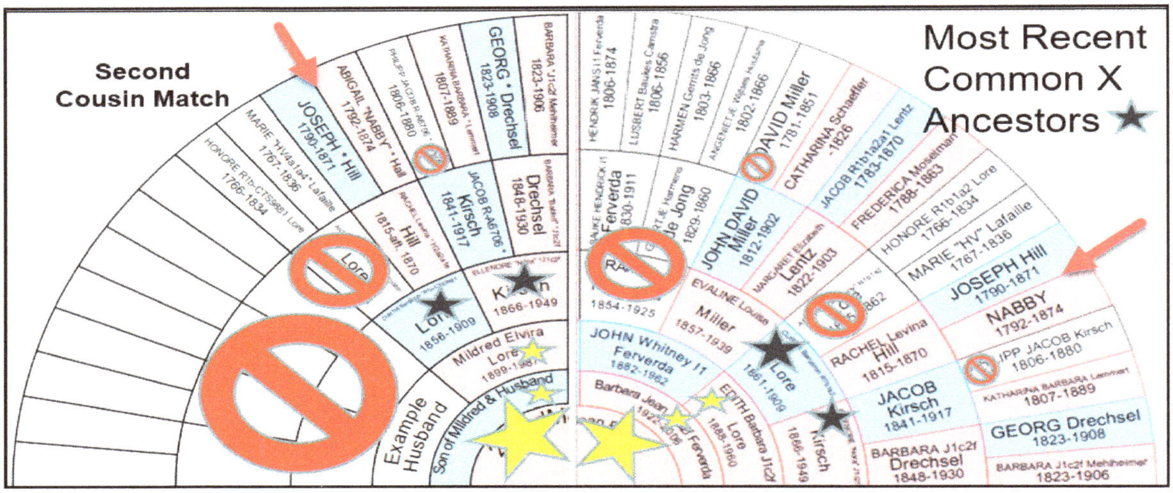

As it turns out, we both inherited most of our X chromosomes from our great-grandparents, marked above with the black stars.

Several lines are blocked, and my grandfather's X chromosome is not a possibility because the common ancestor is my maternal grandmother's parents. My grandfather is not one of my cousin's ancestors.

Having identified this match as my closest relative (other than my mother) to descend on my mother's maternal side, I was able to map that portion of my X chromosome to my great-grandparents Nora Kirsch[200] and Curtis Benjamin Lore[201], then through his mother to her parents Joseph Hill[202] and Nabby Hall[203] through additional matches.

---

200 https://dna-explained.com/2015/10/05/nora-kirsch-1866-1949-quilter-extraordinaire-52-ancestors-92/

201 https://dna-explained.com/2021/04/25/curtis-lore-white-plague-times-two-52-ancestors-329/

202 https://dna-explained.com/2016/03/21/joseph-hill-1790-1871-the-second-joseph-shinglemaker-52-ancestors-116/

203 https://dna-explained.com/2016/03/27/abigail-nabby-hall-1792-1874-pioneer-settler-in-little-fort-52-ancestors-117/

My X Chromosome at DNA Painter

I paint my DNA segments for all my chromosomes at DNAPainter,[204] which provides me with a central tracking mechanism that is visual in nature and allows me to combine matches from multiple vendors who provide segment information.

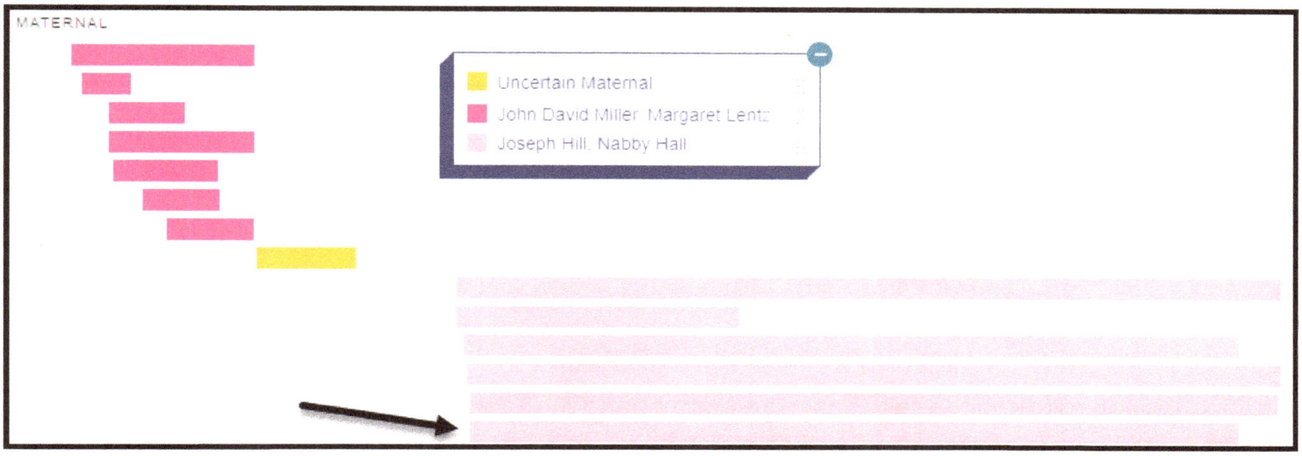

Here's my maternal X chromosome and how I utilized chromosome painting to push the identification of the ancestors whose X chromosome I inherited back an additional two generations.

Using that initial X chromosome match with my second cousin, shown by the arrow at the bottom, I mapped a large segment of my maternal X chromosome to my maternal great-grandparents.

By viewing the trees of subsequent X maternal matches, I was then able to push those common segments, shown painted directly above that match with the same color, back another two generations, to Joseph Hill (1790-1871) and Nabby Hall (1792-1874.) I was able to do that based on the fact that other matches descend from Joseph and Nabby through different children, meaning we all triangulate on that segment.[205]

I received no known X-DNA from my great-grandmother, Nora Kirsch, although a small portion of my X chromosome is still unassigned and "Uncertain."

I received a small portion of my maternal X chromosome, in magenta, at left, from my maternal great-great-grandparents, John David Miller (1812-1902)[206] and Margaret Lentz (1822-1903)[207].

The X chromosome is a powerful tool and can reach far back in time.

TIP: In some cases, the X, and other chromosomes, can be inherited intact from one grandparent. I could have inherited my mother's entire copy of her mother's, or her father's X chromosome based on random recombination, or not. As it turns out, I didn't, and I know that because I've mapped my chromosomes to identify my ancestors.

---

204 https://dna-explained.com/2019/10/14/dnapainter-instructions-and-resources/

205 https://dna-explained.com/2020/04/01/triangulation-in-action-at-dnapainter/

206 https://dna-explained.com/2016/07/04/john-david-miller-1812-1902-never-in-his-wildest-dreams-52-ancestors-125/

207 https://dna-explained.com/2016/06/27/margaret-lentz-1822-1903-the-seasons-and-the-sundays-52-ancestors-124/

X Advanced Matches

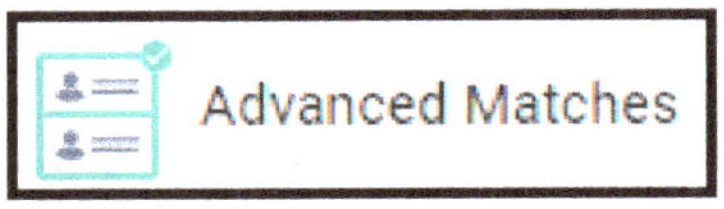

Advanced Matches also include the ability to search for X matches, either within the entire database or within specific projects. I find the project selection to be particularly useful.

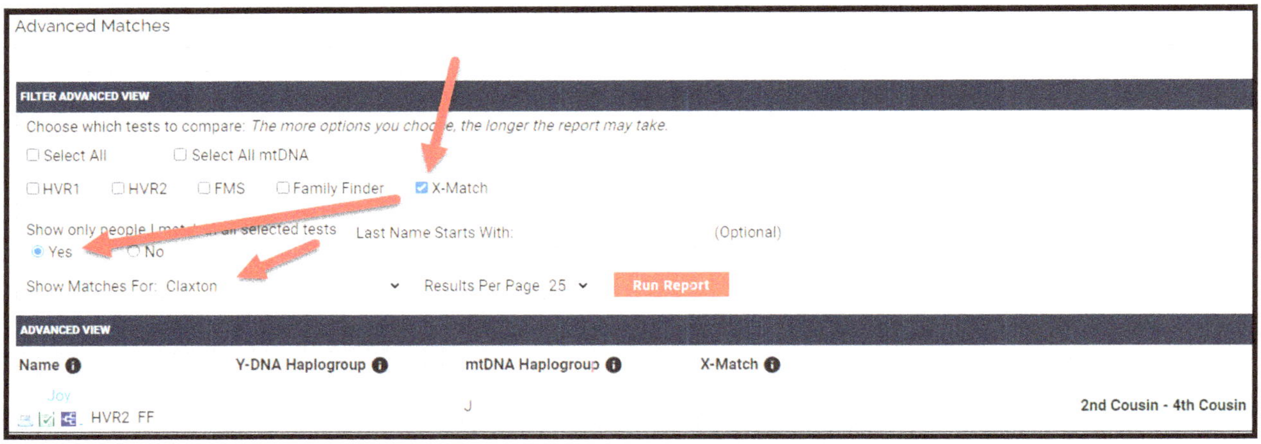

For example, within the Claxton project, my father's maternal grandmother's line, I recognize my match, Joy, which provides me an important clue as to the possible common ancestor(s) of our shared segments.

Joy's tree shows that her 4-times great-grandparents are my 3-times great-grandparents, meaning we are 4th cousins once removed and share 17 cM of DNA on our X chromosome across two segments.

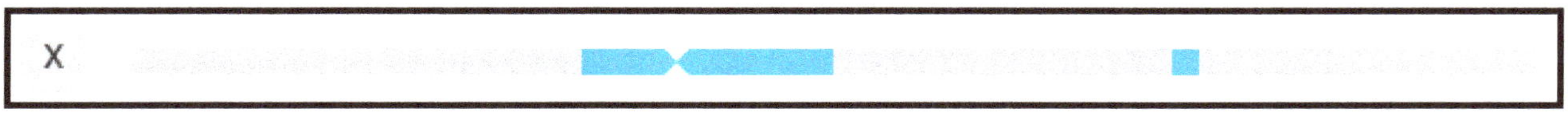

Don't be deceived by the appearance of "size" on your chromosomes. The first segment that spans the centromere, or "waist" of the chromosome, above, is 10.29 cM, and the smaller segment at the right is 7.02 cM. Remember, SNPs are not necessarily evenly distributed along chromosomes, which means that the SNPs in the smaller region may be more densely packed. Don't judge the relevance or comparative size of segments based on how the chromosomes look.

TIP: An X match doesn't necessarily mean the entire match is contained in one segment.

It's worth noting that Joy and I actually share at least two different, unrelated ancestral lines. It's important to evaluate all possible ancestors, plus the inheritance path, to eliminate any lineage that involves a father-to-son inheritance on the X chromosome.

You may match on your X chromosome through a different ancestor than on other chromosomes. Every matching segment has its own individual history.

Chapter 7

ETHNICITY - MyORIGINS

Many people begin their DNA journey by taking a DNA test to discover "who they are" and "where they came from." Ethnicity testing provides them with an estimate of their genetic ancestry.[208] While those types of tests tend to frustrate seasoned genealogists, they attract many people who might never otherwise dip their toe into the genealogy water.

Ethnicity is a lot more than percentages, especially when you're provided with segment information. We're going to learn how to get the most out of population results.[209]

Ethnicity, known as myOrigins at FamilyTreeDNA, provides testers with ancestral population estimates based on the DNA they inherited from their ancestors.

FamilyTreeDNA published a very educational white paper[210] in 2021 that explains generally how population origins are determined, and how your myOrigins 3 results are calculated.

The science of population genetics determines how people from specific regions of the earth, or ethnic populations, are more alike than people from other populations. For example, an aboriginal group of people who live in Australia have, for tens of thousands of years, developed many genetic similarities to each other that are not equally as similar to any other population in the world.

For a population to be detectable as a "population," they have to be different enough from neighboring populations to be identifiable as a unique group. That's not too difficult with barriers like oceans to prevent the mixing of populations.

However, the genetic similarities among France, Germany, Belgium, Netherlands, and Switzerland, for example, that adjoin one another and were settled by many of the same original groups of people, is much more pronounced. Those similarities also mean it's much more difficult to assign someone confidently to one of those population groups, or today's countries.

Add to that the fact that borders are political boundaries that have and do change.

---

208 https://dna-explained.com/2019/07/10/dna-results-first-glances-at-ethnicity-and-matching/

209 https://dna-explained.com/2018/10/30/ethnicity-far-more-than-percentages/

210 https://blog.familytreedna.com/wp-content/uploads/2021/08/myOrigins_3_WhitePaper.pdf

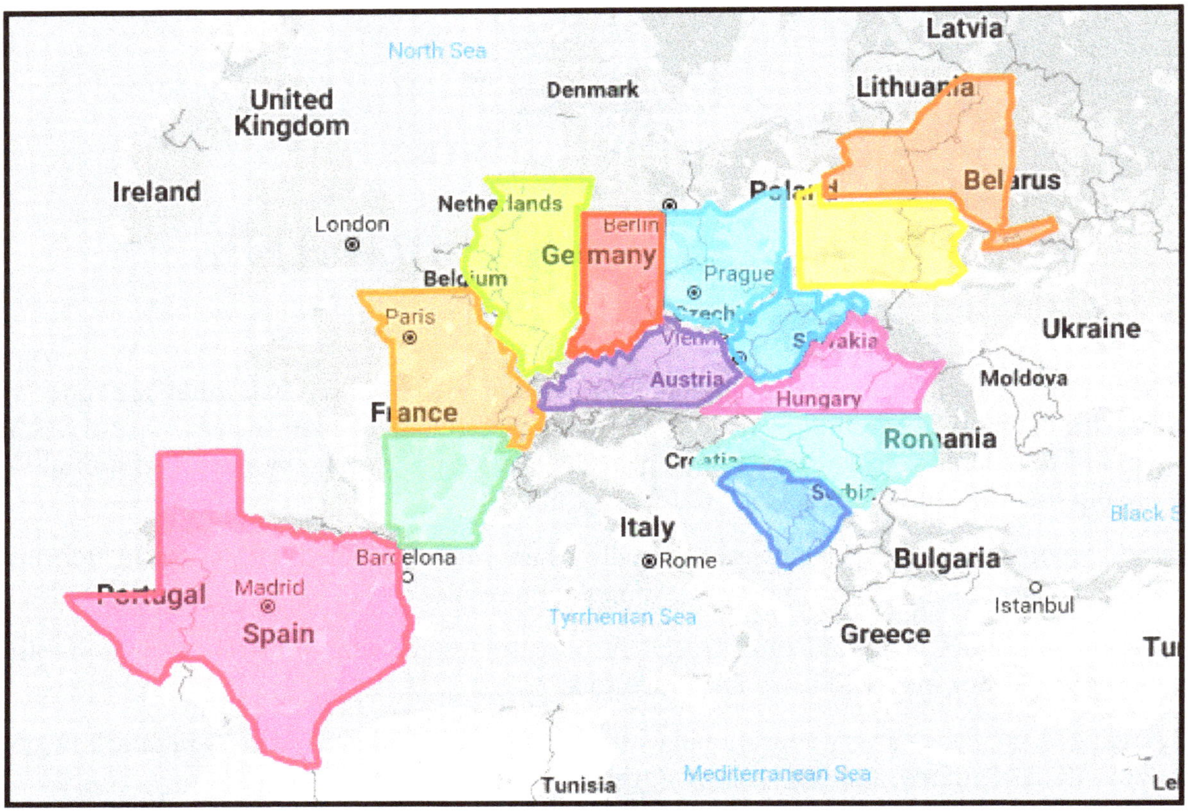

To provide some perspective, here's a map of several US states overlaid over Europe. No one would ask or expect any DNA testing company to be able to genetically discern someone from Indiana from an individual from Illinois, New York, or even Texas, but we hope for exactly that for European countries.

In heavily populated areas that have had a lot of introgression and colonization in relatively recent times, meaning hundreds to a few thousand years, where various populations have intermixed, it's very difficult to discern ethnicity accurately.[211] Ethnicity is an estimate that:

- Is based on the science of population genetics
- Includes publicly available research data
- Is augmented with user-provided ancestral origin data

FamilyTreeDNA and other companies periodically update their estimates based on changes in the above factors.

211 https://dna-explained.com/2018/12/28/ethnicity-is-just-an-estimate-yes-really/

How Are myOrigins Matches Calculated?

Unlike Y-DNA and mitochondrial DNA, which are contributed by only one parent, respectively, autosomal DNA is made up of one copy of each chromosome contributed by each parent. You have two nucleotides at all locations, one contributed by each parent.

This means that you have two allele values - some combination of T, A, C or G at every location on each chromosome – one contributed by your mother and one by your father. Those are labeled "unphased Genotypes" in the image below.

DNA sequencing has no way to determine which nucleotides at any address were received from which parent. There's no convenient zipper[212] to separate the two. The DNA from your parents is mixed in your chromosomes, so it's not like the lab can read one side that physically came from your mom and the other that physically came from your dad. Of course, this means that sorting out which values came from each parent is much like assembling a 700,000-piece jigsaw puzzle without a picture on the box lid.[213]

The good news is that scientists have developed a methodology to "phase" your DNA, meaning to reassemble it in the sequences most likely to have originated from one parent, by chromosome. The phasing of each chromosome is independent.

Some nucleotides are more or less likely to be found paired with or adjacent to other nucleotides, so it's a matter of fitting those pieces together in the most logical manner.

212 https://dna-explained.com/2013/12/15/one-chromosome-two-sides-no-zipper-icw-and-the-matrix/

213 https://dna-explained.com/2019/10/18/hit-a-genetic-genealogy-home-run-using-your-double-sided-two-faced-chromosomes-while-avoiding-imposters/

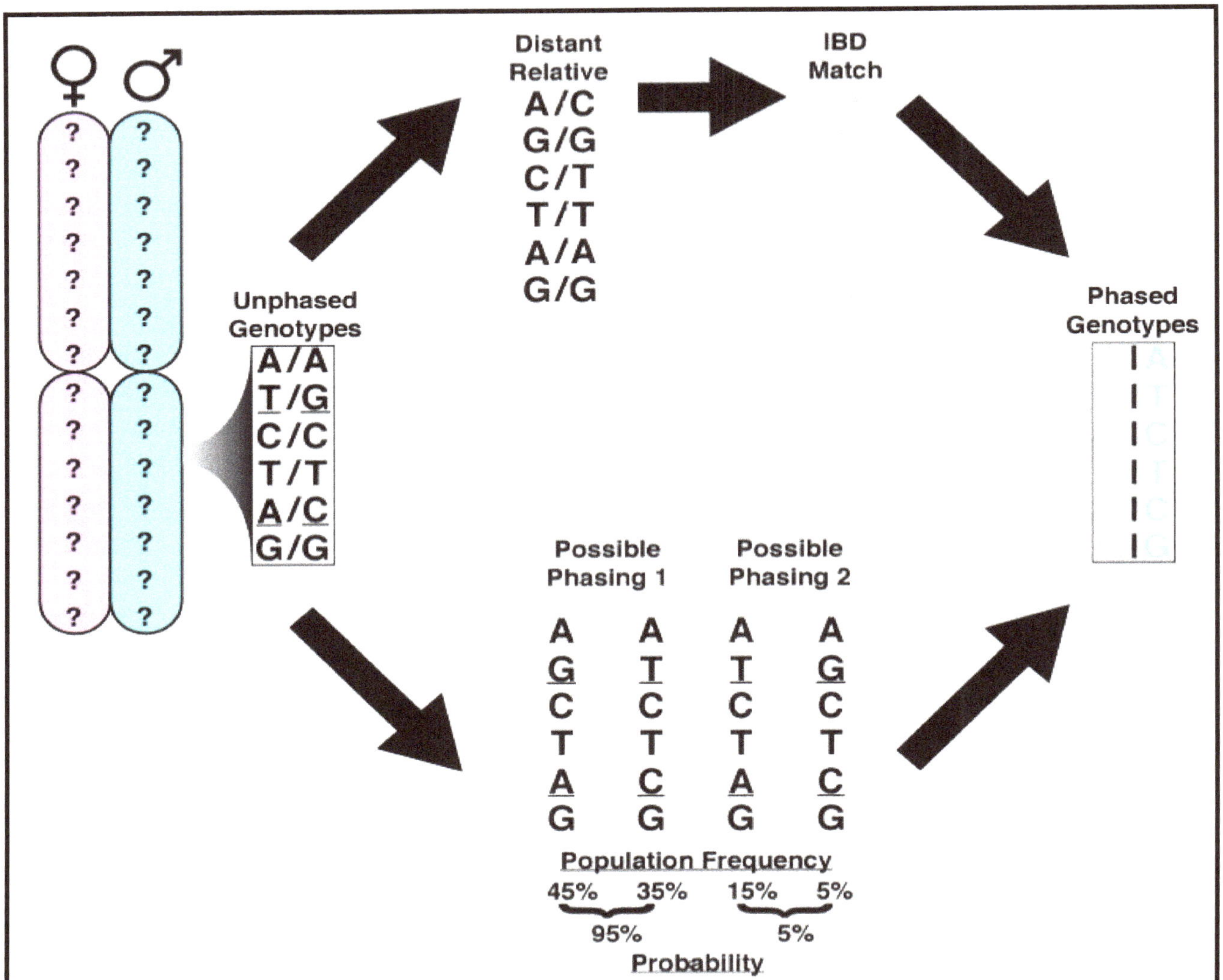

Figure 10. Eagle combines two different methods of phasing: exact IBD matches (top) and haplotype frequencies in a reference panel to generate phasing probabilities (bottom).

This image, extracted from page 22 of the *MyOrigins3 WhitePaper,*[214] shows the steps that occur behind the scenes in order to provide you with the most accurate population origins, attributable to either parent and not mixed between the two. Of course, that's not always entirely possible. It's easiest when the parents are from significantly different continental populations from highly separate world regions.

After your DNA is separated into two chromosomal sides, those sides are matched to reference populations from around the world.

Every single cM is compared individually. One cM could reach back to about 20th cousins, but alone, that's not enough information to be relevant. Therefore, FamilyTreeDNA evaluates 4 cM matching segment windows for population matches. All of your DNA will match some population, more or less closely. The higher the number of matching cMs, the greater the probability of accuracy.

214 https://blog.familytreedna.com/wp-content/uploads/2021/08/myOrigins_3_WhitePaper.pdf

Caveats

Taking that into consideration, I'd like to provide a few caveats to set the stage and expectations appropriately.

- Ethnicity is only an estimate![215]
- Just because you don't show a specific ethnicity doesn't mean you don't have that heritage, unless you're referring to a majority ethnicity. If you think you're half Jewish, and you receive no Jewish percentage, there's a disconnect someplace.
- You don't inherit exactly half of the DNA of your ancestors. In fact, you may or may not inherit any measurable DNA from any specific ancestor(s) from several generations back in time.
- Small amounts of ethnicity can be noise.
- While you cannot legitimately have an ethnicity that neither of your parents have, you may have a population with a different name that is in the same world region or from a population with a common root. Chromosome painting will help unravel this puzzle.
- Your ethnicity profile reported at every vendor will "change" over time as they refine their algorithms and update reference populations. Those changes are sometimes accompanied by great wailing and also cheering within the genetic genealogy community. The people who believe the update to be more accurate will be happy, and those who thought the previous version was more accurate will be equally as unhappy. Some people just take a look, think "Cool," and move on.
- Your population percentage will vary based on the amount of DNA you inherited from the ancestors from that region.
- Your populations will also vary based on the reference population.
- Did I mention that ethnicity is only an estimate?

As a long-time genetic genealogist, my ethnicity estimates have changed so many times that I no longer keep track, with the exception of my minority ethnicity.

By minority ethnicity, I mean minority to me.[216] Let me explain.

The majority of my ancestry is European, which I've extensively documented with both paper trail and genetic genealogy, combined with minority amounts of both Native American and African heritage.

I've tracked my ethnicity amounts from all vendors for years on a spreadsheet, and my German/French/British Isles/Scandinavian/Dutch/Irish/Italian, and Greek have literally come and gone for all of those years. By the way, I don't actually have any Italian or Greek, but one vendor thought I did in their 2019 release. Back in 2012, another vendor "claimed" I had 12% Scandinavian and no German.[217] I'm 25% German. I've changed my kilt and lederhosen so many times I've worn them both out.[218]

215 https://dna-explained.com/2018/12/28/ethnicity-is-just-an-estimate-yes-really/

216 https://dna-explained.com/2020/09/22/familytreednas-myorigins-version-3-rollout/

217 https://dna-explained.com/2012/10/24/ancestrys-mythical-admixture-percentages/

218 https://dna-explained.com/2020/09/20/ancestry-releases-updated-ethnicity-estimates-hope-you-still-have-your-kilt/

By the way, my minority ethnicity has come and gone, too, at some vendors, but the two most reliable vendors for population genetics[219] provide segment mapping, and their minority segments agree and have remained consistent. This provides me with segment-specific tools.

Before we review how to leverage minority ancestry, let's first figure out how much of any specific ethnicity, based on your genealogy, you might expect to see.

Calculating Your Expected Ethnicity

I created a spreadsheet where I detailed the heritage of my 64 4-times great-grandparents, but that spreadsheet is too long to replicate here.[220] However, I've prepared an example of my 16 great-great-grandparents' genealogical ethnicity chart.

Position	Name	Birth Location	Father Y, mtDNA Haplogroup	6.25% Ancestral Heritage	England	Inferred British Isles	Scotland	Ireland	Native	Dutch	African
1	Estes	Virginia	R-ZS3700, need mtDNA	Primarily British Isles, mother 1/4th Scottish, ? African	1.56	4.68					?
2	Dodson	Alabama	R-FT14602, H2a1	Half English, half Scottish	3.125		3.125				
3	Vannoy	North Carolina	I-Y111141, U5a2a1d	Father's line Dutch, mother presumed Dutch						6.25	
4	Crumley	Virginia	I-FT272214, J1c2c	One quarter Irish, the rest inferred British Isles		4.68		1.56			
5	Bolton	England	R-BY70295, K1c2	Both parents English	6.25						
6	Herrell	Prob Virginia	I-FT99343, U5b2b1a1	Irish based on Y and mtDNA				6.25			
7	Clarkson	Virginia	R-JFS2001, H5a1	Inferred British Isles, Native line in here someplace	3.125	3.125			?		
8	Speak	Maryland	I-BY215064, J1c1e	Father's line is English	3.125	3.125					
					17.185	15.61	3.125	7.81	?	6.25	?
					England	French	Germany	Ireland	Native	Dutch	
9	Lore	Canada	R-CTS9881, X2a2	Three quarters French, one fourth Native		4.68			1.56		
10	Hill	New Hampshire	R-M269, H2a2a1e	English	6.25						
11	Kirsch	Germany	R-A6706, J1c2f	German			6.25				
12	Dreschel	Germany	Need Y, J1c2f	German			6.25				
13	Ferverda	Netherlands	I-BY61100, need mtDNA	Dutch						6.25	
14	de Jong	Netherlands	Need both	Dutch						6.25	
15	Miller	Maryland	R-FT182458, need mtDNA	Brethren, German & Swiss			6.25				
16	Lentz	Germany	R-BY62279, T2b	German			6.25				
					6.25	4.68	25	0	1.56	12.5	

The first column is the position of the ancestral line from my fan chart, and the second is the birth surname of the ancestor in that position so I can keep track of who's who.

The birth location may provide all you need in terms of their heritage. That's true for several of my mother's ancestors who were born overseas, but that's not the case for my father's ancestors, although I do know where many originated overseas, just in substantially earlier generations.

219 FamilyTreeDNA and 23andMe

220 https://dna-explained.com/2017/01/11/concepts-calculating-ethnicity-percentages/

The fourth column is particularly important. This column records the relevant Y-DNA and mitochondrial DNA haplogroups. If the ancestor in that lineage position is a male, then it's his paternal haplogroup and his mother's mitochondrial haplogroup.

If the ancestor in that position is a female, then the Y-DNA haplogroup is her father's, and the mitochondrial DNA is hers. Haplogroups, often in combination with the Y-DNA and mitochondrial DNA Matches Maps, provide significant insight into the origins of a specific family line, especially when a genealogist is brick-walled in the US. Haplogroups can be or are often hints, confirmation, or sometimes a "get out of jail free" card.

The total amount of autosomal DNA represented by each one of 16 ancestors is 6.25%, so the 5th column is how that 6.25% is divided for that ancestor. In my case, I can actually subdivide this further, which is why I maintain a 64-ancestor spreadsheet, but for this example, this breakdown is adequate.

The next several columns, above, are the percentages attributed to each geography for the origins of that family line. Note that the column headings are not identical for the paternal upper and maternal lower sections. In some cases, I've inferred relationships based on surnames, marriage customs, or religion, such as Quakers or Brethren/Mennonites and their spouses. It's possible that some of these inferred locations are inaccurate.

In this example, I could expect to receive roughly the following population percentages, in highest to lowest order.

German	English	Dutch	Inferred British Isles	Ireland	French	Scottish	Native	African
25	23.375	18.75	15.61	7.81	4.68	3.125	1.56+	Trace

Of course, this assumes that my genealogy is accurate and that the ancestors who were first found in what is now Germany, for example, hadn't recently arrived from Sweden, or France, or Switzerland, or someplace else.[221] Ditto for English and Irish and anyplace else, especially diaspora regions. There's also the potential for unknown or misattributed parentage, or adoption. Plus, remember, you don't inherit exactly half of any ancestor's DNA in subsequent generations.

However, for someone who has invested substantial work in their traditional genealogy, creating this spreadsheet provides a litmus test of whether or not the population results are in the expected ballpark. Ethnicity results do not and cannot replace traditional genealogy, only augment that research.

By and large, for any significant amount of population ethnicity that you receive from a vendor, you should have some corresponding genealogy research that correlates with the results.

TIP: Sometimes, especially for people with no prior knowledge of their background, ethnicity, or population, results can shed light on majority or admixed heritage from different world regions.

221 Of course we use today's locations and country names, but in the not-too-distant past, Germany, a country formed in 1871 by a political process, was a confederation of Germanic tribes, and they weren't confined to what is today the country of Germany. Of course the same is true throughout the world. Boundaries and countries change over time.

We can't always take things at face value. Although I have 25% German genealogy, I do NOT have one fully German grandparent. I also don't have one fully English grandparent. In fact, I don't have any known English ancestors born in England after 1762, but I have MANY English ancestors in both my maternal and paternal lines. These amounts are cumulative. However, 25% could also be one individual if I did have one German and one English grandparent, and the other two were from elsewhere. Of course, we also have to keep in mind the history of those regions. For example, England is a combination of Germanic and Scandinavian tribes, plus Romans who arrived later bringing enslaved workers. It's no wonder ethnicity can be confounding.

The most accurate genetic ethnicity divisions are at the continental level, and the most challenging regions are populations within those continents.

Results!!!

You've waited long enough. You've swabbed and dropped your test kit in the mail. Now, the big day has arrived, and you're anxious to view your results.

Clicking on the MyOrigins icon displays both your map and your population percentages from a menu of more than 90 populations divided into three categories.[222]

- Continental Regions are the main regions of the world in which one or more Super-Populations are located.
- Super-Populations are regions where one or more Population Clusters are found. Some Super-Populations are the same as Continental Regions.
- Population Clusters are reference populations against which FamilyTreeDNA customers are compared.

222 https://help.familytreedna.com/hc/en-us/articles/4401981569423

Let's take a look!

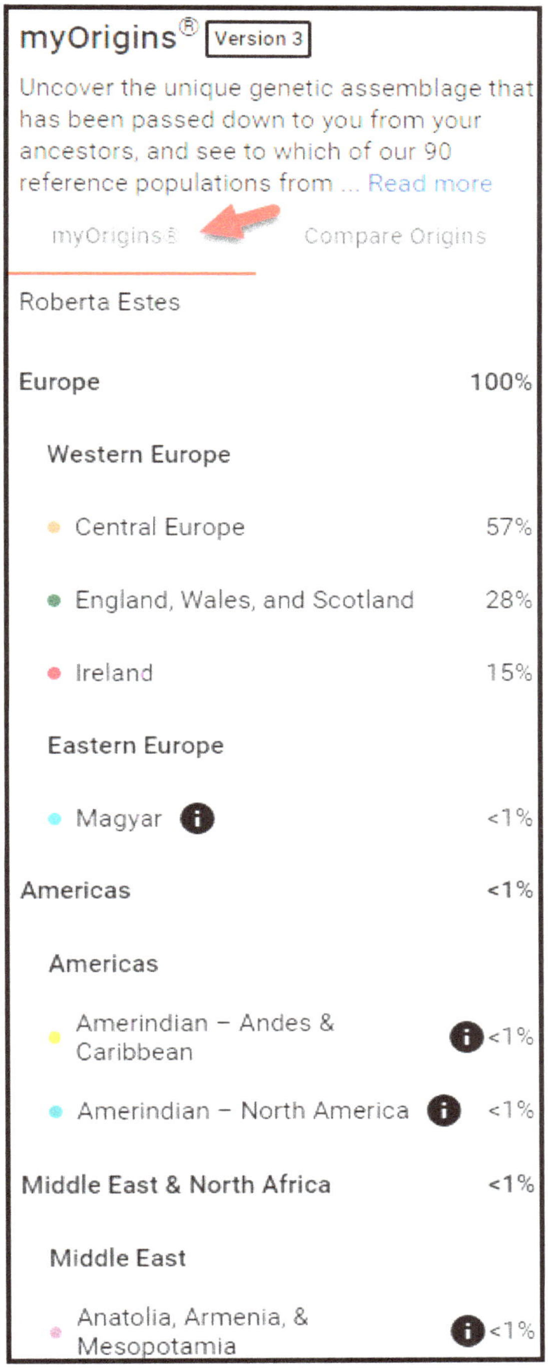

TIP: Because amounts of less than 1% can be reported in several categories, and the percentages are rounded, the total of your individual percentage amounts may not add up to exactly 100%. Don't be concerned, there's no DNA missing or percentages duplicated.

1% of your heritage, which is approximately 70 cMs of DNA, can be quite important.

The accompanying map displays your matching population regions.

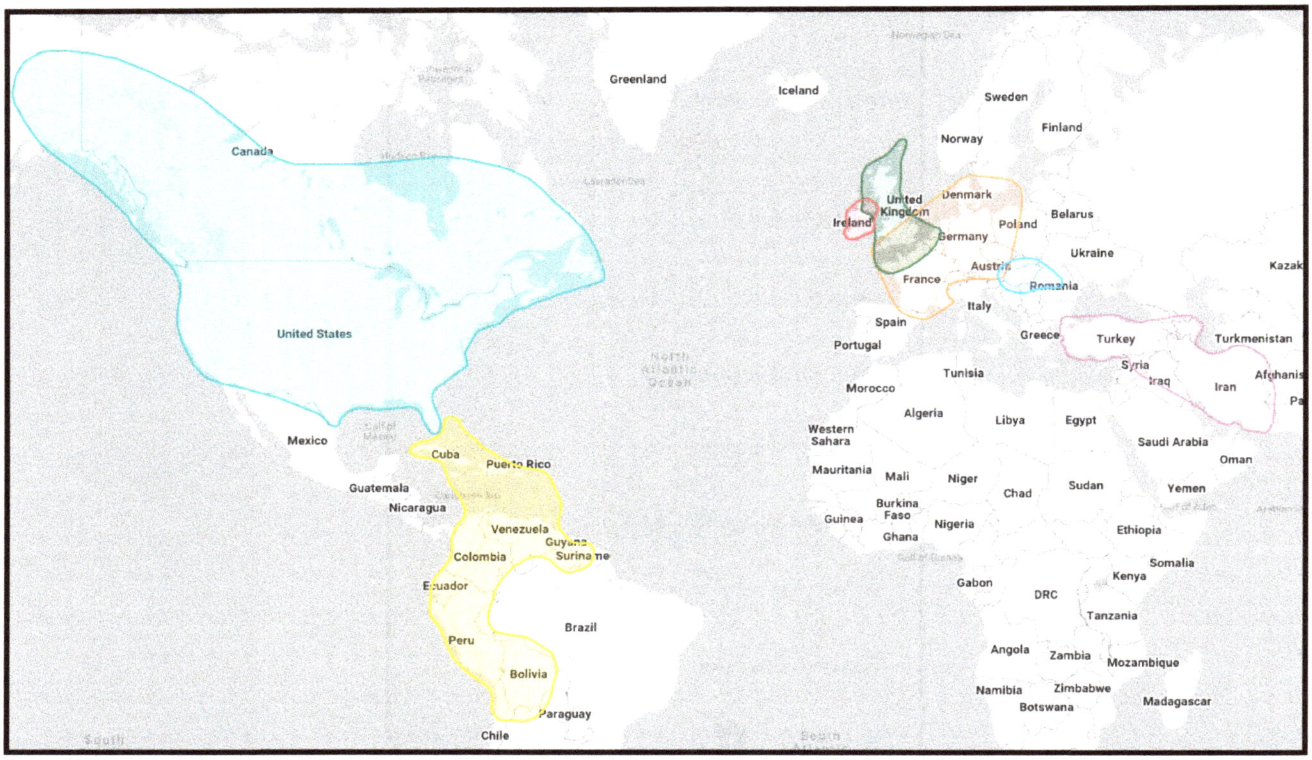

The size or color of the geography is not related to the percentage of DNA detected from that region.

FamilyTreeDNA, thankfully, reports trace amounts, identified as less than 1%, but they also note that "a trace percentage indicates a very small amount of shared DNA in common with the corresponding population. Smaller DNA segments are more likely to be misattributed."

The smaller the amount of ethnicity found, the larger the grain of salt required.

However, and this is an incredibly important "however," minority segments can be the only link we have to ancestors for whom records do not exist. This is especially true for people with minority admixture from more than one population that reaches back more than 6 or 7 generations, prior to 1800 or so. Minority segments are also particularly important for oppressed, marginalized, and enslaved populations such as both Native and African people during the colonial period, through the mid-1800s, in the Americas.

TIP: In densely populated regions like Europe, where some regions overlap, people have moved across that part of the world fairly freely for millennia, making population assignment very challenging.

Compare Origins

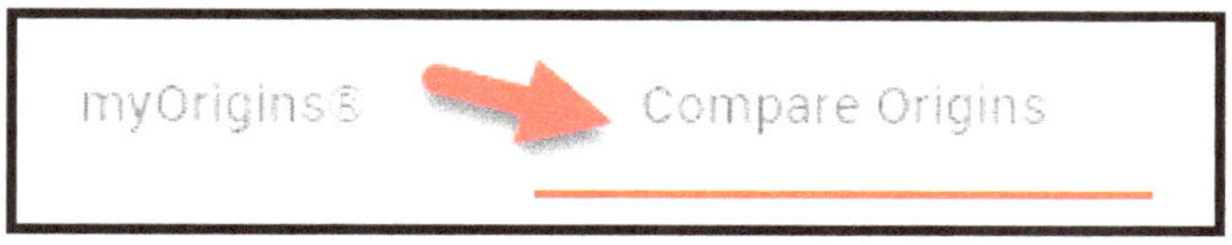

The Compare Origins feature compares your population results to those of your Family Finder matches who opt in for Compare Origins.

If you are not opted-in, you'll be prompted to opt in when you click on Compare Origins. If your matches aren't opted-in, you simply won't see them on your Compare Origins list. About half of my matches have opted in.

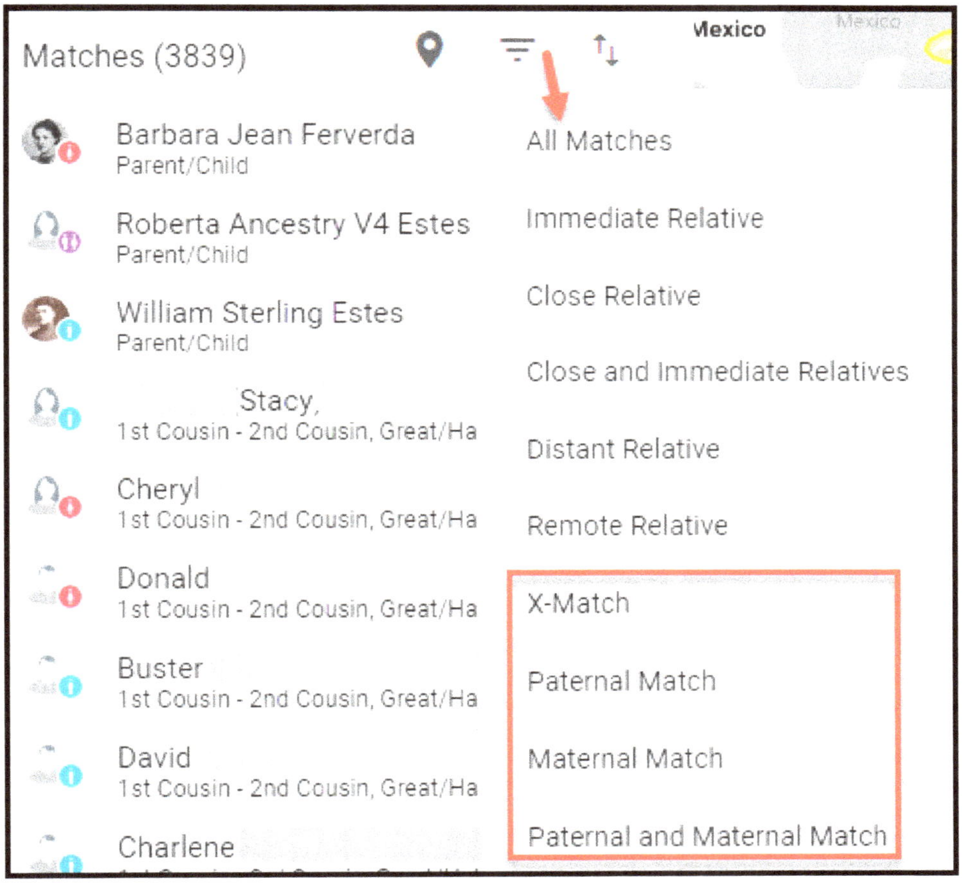

You can filter and display your myOrigins matches in a variety of ways.

To view your MyOrigins results compared to another person, click on their name.

Your origins compared with Buster

	Buster	Roberta Estes
Europe	**100%**	**100%**
Western Europe	**92%**	**100%**
Central Europe	<0%	57%
England, Wales, and Scotland	51%	28%
Ireland	32%	15%
Scandinavia	9%	<0%
Eastern Europe	**0%**	**<1%**
Magyar	<0%	<1%
Southern Europe	**8%**	**0%**
Greece & Balkans	8%	<0%

You will see regions where you share the same ethnicity, where you have a percentage of ethnicity, and your match does not, and vice versa.

TIP: Having the same population as a match does NOT mean that the population is attributed to the same segment of DNA, nor the same ancestor. It can be unrelated and circumstantial.

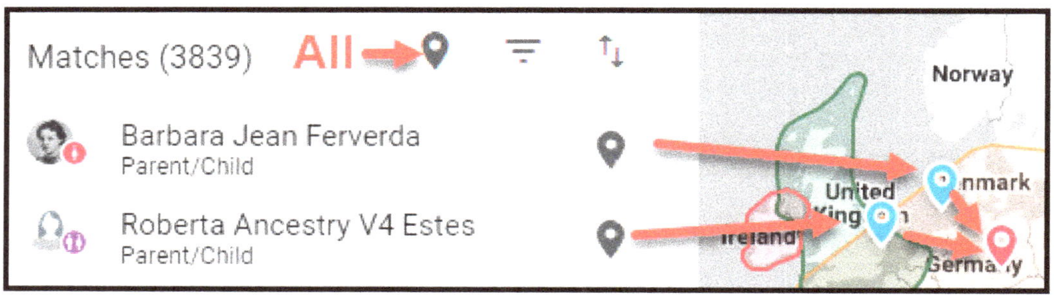

By clicking on the pins beside each match's name, their earliest known maternal and paternal ancestor will be placed on the map if they have provided that information. You can pin any number of matches' locations on the map, or even all maternal or paternal matches.

If you click on the pin at the top, you can select to display all maternal or all paternal pins.

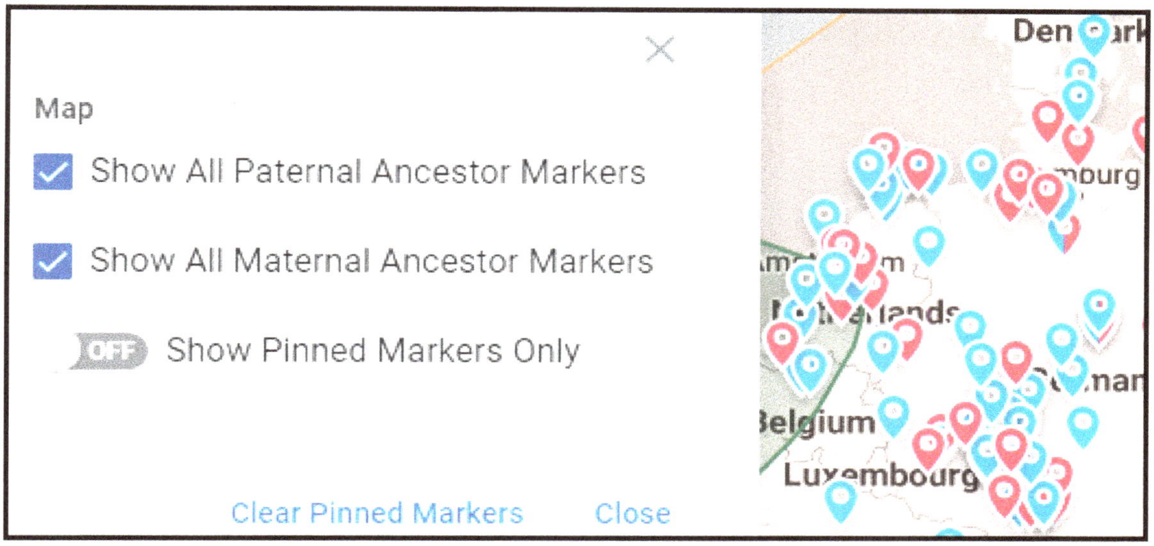

By hovering over any specific match's pins, you can view their direct paternal and maternal ancestor's lines which will turn black until you stop hovering. My maternal grandfather's ancestral location is the black pin, in the Netherlands, below. There are several other pins located nearby that may provide hints as to why I match that person.

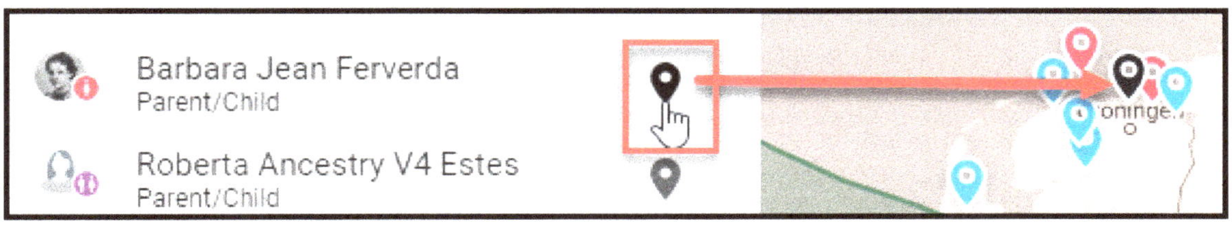

TIP: Note that this is the only avenue available for viewing the mapped locations of BOTH the direct maternal and paternal ancestors of your Family Finder matches.

If you match someone on a mitochondrial DNA test, you'll see their matrilineal ancestor on your mitochondrial matches map, and if you match them on a Y-DNA test, you'll see a male's earliest known paternal ancestor on the Y-DNA Matches Map.

If you match these people autosomally:

- A biological male's mitochondrial and Y-DNA pins will be displayed
- A biological female's mitochondrial DNA pin will be displayed, even if she has provided her direct paternal line information.

While your connection may not be through their patrilineal or matrilineal lines, finding someone whose ancestors are located near your ancestors might provide you with a critical clue. Clicking on your match's pin displays additional information.

The great news is that you can view the location of the various populations on your actual chromosomes.

Chromosome Painter - Ethnicity Chromosome Painting

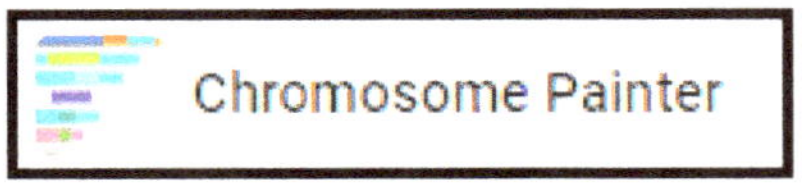

I love this feature. The Chromosome Painter literally paints your population segments on your chromosomes.

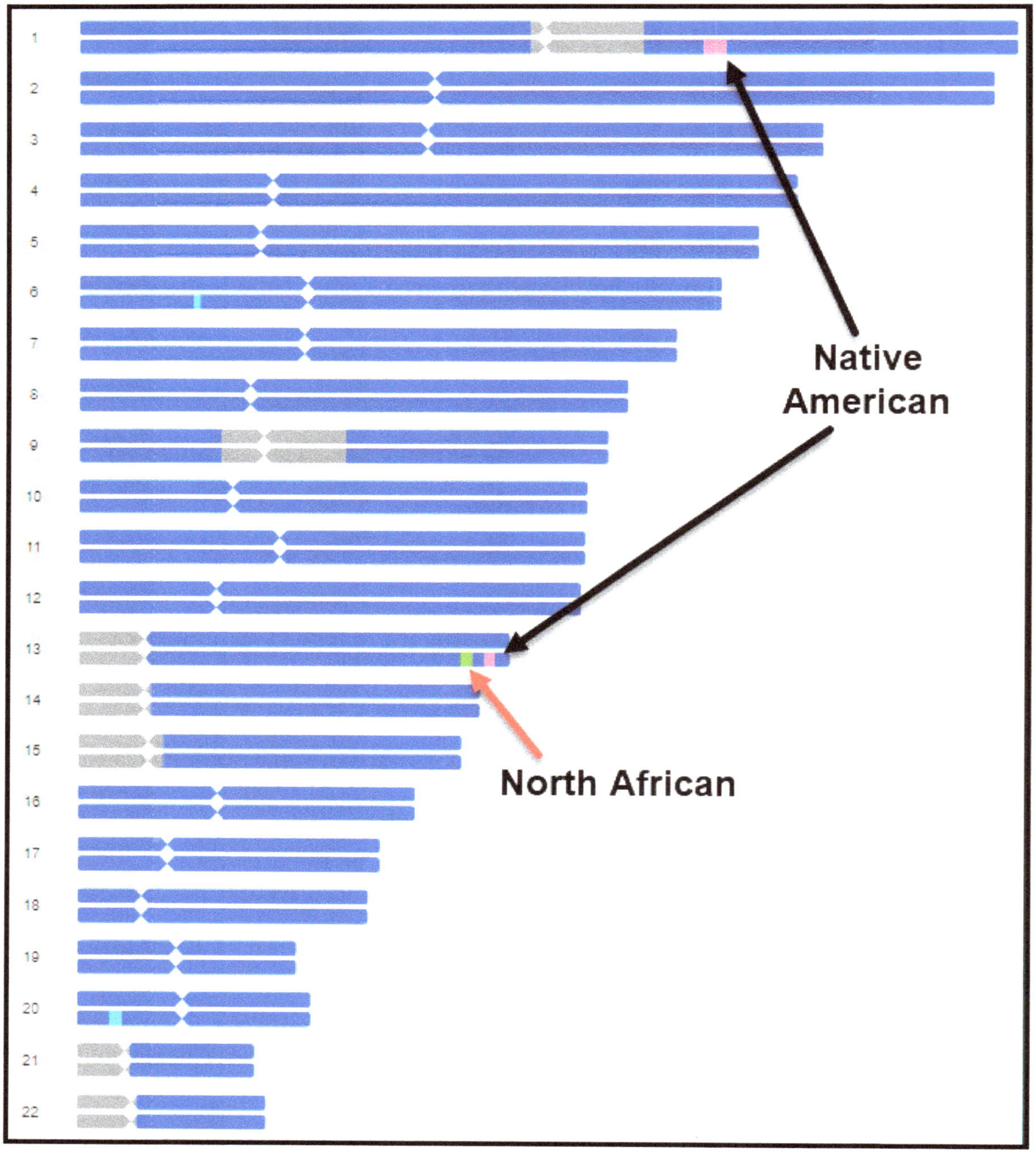

While the majority of my chromosomes are Western European, I do have some minority segments, meaning minority to me. My Native American and Middle East/North African segments are of particular interest. Identifying those segments may well be the key to unraveling which of my ancestral lines contributed those segments, which means I may be able to unveil the identity of my Native American and African ancestors.

It's worth noting that both the Native and African segments are:

- On the same parent's side on Chromosome 13
- Located in close proximity to each other

This raises the possibility that if I can identify which parent, and find matches that span both segments, it may indicate that both came from the same ancestor(s). Based on my genealogy, I have a suspicion of which line that might be.

In both cases, colonization and slavery were responsible for both African and Native American people being enslaved side by side. In many cases, no records exist and neither did surnames. In order to survive, individuals of mixed-race ancestry often omitted that information. In more recent generations, people simply weren't aware or continued omitting information to escape engrained systemic discriminatory practices.

Today, our DNA may be the only clues left to lead us back to the ancestral line to research for that minority ancestry.

Everyone can take this approach with their minority ancestry. By minority, I'm referring to minority-to-you. Minority ancestry is more likely to be valid and traceable to an ancestor when it originates on separate continents. Continental differences are more readily distinguishable than neighboring countries.

The top and bottom copies of different chromosomes displayed are NOT necessarily attributed to:

- Either the mother's or father's chromosome
- The same parent on each chromosome

Said another way, I happen to know that my Native segment on Chromosome 1 descends from my mother. That segment happens to be displayed on the bottom copy of Chromosome 1. However, on Chromosome 2 or any other chromosome, my mother could be displayed on top. Each chromosome is phased independently.

Furthermore, the Native segment on Chromosome 13 may NOT descend from my mother. It can **NOT** be assumed that because:

- The Native Segment is displayed on the bottom copy of Chromosome 13, it descends from my mother
- The Native segment on Chromosome 1 is from my mother, that my other Native segment is also from my mother
- The bottom copy of Chromosome 1 is my mother, that the bottom copy of other chromosomes are also from my mother

Notice that the African segment also appears on Chromosome 13, near the Native segment, which suggests that those two segments originated in the same parent. I say "suggests" because it's possible that due to a phenomenon called "strand swap," a portion of the DNA from both parents could be displayed on the same side of a chromosome – in other words, switched mid-chromosome - although it's unlikely.

It's tempting to conclude that both segments of Native DNA originated with the same ancestor, but in this case, they may not. It's very likely, based on my genealogy and assigning my segments to ancestors, that the Native and African segments on Chromosome 13 may have been inherited from my father's side. At this point, which parent's side is inconclusive. My maternal ancestors on that same segment are also Acadian, my father's ancestors on that segment have Native roots in the Virginia/North Carolina border region, and neither parent's ethnicity matches exactly.

TIP: Your population segments may not match your parents exactly, meaning that your Native American segment might be labeled as Amerindian-North American and their corresponding segment, or a portion thereof, might be labeled Amerindian-Andes & Caribbean. In other words, compare for similarities in addition to an exact population match.[223]

How can you determine the locations of your population segments?

Population Segments

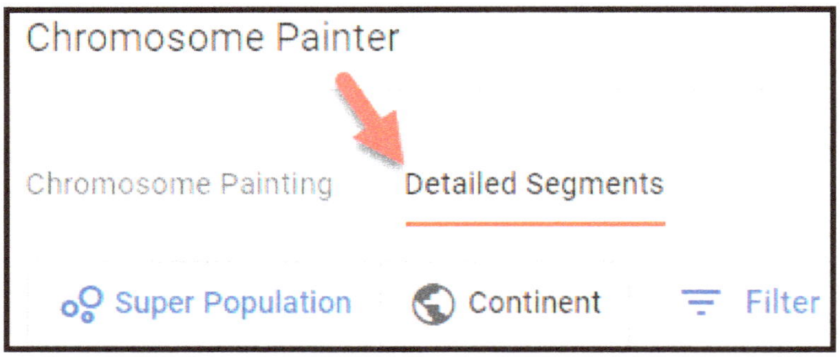

By selecting Detailed Segments, your population segment addresses will be displayed.

223 Populations and ethnicity does not always phase well to parents. The system does not actively compare children and parents to correlate or align population segments. Looking at differences at the same location can provide insight as to possible origins.

Download Segments

Super Population	Chromosome	Haplotype	Start Position	End Position	Centimorgans (cM)
Western Europe	1	1	752,721	120,309,868	151.24
Western Europe	1	1	150,204,731	249,218,992	127.64
Western Europe	1	2	752,721	120,309,868	151.24
Western Europe	1	2	150,204,731	166,010,221	20.02
Americas	1	2	166,010,221	172,069,641	7.91

All of my population segments on Chromosome 1 are shown, above, with the haplotype column indicating the copy of the chromosome where those segments are displayed. My Native American segments are found on the second copy of Chromosome 1, with the beginning and ending positions displayed, for a total of 7.91 cMs.

While the FamilyTreeDNA matching threshold to other testers is 7 cMs, population segments are reported below that level.

Two people may match on the same segment location, but in order to attribute it to the same ancestor, the two people must triangulate to eliminate:

- One person matching from their mother's side and the other from their father's side.
- Segments that are identical by chance

You can download a csv-format file by clicking on "Download Segments."

Painting Ethnicity Segments

In order to determine which people I match on my Native American and African segments, I painted my ethnicity segments at DNAPainter.

Segments are assigned to ancestors at DNAPainter when I can identify common ancestors with my matches, so it makes sense to paint my population segments as well – especially since I'm searching for the source of my minority ancestry.

DNAPainter provides instructions for importing your myOrigins download file.[224]

After you've imported your myOrigins populations into DNAPainter, your ethnicity segments will show in the same way that matches to other people appear.

224 https://dnapainter.com/blog/painting-your-populations/

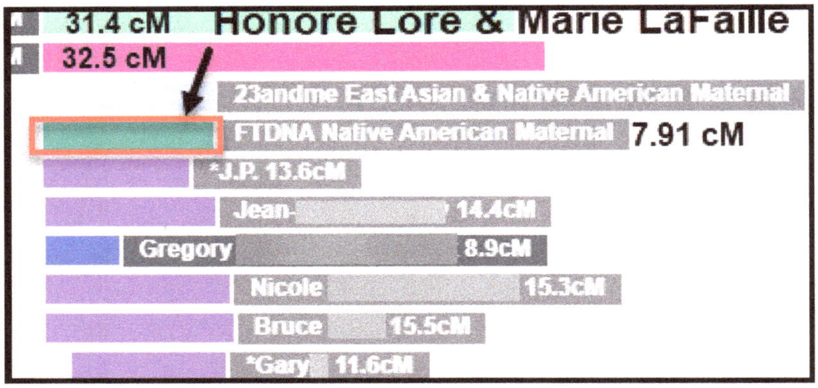

On the relevant portion of my Chromosome 1, above, you can see that:

- I've renamed the segment FTDNA Native American Maternal, so I know exactly where it came from.
- 23andMe also found the same Native segment, which tends to confirm smaller cM population amounts.
- I have several matches to testers on the same area of my mother's chromosome.

The different colors correspond to different ancestors in the same lineage.

Honoré Lore/Lord and Marie LaFaille are my 6th-generation ancestors.

The other matching people share common ancestors with me in closer generations. Several matches span the entire Native segment. Two, however, at the top, match on a larger segment. The top match descends from Honoré and Marie, and the second match that's just slightly larger descends from one generation closer in time.

Each of these people should have (at least) this portion of their DNA assigned as Native American. If you only match on one segment with someone, and it's your Native segment, you know there's a common Native ancestor involved, and they contributed this segment to you both. You can confirm that you and your match share Native American ethnicity by using the Compare Origins feature.

What About Confirming Evidence?

Now, of course, we need to ask if we have any documentary evidence or proof that the Native American designation is accurate.

As it turns out, we do. In historical records, a record from a priest to his bishop reports that Philippe Mius d'Azy[225], an Acadian settler, had two Amerindian wives.[226] Honoré Lord's[227] paternal grandmother is the granddaughter of Philippe Mius d'Azy with his first Native wife.

225 https://www.wikitree.com/wiki/Mius-24

226 https://www.wikitree.com/wiki/Mi'kmaq-17

227 https://dna-explained.com/2023/04/02/honorius-lord-1768-1834-catholic-church-records-illuminate-migration-along-the-richelieu-river-52-ancestors-393/

Testers who are maternally descended from this couple have taken a full sequence mitochondrial DNA test, and the resulting haplogroup X2a2 is consistent with known Native American haplogroups and other known Native American individuals.[228]

Ancient European Origins

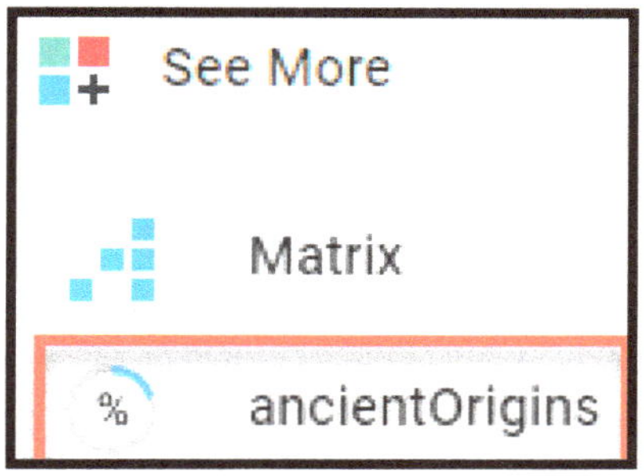

Some people are disappointed when their results reflect a majority of European heritage, with little differentiation. The good news is that ancientOrigins provides additional enlightenment about European heritage, breaking your ethnicity down into approximate percentages of the founding settler groups based on ancient DNA.

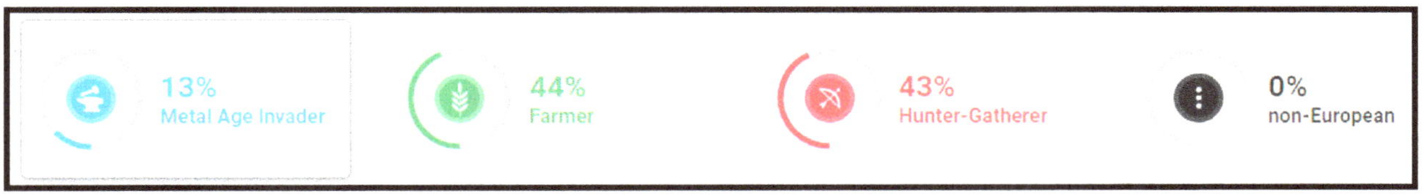

Clicking on the map reveals the migration routes for each category, along with the location of remains used to designate Metal Age Invader, Farmer, or Hunter-Gatherer.

Clicking on the placard reveals information about the Metal Age Invaders, for example, what defined that age, who they were, when they arrived, and where they lived. Their migration path is shown on the accompanying map.

Clicking on the map shows all three migration paths.

228 https://dna-explained.com/2013/09/18/native-american-mitochondrial-haplogroups/

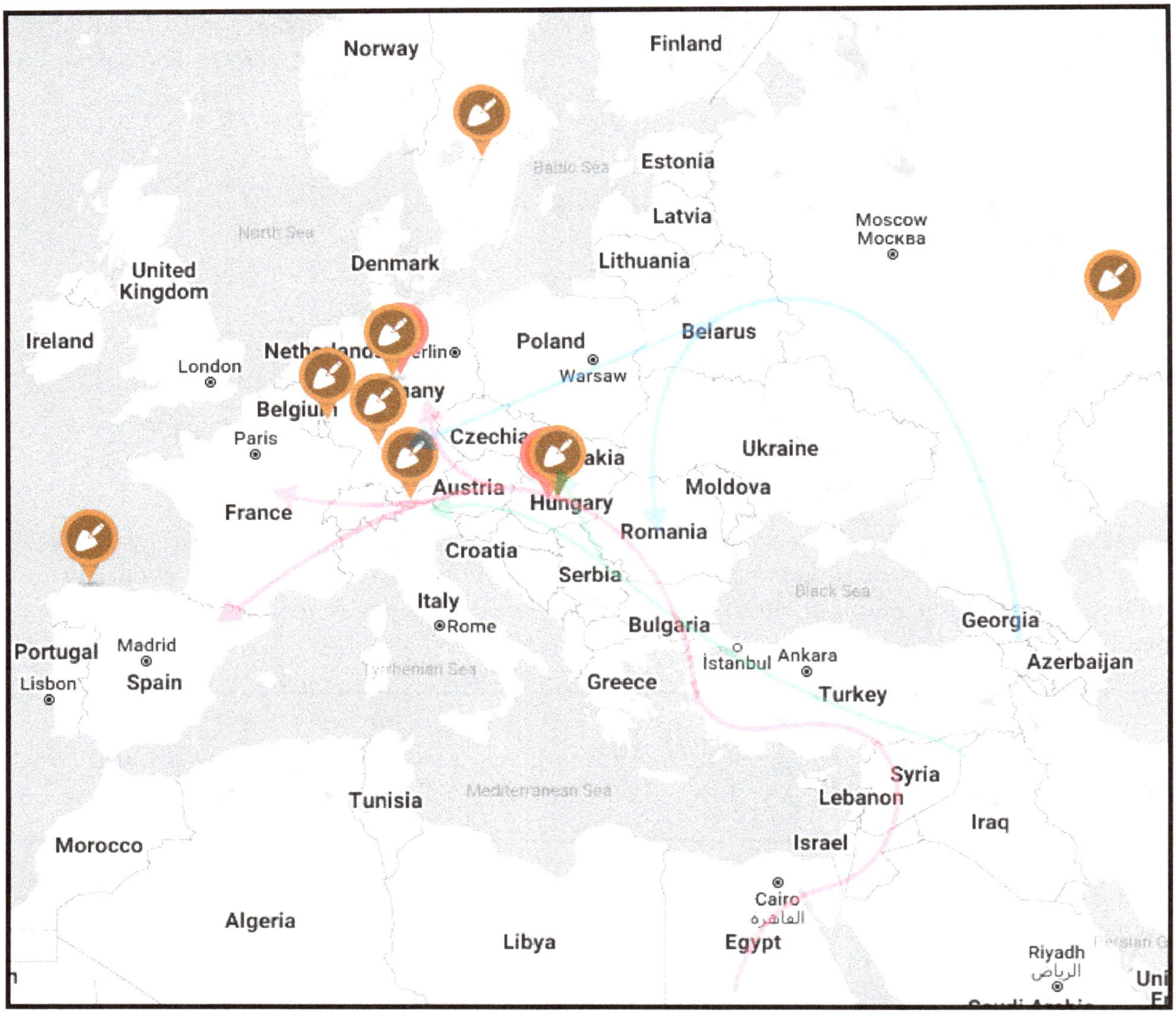

Clicking on a shovel provides information about that archaeological excavation.

Our ancestry reaches back in time beyond surnames, and ancientOrigins helps shed light on deeper European autosomal ancestry.

Chapter 8

ADVANCED MATCHING

We touched on Advanced Matching in specific instances, but it's an often-overlooked tool that can be very useful in a number of ways.

Testers can combine matching criteria from multiple types of tests and projects, in various ways, to view selectively filtered matches.

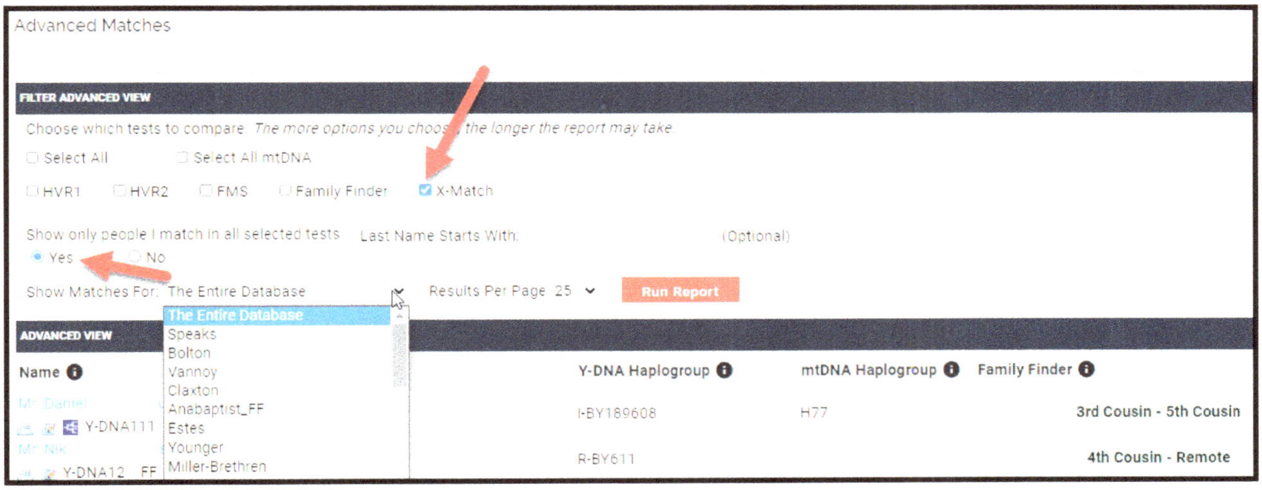

For example, I'm filtering for only X matches in the entire database.

Be sure to select "yes" to "show only people I match in all selected tests." Otherwise, you will see your matches to "everyone," not just people in both or all the tests you've selected.

I often utilize Advanced matching for:

- Mitochondrial plus Family Finder to see which mitochondrial DNA matches, if any, match me on Family Finder as well
- Y-DNA plus Family Finder
- X Matches
- Matches within projects that I've joined

One of my favorite uses of Advanced Matching is being able to select matches by project. Testers join projects because they have some genealogical connection to other people who might be interested in joining that specific project.

Discovering that you match someone within a project is a hint that perhaps you share a common ancestor from that surname line, or from that region, or whatever project you've selected.

Not all projects are created equal. Some surname administrators don't accept females or males who don't descend paternally through the surname line and haven't taken a Y-DNA test. Volunteer administrators who invest time into the project setup and management determine the parameters for the projects they manage.

TIP: Just because you match someone in a specific project does NOT mean that your common ancestor is from that surname line or associated with that project – but it's a great place to begin. All hints are welcome!

Chapter 9

FINDING, JOINING AND UTILIZING PROJECTS

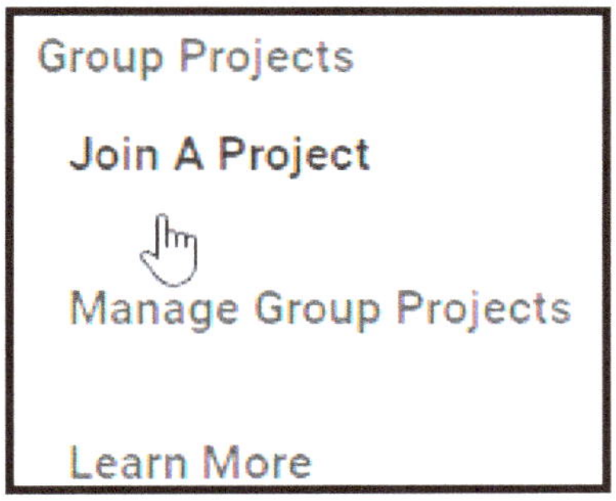

In the top bar on your personal page, you can click on Group Projects to:

- Find a project to join
- Manage projects you've already joined
- Learn more about projects

Group Projects, also known as just Projects or just Groups, are hosted by FamilyTreeDNA and are free for everyone – meaning free to set up, to run and to join.

Joining one of the more than 11,000 available projects is one of the best ways to leverage your investment and collaborate with others. You may also want to volunteer to assist with a project of your choosing. Volunteer administrators often split their duties in various ways. Many people turn to administrators for assistance with genealogy, understanding results, or requesting upgrade advice.

You can search for projects that are relevant to you by entering a surname, sometimes a location, haplogroup, or keyword. Some administrators know that entering other words as "surnames" allows them to be found in searches. For example, as an administrator for the American Indian project, I have entered keywords such as tribal names, as well as the words "Native" and "Indian." Clearly, I can't enter all of the surnames that are Native American, but I can help people find those projects by adding relevant keywords.

Testers can search for "Geographic" projects, meaning non-surname projects, that are relevant to them and can also browse projects that are grouped alphabetically by type.

TIP: You can join an unlimited number of projects, but FamilyTreeDNA does reserve the right to limit the number of projects you join to which you have no genetic or geographic connection. Joining projects to mine data from them violates the Terms of Service

What to Expect When Joining a Project

Generally, projects are grouped or organized in a manner that is useful to the testers. How projects are organized, however, is usually a factor of the type of project.

Projects fall into various categories:

- **Surname** – Based on surnames and generally focused on Y-DNA testing, these projects may or may not accept females by that surname or people with that surname in their family tree.
- **Y-DNA Geographical Projects** – Geographical Projects, in this context, may refer to an actual physical geography, such as France, but also includes projects that are more topic or group-focused, such as Jewish Prussia, Cossaks, Mennonites, or Hungarian Magyars.
- **MTDNA (Mitochondrial) Geographical Projects** – Same as Y-DNA, except mitochondrial DNA focused.
- **Dual (Y-DNA and mtDNA) Geographical Projects** – Same, but for both Y-DNA and mtDNA. You may wonder why the differences. If an individual joins the American Indian project, for example, and has taken both the Y-DNA and mitochondrial DNA test, BOTH their Y-DNA and mitochondrial DNA test results will show in those respective portions of the project, even though one parent may be Native, and the other may be European. The administrators can suppress either test from showing, but they have to both be aware of it, and do that for every member with similar results. If the administrator creates a Y-DNA **or** mtDNA Geographical project, instead of a Y-DNA **and** mtDNA project, only the relevant type of DNA is displayed in the public-facing portion of the project. It's also worth noting that many geographical projects DO welcome everyone with an interest in the topic and are not restricted to Y-DNA and mtDNA only. There just isn't a category for "everything," and there's nothing to "show" publicly for autosomal testers. Make sure you understand the focus and parameters when you are viewing project information and results.
- **MTDNA Lineage Projects** – The category of mtDNA lineage projects was established to facilitate something similar to Y-DNA surname projects, but the female's surname in Western culture often changes in every generation, so one can't give their mitochondrial lineage a specific surname. Fortunately, each project has a description and projects have a search feature.
- **Y-DNA Haplogroup Projects** – Generally, Y-DNA haplogroup projects begin with the beginning letter of the haplogroup, but not always. For example, under "A", we find Y-DNA haplogroup A, but we also find several others, including several Arab projects and an Ashkenazi Levite project. I sometimes find administrators have requested their haplogroup projects be categorized under Y-DNA Geographic Projects, so be sure to check in that category as well.

- **MTDNA Haplogroup Projects** – Same as above except for mitochondrial DNA.
- **Family Projects** – Many family projects are private, meaning they don't publicly display and/or aren't searchable, because they are designed to allow for grouping several kits together. For example, let's say I wanted to test and manage the autosomal, Y-DNA, and mtDNA tests of several family members who descend from common great-grandparents. That's not a good fit for any of the other project categories, but it would be a wonderful Family Project. Based on matches, newly discovered cousins can be invited to join.

Projects, their goals, and how they are managed vary widely. Some projects are private, meaning they have no public-facing page, and only members can view groupings and results. Others display non-identifying information publicly.

FamilyTreeDNA prevents private information, such as the tester's name or personal information, from ever being accidentally displayed in a project by administrators. Displayed information is quite useful, but limited to categories that you see on this public page and the corresponding one for mitochondrial DNA.

Kit Number	Name	Paternal Ancestor Name	Country	Haplogroup	DYS393	DYS390	DYS19
Estes - Autosomal, Not Y DNA							
102259	Magner	Edward Magner, 1815 - 1890	Ireland	J-M67	12	23	14
146880	Scott	joseph scott b.abt 1748. lived in madison co KY US	Unknown Origin	R-M269	13	24	14
252759	Stamper	Jacques Jacob Ramey/Remy B 1630-	France	R-BY67773	13	24	14
101466	Simmons	Jonathan Simmons (Symmons) b. bef. 1684, England.	England	R Z253	13	24	14
N60267	Arias	Antonio Mª Arias Quirós, b.1828 Mondoñedo, Spain	Spain	R-Y61135	13	24	14
249804	Jackson		Unknown Origin	R-M269	13	25	14
118647	Headen (Ó h-Éideáin in Gaelic)	Patt Headen Bendenstown Ballon Co Carlow b.1770	Ireland	R-FGC5939	13	25	14
157414	Pitchford		Unknown Origin	R-M269	14	24	14
Estes 1 - Abraham - Abraham Jr. c 1697-1759 + Ann Watkins and Elizbaeth Jeeter, Caroline Co., Va							
92743	Estes		Unknown Origin	R-M269	13	25	14
46167	Estes	Abraham Jr 1697-1759 m Ann Clark, Phillip bef 1720	Unknown Origin	R-M269	13	25	14
45614	Estes		Unknown Origin	R-M269	13	25	14
43144	Estes	Abraham Jr 1697-1759 m Ann Clark, Phillip bef 1720	Unknown Origin	R-M269	13	25	14
51909	Estes	Thomas Estes	United Kingdom	R-M269	13	25	14
49592	Estes	Abraham Jr 1697-1759 m Ann Clark, Samuel b 1727	England	R-M269	13	25	14
Estes 10 - Abraham - Sylvester 1684-1754 Bertie and Granville Co., NC							
199378	Estes	George Washington Estes, abt. 1845 - 1923	United States	R-BY490	13	25	14
17420	Estes	Abe b 1647, Sylvester, Thomas, Thomas, Burroughs	England	R-M269	13	25	14
13805	Estes	Nathaniel Estes, b. 1770 and d. 1845	England	R-BY490	13	25	14
235622	Estes		Unknown Origin	R-M269	13	25	14

The Estes DNA project[229] is public, and we welcome all Estes descendants. Estes males are grouped accordingly, and the rest (non-Estes Y-DNA testers) are grouped together.

The American Indian Project[230] is also public and open to all, but is grouped by haplogroup category, meaning European, African, Asian, and Native American haplogroups, and then by haplogroup within those categories.

229 https://www.familytreedna.com/public/Estes?iframe=yresults

230 https://www.familytreedna.com/public/AmericanIndian?iframe=yresults

Administrators utilize your earliest known ancestor, your trees, and sometimes correspondence to group your test appropriately.

If the projects you choose to join are public, and most are, you can opt to not have your results displayed in the public-facing part of the project. You can modify your "Sharing" setting, as well as other options under your account settings drop down by your name in the upper right-hand corner, then click on Project Preferences.

I encourage you to share your results on the public pages, as projects are a wonderful recruitment tool. The more people who test, the better for everyone.

Many people check surname projects before ordering a test to see if their line is represented. Everyone wants someone to compare to, if possible. But remember, just because a tester from your line hasn't joined a project, or doesn't have public results, doesn't mean that they're not in the database just waiting to match you.

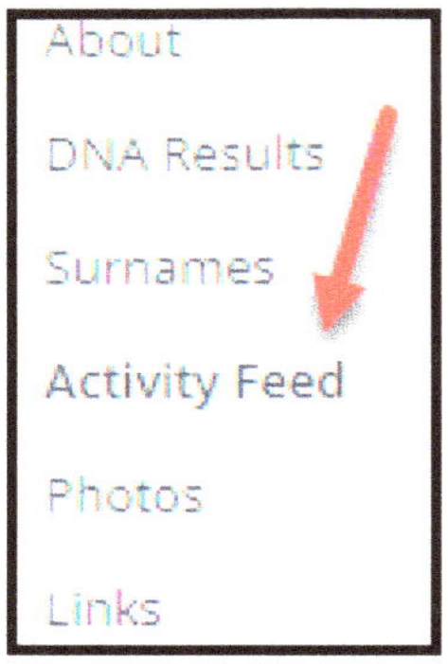

TIP: If you're searching for additional information about your ancestors, don't forget to periodically check the Activity Feed for projects you've joined. For projects that have enabled the Activity Feed, members can post information or questions about their ancestors or genealogy. There's no search function today, but hopefully, one will be added soon.

Public Project Search

In addition to the internal Project features, FamilyTreeDNA provides a public project search on their main page[231] and also by clicking on "Group Projects" in the footer of most pages.

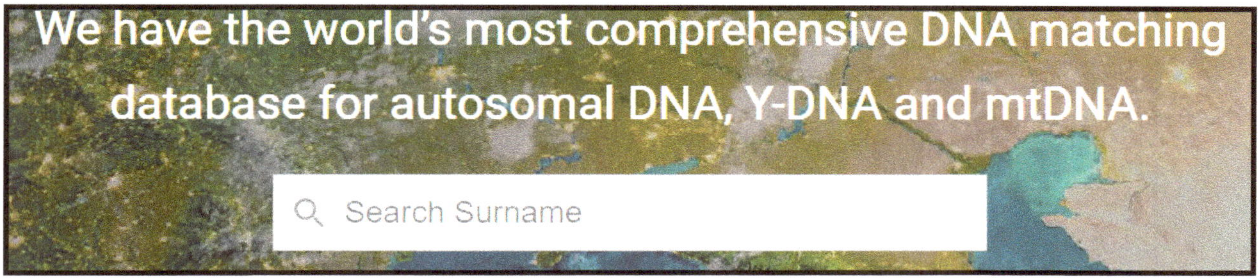

Scrolling down and entering a surname in the search box provides the ability to see how many people in the database with that surname have tested. You can view the various projects that have listed that surname as potentially being of interest within that project, or, conversely, their project being of interest to people with that surname.

A search for McNeil shows that 296 people with the McNeil surname have tested.

231 https://www.familytreedna.com/ or by going directly to this link: https://www.familytreedna.com/group-project-search

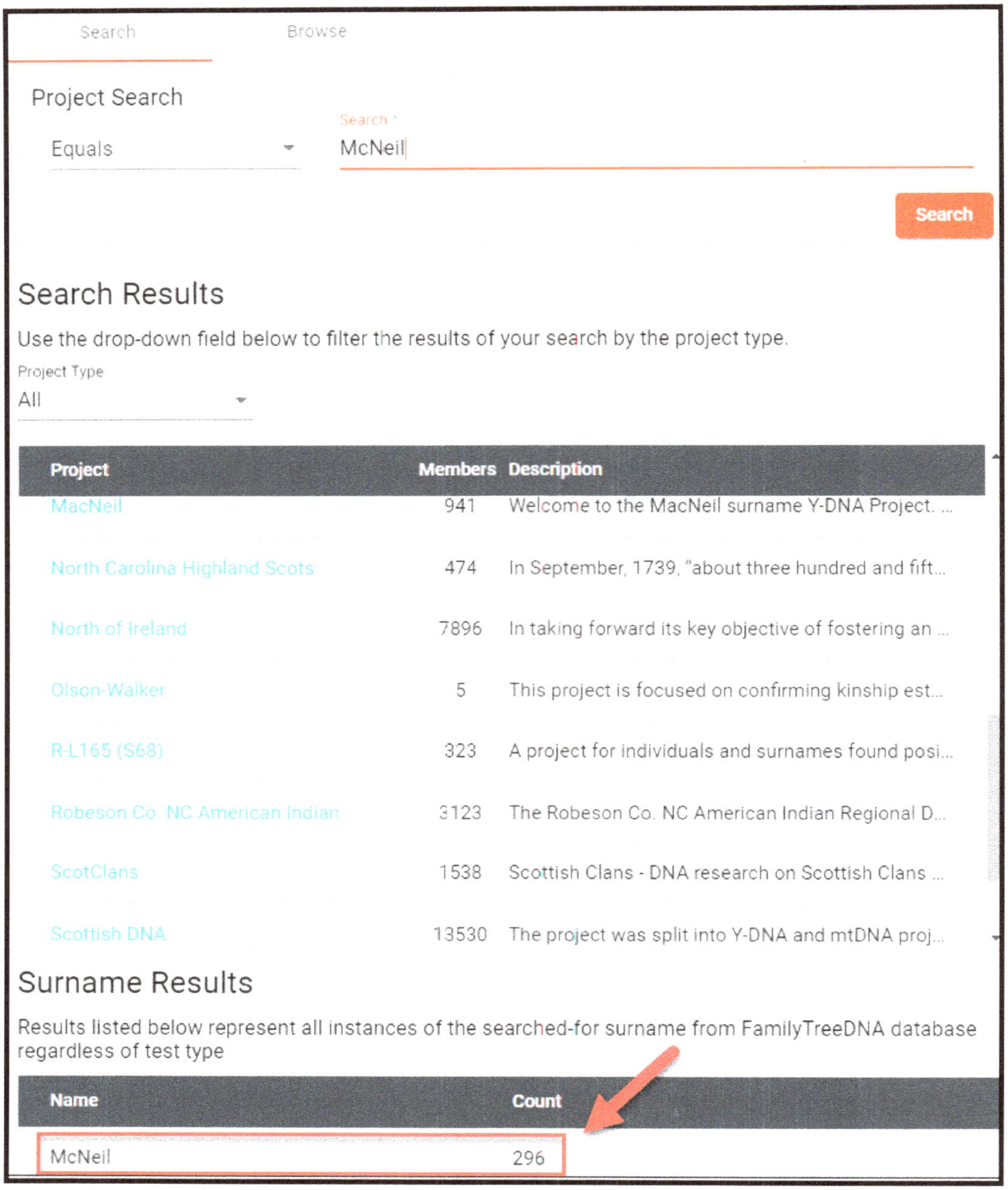

Of course, not all 296 McNeils who have tested would be males, but many are, and by clicking on the McNeil or other projects, one can see if perhaps a male from the relevant line has tested.

Check alternate surname spellings as well.

TIP: Administrators add surnames of interest, so not all projects that list your surname may be relevant to your surname line.

File Downloads

I'm truly grateful that FamilyTreeDNA provides so many download files for their customers, but I have a difficult time remembering where each download is found and what's included. [232]

I've created a table to provide the download location path, file name, and purpose of each file download available.

Type	Download Location Path	File Name	Description & Comment
Y-DNA SNPs	Y-DNA Results & Tools, See More, Data Download, SNP Results, Download All SNPs	SNP_Results + kit number.csv[233]	Only available if the tester has taken a SNP test of some kind, including individual SNPs, SNP packs, a Big Y of any iteration, and obsolete tests no longer offered such as "Walk Through the Y," Deep Clade, and Genographic transfers
Y-DNA matches	"Export CSV" at upper right on Y-DNA Matches page	Kit number + Y_DNA_Matches.csv	Select "All Matches" or "Filtered Matches"
Y-DNA STR Marker values	Y-DNA Results & Tools, See More, Y-STR Results, lower right-hand corner, "Down-load CSV"	Kit number + Y_DNA_DYS_Results + date.csv	STR marker values

232 The download option for some files has been paused due to the 23andMe data exposure and will be resumed after 2FA is implemented in 2024.

233 An example of this format would be SNP_Results6696.csv for kit number 6656.

Big Y	Big Y, Results, "Download Files" in upper right-hand corner	6 choices >	Export Matches (CSV), Export Derived SNPs (CSV), Export Ancestral SNPs (CSV), Export No Call SNPs (CSV), Download VCF, Download BAM[234]
MtDNA FASTA	mtDNA Results & Tools, See More, Mutations, lower right-hand corner, "Download FASTA file"	Kit number + FASTA.fasta	This is only readable with a FASTA file viewer and is only needed if you're going to upload to another mitochondrial DNA site
MtDNA matches	Download CSV at bottom right of mtDNA Matches page	Kit number + mtDNA_Matches + date. csv	
Family Finder Y-DNA haplogroup	Y-DNA Results & Tools, Haplotree & SNPs, SNP Results, download	SNP_Results_kit number+date.csv	Includes Y-DNA SNPs from the Family Finder test - only relevant for Y-DNA STR testers or Family Finder testers - Big Y test is more refined
Family Finder Autosomal matches[235]	"Export CSV" upper right at top of Family Finder Matches Page	Kit number + Family_Finder_Matches + date.csv	Select "All Matches" or "Filtered Matches" if you've applied filters
Family Finder Autosomal segment[236]	Chromosome Browser, Download All Segments	Kit number + Chromosome_Browser_Results + date.csv	Be sure to select "All Segments" without selecting individual matches to compare

234 Please note that the Big Y BAM file is not free. It is not generated until needed and the cost of generation and storage (it's a massive file) was initially rolled into the price of each test. However, since few testers actually want this file, in November 2019, FamilyTreeDNA uncoupled the file from the test and reduced the cost of all Big Y tests by $100. If you want to order the BAM file, it's $100, but there is really no reason to purchase this file. BAM files require special programs to view the file.

235 Paused after the 23andMe data compromise.

236 Also paused.

Family Finder Autosomal selected segments	Chromosome Browser, select matches to compare, click compare, "Download Segments" at upper right	Kit number + Chromosome_Browser_Results + date.csv	Downloads only selected matches' segments – same file name as above
Autosomal Raw data download	Autosomal DNA Results & Tools, See More, Data Download	37_R_Estes_Chrom_ Autoso + date.csv.gz	Build 37 - file is zipped, you don't need to unzip before uploading elsewhere
myOrigins3 segments	Chromosome Painter – Download Segments in the upper right-hand corner	Kit number + detailed_segments_data	

Chapter 10

THIRD PARTY TOOLS

Two well-known third-party tools enhance the capabilities of FamilyTreeDNA and are widely used by genealogists.

Genetic Affairs

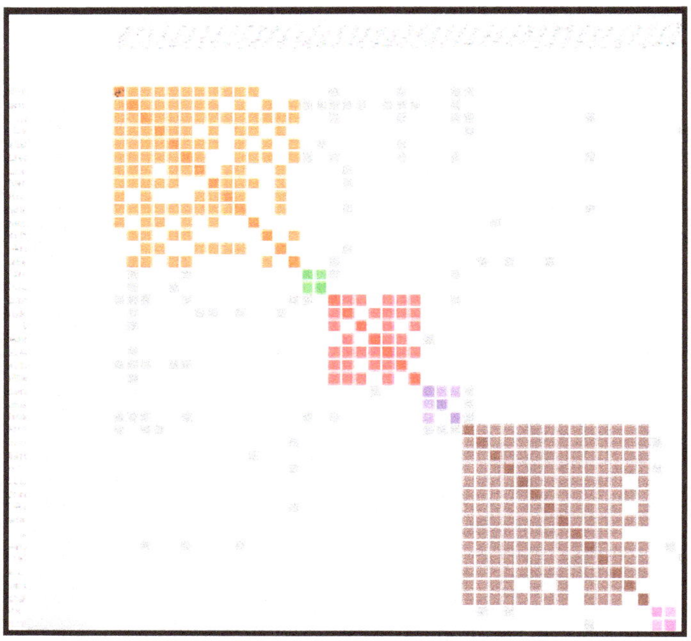

Genetic Affairs[237] is a third-party tool that enhances Family Finder, and in some cases, Y-DNA and mitochondrial capabilities[238] by providing:

- AutoClusters[239] – Automated clustering of shared autosomal matches organizes matches into colorful clusters based on shared matches. Clusters represent people with common ancestors.

---

237 https://geneticaffairs.com/

238 https://dna-explained.com/2020/08/13/genetic-affairs-instructions-and-resources/

239 https://dna-explained.com/2018/12/04/autoclustering-by-genetic-affairs/

All Genetic Affairs tools below include an AutoCluster, pictured above, plus additional features:

- AutoTree[240] – Automated tree reconstruction compares trees of you and your matches to find common ancestors. Reconstructs trees based on the trees of matches. Works without having a tree yourself by comparing the trees of your matches.
- AutoPedigree – An option of AutoTree, AutoPedigree generates hypotheses about how the tester fits into the auto-generated trees based on shared matches and relationships to other testers.
- AutoSegment – Uses the Chromosome Browser Results segment download file[241] to cluster based on overlapping segments.
- AutoSegment ICW – Downloads the Chromosome Browser Results segment file automatically and improves on regular AutoSegment by using "in common with" match data to discard overlapping segments for which the underlying matches are not a shared match with each other.[242]
- Hybrid AutoSegment - Identifies overlapping segments between segments of different companies, for example, segments from FamilyTreeDNA, MyHeritage, and 23andMe from their downloaded segment files.[243]
- AutoTree + mtDNA or Y-DNA – By selecting the AutoTree feature and checking the "Y-DNA" or "mtDNA DNA" option, along with "AutoTree identify common ancestors from trees," Y-DNA or mitochondrial DNA results will be read first and given tree-building priority, followed by autosomal matches. Wonderful way to search for mitochondrial tree matches to your tree, and your matches to each other.

TIP: All Genetic Affairs runs are time-limited or CPU-limited, meaning that the run may not complete if it's too complex or there's too much data. With all AutoClusters, select features one at a time, like only mtDNA with AutoTree, not every option combined with AutoTree, or the process may not complete. There's no way to know if the process actually worked all the way to the end.

One of the best features of Genetic Affairs, aside from the clusters themselves, is the AutoSegment and AutoSegment ICW tools because they cluster your matches, by segment, into maternal and paternal sides for each segment. The ICW version removes matches that are identical by chance. This means, in essence, that if you can figure out your common ancestor with one person in any specific segment cluster, you should share that same genetic line with all the people in that cluster, one way or another, someplace back in time. It's easy to figure out which side is which if you have bucketed matches.

---

240 https://dna-explained.com/2019/12/02/genetic-affairs-reconstructs-trees-from-genetic-clusters-even-without-your-tree-or-common-ancestors/

241 The ability to download this file at FamilyTreeDNA is currently paused, although you can still use a previously downloaded file.

242 https://dna-explained.com/2022/12/13/concepts-your-matches-on-the-same-segment-are-not-necessarily-related-to-each-other/

243 Downloads are currently disabled at all three companies as a result of the data compromise at 23andMe. Hopefully this feature will be returned in 2024 at all companies.

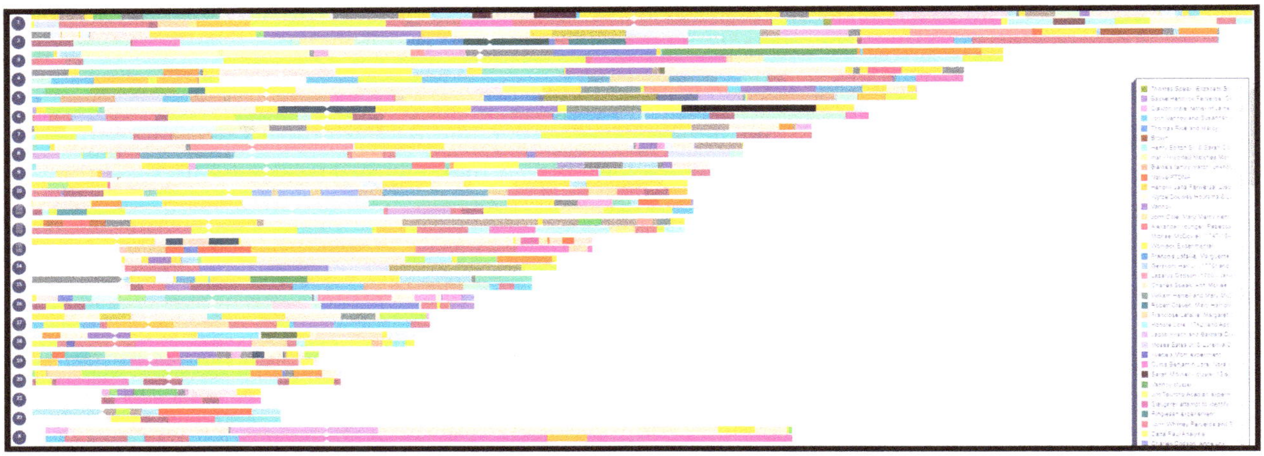

DNAPainter

I've mentioned DNAPainter several times in specific sections of this book, but I'd like to explain why I use DNAPainter extensively to paint:

- Segments from matches whose common ancestors I can identify at vendors who provide segment location information for your matches; FamilyTreeDNA, MyHeritage, 23andMe[244] and GEDmatch.
- Ethnicity/population segments from both FamilyTreeDNA and 23andMe, who provide segment address information for ethnicity segments.

DNAPainter allows users to paint segments by associating them with specific ancestors, or ancestral couples. Initially, you'll only be able to identify a common ancestral couple, until you match with someone who descends from the next generation further back in time, which allows you to identify which person of the pair contributed that particular segment.

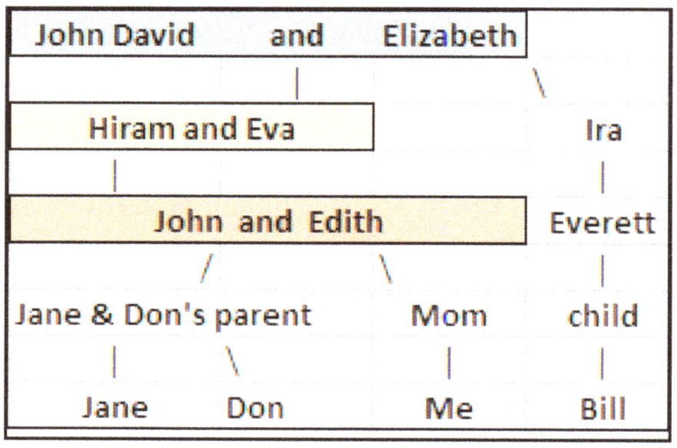

Let's look at an easy example.

244 Currently not available at 23andMe..

Let's say I match my first cousin, Jane, and her brother, Don, on a particular segment. I know that segment descended to all three of us from our common grandparents, John and Edith.

Who contributed that segment, or parts of that segment to our grandparents? Which grandparent gave that segment to us, or, is it a combination of segments from both grandparents?

Next, I match Bill on that same segment, and so do Jane and Don. We know that Jane, Don, and I are all related to Bill through the ancestor who contributed that segment to all four of us. But Bill doesn't descend from our grandparents so that common ancestor has to be further back than John and Edith.

Bill descends from my great-great-grandparents, John David and Elizabeth, through their son, Ira. Therefore, we know that our shared segment with Bill descends from John David and Elizabeth through their son Hiram through their son John's two children to Jane, Don and me.

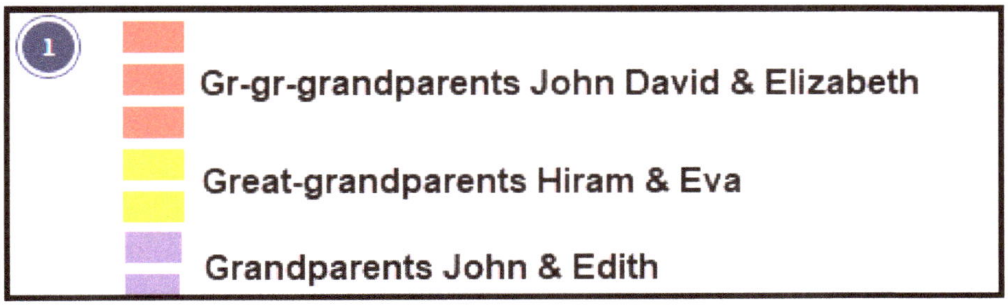

In this example from DNAPainter, the two bottom segments are the painted segments from Jane and Don. Our most recent ancestors are our grandparents, John and Edith.

The next two segments from the bottom are the same segments, attributed to Hiram and Eva. The top three segments are the three segments from Jane, Don, and Bill. We know this segment, represented by several matches, descends from John David and Elizabeth, based on the match between me, Jane, Don (and others) with Bill on this segment. It's our match with Bill that cements **where** this segment originated, because we all share the entire segment **and** those ancestors, both.

As I continue to evaluate each of my matches for our common ancestors, eventually, I'll find another person who matches me, Jane, Don, and Bill on that segment, or a significant portion of that segment (generally 7 cMs or larger), and they will descend from the parents or grandparents of John David or Elizabeth. Then I'll have pushed my knowledge of where this segment originated back another generation or two.

That's how we "push segments back in time," associating those segments with specific ancestors through our matches with testers.

Before DNAPainter, genetic genealogists maintained a massive spreadsheet where we formed triangulation groups of people. Now we don't need to do that anymore, because we can paint those segments at DNAPainter, where they are stored and displayed visually by ancestor on each one of our chromosomes. Triangulation groups are formed automatically and visually.

Once we associate a particular segment with the most distant ancestor in the lineage, then we know that all matches downstream who share that segment descend from that ancestral couple.

Our goal is to continue to identify more distant ancestors by matching with more than one individual who descends from the same ancestral couple through different children. Sharing matches with people who descend from the same couple through different children confirms that the couple actually contributed that particular segment.

Pulling It All Together

FamilyTreeDNA customers are fortunate because they have four distinct tools to utilize that reveal clues about several aspects of ancestors that could never be discovered any other way.

- Mitochondrial DNA – everyone's mother's direct maternal, or matrilineal, line – infinitely deep, but can also be used successfully for genealogy. One line only
- Y-DNA – every male's direct paternal, or patrilineal, line – infinitely deep, but can also reveal or confirm relatively close relationships. One line only.
- Family Finder Autosomal DNA – testers carry DNA from all ancestral lines for the first 5 or 6 generations, then the amount of DNA inherited from each ancestor, and the ability to identify those ancestors diminishes with each generation.
- X-DNA – similar to the autosomes, but with a unique inheritance path that precludes inheritance from some ancestors but increases the amount of X-DNA inherited in each generation from those ancestors who do contribute X-DNA to descendants. X-DNA is included in the Family Finder test at FamilyTreeDNA, but not at all other vendors.

FamilyTreeDNA provides numerous download files that can be utilized in a variety of ways. Many people upload their raw autosomal DNA file to either MyHeritage or GEDmatch, or both. Neither Ancestry nor 23andMe accept uploads, but some customers from those vendors upload elsewhere. Serious genealogists should test or upload at all four primary vendors.

Ancestry does not provide segment information for your matches. Genealogists who utilize segment matching to identify and confirm ancestors hope that their Ancestry matches will test at or upload their DNA file to other testing vendors, or GEDmatch. I've written several articles, one per vendor, to encourage people to upload. Please feel free to share widely.[245]

FamilyTreeDNA provides many features and tools for each type of DNA to assist genealogists and accepts uploads from 23andMe[246], Ancestry, and MyHeritage.

TIP: Don't forget that if you have questions or challenges using the FamilyTreeDNA products, you can call, email, or computer chat with their support department.

In addition to tools provided by FamilyTreeDNA, I utilize both DNAPainter and Genetic Affairs extensively, although they are not the only third-party tools available.

That said, how do we weave these threads together?

I suggest you begin by creating a DNA Pedigree Chart.

245 https://dna-explained.com/2019/11/04/dna-file-upload-download-and-transfer-instructions-to-and-from-dna-testing-companies/

246 Uploads are currently paused from 23andMe.

Creating a DNA Pedigree Chart

Every genealogist has embarked on an ancestral journey of discovery, and every ancestor has a story. Who doesn't want to know more about the people who, quite literally, contributed the ingredients in the recipe of who we are?

Significant chapters of that story, Y-DNA and mitochondrial DNA, cannot be discovered without those specific DNA tests. Both of those tools provide numerous features.

Matching may help you break down brick walls, and other tools show you where your ancestors came from, both recently and further back in time.

Remember that both Y-DNA and mitochondrial DNA do not dilute in each generation, so they reach back much further than autosomal DNA, which means you may not recognize matches, especially with mitochondrial DNA, where the surname changes in each generation. However, when you do establish a connection, the victories are huge because so many female ancestors have lost their birth surnames, creating seemingly insurmountable brick walls.

Additional answers may emerge as more people test, and testers correlate their ancestral trees. That's one of the reasons I use Genetic Affairs, where the construction of matching trees is one of their features.

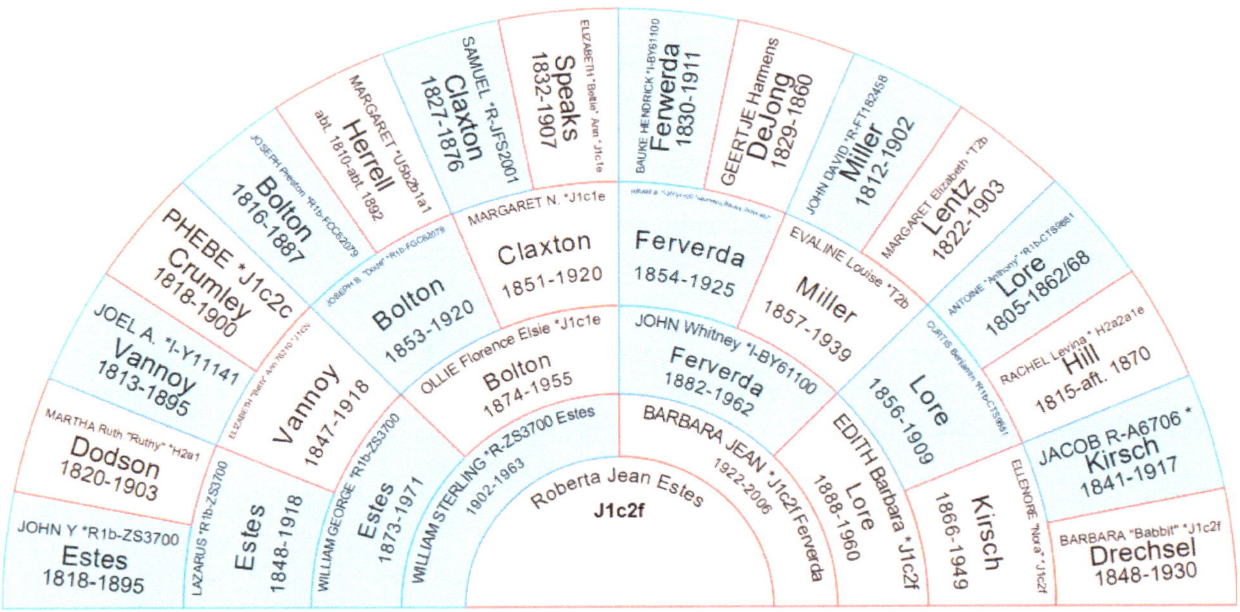

In my genealogy software on my computer, I store my ancestor's haplogroups as a middle name, then display my tree as a fan or other chart. Alternatively, you could use the haplogroup as a name suffix.

Never include haplogroup information as any part of a name in a tree in a public database. Using a haplogroup as part of the name in a public tree interferes with name searches, which in turn will interfere with that vendor's tools. That doesn't help you or anyone else.

To create a DNA pedigree chart, I recommend beginning by testing your own mitochondrial DNA, which everyone inherits from their mother. If you're a male, take the Big Y test to obtain your most granular and specific results.

Then, by working your way back in your tree, I suggest that you test relatives who descend appropriately from ancestors whose Y-DNA or mitochondrial DNA you don't have.

For example, if you're a female, you need your father's Y-DNA, which he inherited from his father, and his mitochondrial DNA, which he inherited from his mother.

If your father is available to test, he can take both tests for you and will receive matches, haplogroups, and more. If your father isn't available, his full brothers also carry the same Y-DNA and mitochondrial DNA as your father.

For each ancestor in your tree, view downstream descendants[247] to see who carries their Y-DNA or mitochondrial DNA. I utilize public databases to peruse trees to identify relevant living testers:

- WikiTree, which includes both Y-DNA and mtDNA information, along with the ability to message those descendants[248]
- Geni
- FamilySearch
- MyHeritage trees, SmartMatches and Theories of Family Relativity[249]
- Ancestry trees and ThruLines[250]
- Relatives at RootsTech before and during RootsTech[251]

I offer DNA testing scholarships for the appropriate descendants of ancestors whose Y-DNA and mitochondrial DNA information I don't yet have. I request that they join a family project so that I can view their results and explain those results to them when testing is complete.

When I provide DNA testing scholarships for my family members, I also add a Family Finder test. I fully believe in testing as much as possible and striking while the iron is hot. You may not be able to obtain permission to upgrade later, or they may pass away, and the stored DNA may no longer be viable.

TIP: With autosomal testing, you will match all 2nd cousins or closer, along with many people who are related more distantly.

247 https://dna-explained.com/2020/08/20/search-techniques-for-y-and-mitochondrial-dna-test-candidates/

248 https://dna-explained.com/2014/11/07/wikitree-makes-finding-relationships-with-dna-matches-easier/

249 https://dna-explained.com/2022/07/08/tips-tricks-for-working-with-theories-of-family-relativity/

250 https://dna-explained.com/2020/02/22/optimizing-your-tree-at-ancestry-for-more-hints-dna-thrulines/

251 https://dna-explained.com/2022/03/16/hurry-relatives-at-rootstech-ends-march-25-search-for-y-mitochondrial-dna-cousins-while-you-can/

Chapter 11

CREATING YOUR STEP-BY-STEP ROADMAP

What are the steps in your DNA journey at FamilyTreeDNA? Why is each step necessary, both in terms of testing and utilizing third-party tools for genetic genealogy? Let's make a list.

- Take a Family Finder autosomal and a full sequence mitochondrial DNA (mtFull) test. Everyone, males, and females, can take both of these.
- If you've already taken an autosomal DNA test elsewhere, you can upload your DNA raw data file to FamilyTreeDNA and then just pay $19 to unlock the advanced features.
- To obtain all matches possible, upload your raw DNA file to MyHeritage and GEDmatch.
- If you're a male, order or upgrade to the Big Y-700 DNA test.
- Create your DNA pedigree chart by testing your relatives to obtain your ancestors' Y-DNA and mitochondrial DNA information.
- Create a tree at or upload a tree to FamilyTreeDNA.[252]

Mitochondrial and Y- DNA

- View your matches, noting their earliest known ancestor.
- Review your matches' trees.
- View the matches map beginning with the closest, GD 0, mtFull test results, then view increasingly distant matches to determine where your matches' ancestors were from.
- Correlate possible history associated with the map pattern, above.
- Utilize various methods to increase Y-DNA and mtDNA match information.[253]
- View haplogroup information on the public mtDNA tree and Discover, once mitochondrial information is added there.

---

252 In November 2023, FamilyTreeDNA announced that they will integrate their trees with MyHeritage. https://dna-explained.com/2023/12/11/familytreedna-2023-update-past-present-and-future/

253 https://dna-explained.com/2019/07/03/mitochondrial-dna-part-4-techniques-for-doubling-your-useful-matches/

- Record your ancestors' haplogroups in your personal tree and check periodically to see if they have been upgraded.
- Utilize Advanced Matching to determine Y-DNA and mitochondrial DNA matches that also match autosomally.
- Review group projects for lineages and ancestors.
- Check your ancestors at WikiTree to see if other genealogists report having taken either Y-DNA or mitochondrial DNA tests that represent that ancestor.
- For Y-DNA, utilize the Discover™ Haplogroup Reports tool. A similar mitochondrial DNA Discover™ tool is anticipated soon.

Autosomal DNA

- Test close relatives, but not your descendants, who only have the DNA you gave them.
- Test both of your parents, if possible. This provides you with the ability to see if your matches match you, plus a parent, which immediately identifies which side they match you on.
- If both of your parents have tested, you don't need to test siblings.
- If both of your parents **have NOT** tested, test all of your full in addition to any half-siblings from the parent(s) who have not tested.
- Test all aunts and uncles unless both grandparents from that side have tested.
- If your family member has tested, testing their child won't help you genealogically.
- Link identified family members to their profile card on your tree to enable paternal and maternal family matching, aka bucketing.
- Review shared matches to determine who you share with known matches.
- Utilize the Matrix to determine if your matches also match each other.
- Utilize the Chromosome Browser to view matching segments. If your matches are all bucketed to the same parent, then segments are automatically phased, and people matching you on the same segment on that parent's side should all triangulate. This is only true for bucketed or phased matches on the same segment on the same parent's side.
- To download your matching segments for painting at DNAPainter, click on "Download Segments" on the Chromosome Browser while displaying those matches.[254]
- You can also paint your segments easily for each individual match. I paint each of mine as I identify our common ancestors.

254 This feature has been temporarily paused due to the 23andMe data exposure.

- To sort and view matches by segment for all matches, download your segment file by clicking on the Chromosome Browser WITHOUT selecting matches and then clicking on "Download All Segments."[255]
- To identify segments by maternal or paternal side if bucketed, download your Match file[256] and integrate it with the Chromosome Browser Results segment file, as instructed.
- After identifying your MRCA, most recent common ancestor, or ancestral couple, make a note on your match, and paint the match at DNAPainter.
- View myOrigins to identify your population segments, paying particular attention to minority segments which may help you identify specific ancestors.
- Use Compare Origins to compare with matches to identify common minority ancestry with other testers.
- Paint chromosome segments, including myOrigins population segments, at DNAPainter.

X-DNA

- Review X matches to see if the inheritance path provides clues as to how your match is related to you.
- Refer to the X-inheritance chart to eliminate possible common ancestors.
- When X-ancestors are identified for a match, use shared matching and advanced matches to determine if other X matches descend from that same ancestor.
- The X chromosome of males is already phased because males only inherit their mother's X, so all people who match a male tester on a valid (not IBC) segment must be related to him on his mother's side.
- Leverage X matches to find more X matches from the same ancestor.

255 This feature is currently paused.

256 This download is currently paused.

Genetic Affairs

I created a Genetic Affairs Instructions and Resource article to provide a centralized repository for articles about using Genetic Affairs.[257]

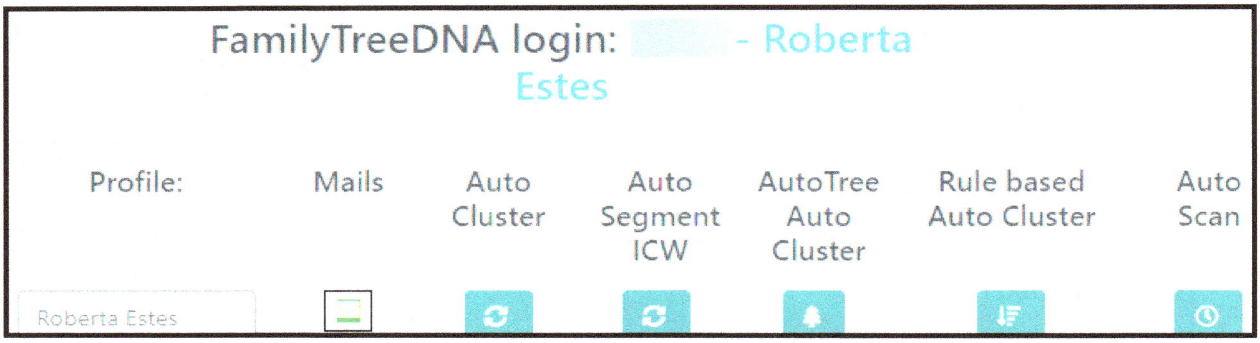

Genetic Affairs provides features and tools based on the vendor where you tested and the features they provide. Genetic Affairs automates the analysis process with several advanced tools. Roadmap steps to take include:

- Run an AutoCluster to determine groupings of people who carry the same DNA and therefore descend in some way from the same ancestral line, barring identical by descent inheritance on their side.
- Generally, your first four large clusters indicate your grandparents, although that may not be true if your grandparents are from a significantly under-sampled population, causing disproportionately fewer matches on that side.
- Grey cells indicate people who match in two (or more) clusters. Don't disregard them, as they are important and connect your lineages. They also provide clues about how your clusters are interrelated.
- Endogamy makes clustering more difficult and often results in a very large single cluster because, literally, everyone is somehow related to everyone else. AutoCluster at MyHeritage is optimized for endogamy.
- Run AutoTree, including Y-DNA and mtDNA (mitochondrial) selections to automatically construct trees with common ancestors among your matches, even if the people in their tree aren't in yours. This is an absolutely wonderful tool and is the only way to achieve automated DNA matching plus "tree matching" for common ancestors at FamilyTreeDNA.
- Run AutoSegment ICW, which clusters overlapping segments, then removes people who do not match in common with each other as being identical by chance. Generally, what is left will be triangulated segments, and based on who is in the cluster, you should be able to assign the DNA to an ancestral couple.
- Paint your various clusters to their appropriate ancestor at DNAPainter, which imports Genetic Affairs cluster files.

257 https://dna-explained.com/2020/08/13/genetic-affairs-instructions-and-resources/

DNAPainter

The purpose of DNAPainter is to paint and organize your DNA matches, attributed to ancestors by segment, from multiple vendors. DNAPainter stores these segments, by match, in one location, superimposed on images of your chromosomes. I created a DNAPainter Instructions and Resources article to provide a centralized repository for articles about how to use DNAPainter.[258] Roadmap steps to take are:

- Identify your matches as maternal or paternal, minimally, and paint them to the appropriate side. DNAPainter does provide a "both" or "unknown" side.
- If I have a match that I know descends from two unrelated lines, I paint them twice, once to map them to each couple, noting that in the DNAPainter description. One or the other painted match will eventually conflict with other identified ancestors on that segment and will need to be removed. It's also possible that if the match matches me on multiple segments, one or some segments will be from one ancestral line, and others will be from the other.
- Upload maternal and paternal bucketed matches[259] from FamilyTreeDNA to paint in bulk, assigning to the proper side.

Painting matches at DNAPainter is fun, but it's also an investment in the long haul and provides a single, one-stop, one-source reference for identified ancestors and segments.

You Don't Know What You Don't Know

The wonderful news is that there's a lot of information available at FamilyTreeDNA and in this book, but I also know that this journey can be a bit overwhelming from time to time. That's why I've broken this process into steps you begin by testing your Y-DNA and mitochondrial DNA, taking a Family Finder test, or transferring your DNA file from another vendor.

Begin this process wherever you are today, then add various tests for yourself, and other family members.

We are never truly "done" with genetic genealogy, just like we are never "done" with traditional genealogy. The genetic aspect provides us with many additional tools that allow us to scale, and then crash through brick walls that were previously insurmountable.

Unlike paper records, as more people test, our genetic investment continues to grow and contributes to information and answers. It's evergreen.

We test ourselves with every test possible and test others to focus on our ancestors because you don't know what you don't know.

Is there someplace you need to focus? An ancestor who is eluding you? If so, review the Roadmap steps with your roadblock in mind and evaluate what you can do to provide evidence or garner new information.

Remember, the longest journey begins with a single step.

Best of luck to you on your journey of joy. May you be rewarded with many newly revealed ancestors.

---

258 https://dna-explained.com/2019/10/14/dnapainter-instructions-and-resources/

259 This download is currently paused.

GLOSSARY

23andMe – Autosomal DNA testing company founded in 2006. Began DNA testing for genealogy matching in 2007. 23andMe focuses on health and provides both genealogy and health/traits testing, either together or separately. The number of matches is limited, but up to 5000 matches can be viewed with an annual membership subscription. 23andMe does not accept uploads from other vendors and is the only vendor that does not support family trees.[260] FamilyTreeDNA accepts 23andMe DNA file uploads.[261]

Adenine - Adenine, Cytosine, Guanine, and Thymine are the four base nucleotides, or DNA words, that comprise your DNA and are represented by the letters, A, C, G, and T.

Admixture – In the genetic genealogy world, admixture occurs when a person has more than one discrete population in their makeup. For example, someone who is 100% Swedish has no admixture. The NCBI[262] definition is, "Admixture occurs when individuals from two or more previously isolated populations interbreed.".

Advanced Matches - A tool at FamilyTreeDNA that provides the ability to filter for the intersection of several different kinds of matches, including different levels of Y-DNA, mitochondrial DNA, Family Finder autosomal, X-DNA, projects, and surnames.

Age Estimate - In the Discover™ Haplogroup Reports, also known as the Discover™ tool, under Scientific Details, the probability plot shows the range of most likely times when the haplogroup you are viewing was formed.

Allele - Either A (Adenine), C (Cytosine), G (Guanine), or T (Thymine) that is found at a specific DNA location. Every person will have two at each location, one from each parent, although the two can be the same value.

Ancestral Haplotype – Specifically in Y-DNA, reconstructing the original STR markers that your ancestor carried. Some genetic genealogists also seek to reconstruct the autosomal haplotype of ancestors through their descendants.

Ancestral Locations - Location where your ancestor in a specific lineage is known to have originated. It's important to complete this information at FamilyTreeDNA because ancestral locations are used in multiple ways to increase accuracy and enhance your experience.

---

260 https://www.23andme.com/membership

261 This feature is currently on pause due to the data exposure at 23andme, but expected to resume in 2024.

262 National Center for Biotechnology Information https://en.wikipedia.org/wiki/National_Center_for_Biotechnology_Information

Ancestral Origins – For Y-DNA and mitochondrial DNA, FamilyTreeDNA compiles the location information provided by your matches about their ancestors and reports by country.

Ancestral Path - In the Discover™ Haplogroup Reports, also known as the Discover™ tool, the haplogroup path, or steps, between the haplogroup you are viewing, and the foundation or genesis of the base haplogroup for that major haplogroup branch. For example, R-M207 is the base or beginning of Y-DNA haplogroup R.

Ancestral Surnames - List of ancestral surnames to be entered so that the system can match surnames between you and your autosomal matches. Ancestral surnames were NOT always harvested from your tree, but FamilyTreeDNA introduced a feature at some time that harvested direct line ancestors only when you upload a GEDCOM. Check your Ancestral Surnames and update them as necessary. Ancestral surnames allow matches to quickly scan names with locations for commonalities.

Ancestral State – In DNA, the original or unmutated state. As compared to Derived or mutated values.

Ancestry – Ancestry.com is a genealogy company that offers both genealogical records for research and AncestryDNA autosomal DNA testing. To fully utilize DNA results, including advanced tools, the ability to view other tester's complete trees and other benefits, a subscription to their genealogical services is required.[263] Some DNA features fall under the "Plus" category, requiring a subscription.[264] Ancestry does not accept uploads from other vendors. FamilyTreeDNA accepts Ancestry uploads except for Ancestry's Health product.

Ancestry Chromosome Painting – At 23andMe, painting the tester's different ethnicity segments on their chromosome pairs.

Ancient Connections - A fun feature provided by FamilyTreeDNA through Discover™ that shows ancient connections, based on archaeology digs and academic publications, along with how closely in time you share a common ancestor.

Ancient DNA – DNA retrieved from burials at archaeological sites.

ancientOrigins - In Family Finder results, testers' European origins (for those who have them) are divided between Metal Age Invaders, Farmers, and Hunter-Gatherers based on archaeological digs.

AutoCluster – A visualization tool created by Genetic Affairs using cluster technology that groups your matches into colorful clusters based on common matching, including who matches each other in addition to who matches you.

AutoPedigree - The option at Genetic Affairs to create an AutoTree based on your matches' common ancestors and include hypotheses about how the tester fits into the auto-generated trees.

AutoSegment – At Genetic Affairs, uses the Chromosome Browser Results file to cluster based on overlapping segments. AutoSegment+ICW also enriches the results by discarding data where the matches do not also match each other, removing identical by chance matches.

---

263 https://support.ancestry.com/s/article/AncestryDNA-with-an-Ancestry-Subscription-US-1460090085520-3160

264 https://dna-explained.com/2023/09/27/ancestry-updates-ethnicity-introduces-new-features-pushes-some-behind-paywall/

Autosomal DNA – 50% of autosomal DNA is inherited from each parent for Chromosomes 1-22, which are referred to as the autosomes. Although not an autosome, the X chromosome is sometimes included in autosomal DNA discussion and products (FamilyTreeDNA and 23andMe,) but not always (Ancestry and MyHeritage) due to its unique inheritance path.

Autosomes – Chromosomes 1-22

AutoTree - The option at Genetic Affairs to create an AutoCluster, then assemble the trees of your matches with common ancestors, even if you don't share those ancestors or have them in your tree. Can select options to include either or both Y-DNA and mitochondrial DNA in the tree generation.

Back Mutation – When a mutation has occurred at a specific location, then in a subsequent generation mutates back to the original value.

BAM File - A specialized file that can be ordered for $100 after taking the Big Y test that contains all of the NGS scan data for the entire Y chromosome. This massive file requires specialized software to read the contents and is of no use unless you are uploading Y-DNA results to a third-party vendor who requires a BAM file, or you have and can use that special software.

Base Pair – A base is a single location in your DNA. A base pair is found in autosomal DNA when a pair of nucleotides – one from your father and one from your mother - is found at a single location. A base or base pair is the smallest measure in your DNA.

BCE - Before Current Era (BCE) has the same meaning as BC but is expressed in a more secular way preferred by scientists and scholars. 1000 BCE is the same as 1000 BC, or approximately 3000 years ago.

Beneficiary Information – Under your Account Settings, FamilyTreeDNA provides the ability for you to designate either an individual or a specific group project administrator as your beneficiary for your tests at FamilyTreeDNA after your decease.

Big Y, currently the Big Y-700 – At FamilyTreeDNA, a Y-DNA test of discovery that sequences the majority of the Y chromosome in order to determine the most refined haplogroup and discover mutations that provide additional refined family genealogical information. Known as the Big Y test, previously known as the Big Y-500. The current version is the Big Y-700 test.

Big Y Matches - Big Y matches are SNP matches, not STR matches, which are separate. Men will be matched on the Big Y if they have 30 or fewer SNP mutation differences, which equates to approximately 1500 years.

Block Tree - A feature of the Big Y test that provides a unique family-style pedigree type tree showing nearby haplogroups, matches, and the country where their earliest known ancestor was found.

Bucketing - Also called Family Matching. Based on uploading or creating a tree and linking known matches to their profile cards on that tree, FamilyTreeDNA can bucket (at least some of) your matches maternally, paternally, or both. Testing and linking both parents produces the best result. The number of people that can be assigned maternally or paternally (or both) is a direct result of how much of your chromosomes are covered by a match that you linked in your tree maternally or paternally.

CE - Common Era (CE) is the same as AD but expressed in a more secular way preferred by scientists and scholars. 2000 CE is the same as 2000 AD, or just the year 2000.

Centimorgan (cM) – Written as cM, a centimorgan is a unit of measure on a chromosome. Vendors establish a minimum cM distance, as well as a minimum number of SNPs within the segment of DNA that qualifies as a match for autosomal DNA matching.

Centromere – The "waist"[265] of the chromosome that joins the two arms. The DNA found in the centromere is often of inferior quality and cannot be used for genetic genealogy matching. That region is omitted, and matches spanning the centromere are counted as a contiguous matching segment.

Chromosome Browser - Using your 23 chromosomes as the palette, your shared segments with individual matches are painted onto each chromosome. FamilyTreeDNA provides for up to 7 matches to be displayed simultaneously.

Chromosome Painting – The third-party tool, DNAPainter, facilitates two types of chromosome painting. Users can paint segments of their chromosomes with matches in order to associate segments of their DNA with specific ancestors, or they can upload their ethnicity results from either 23andMe or FamilyTreeDNA, both of whom provide chromosome painting as part of their autosomal DNA product. Combining the two types of chromosome painting provides the ability to match specific ethnicity segments with the ancestor from whom the segment descended.

Chromosome Painting, myOrigins3 - A chromosome painting is provided for myOrigins3 customers, which paints the various population-assigned segments on the tester's chromosomes.

Coding Region - In mitochondrial DNA, a stretch of approximately 15,425 base pairs outside of the hypervariable regions. This stretch of DNA contains some genes - hence the description, "coding region." The HVR1, HVR2, and Coding Region are tested with the full mitochondrial sequence (mtFull) test.

Compare Origins – At FamilyTreeDNA, a tool that allows customers to compare their ethnicity with their Family Finder matches and also displays the locations of their matches' Y-DNA and mitochondrial DNA earliest known ancestors (EKA) on a map.

Country Frequency - In the Discover™ Haplogroup Reports, also known as the Discover™ tool, a heat map and table view show how frequently a specific haplogroup is found in countries around the world in the FamilyTreeDNA database.

Country Report - For both Y-DNA and mitochondrial DNA, on the Public Haplotrees, the Country Reports provide statistics and totals about countries around the world where specific haplogroups are found.

CRS (Cambridge Reference Sequence) - The mitochondrial DNA reference sequence known as the CRS was first published in 1981 using the DNA of a volunteer in Cambridge, England. That sequence was subsequently updated to correct errors in 1999 and is designated as the rCRS, or revised Cambridge Reference Sequence. The rCRS haplogroup is H2a2a1.

265 https://learn.familytreedna.com/autosomal-ancestry/universal-dna-matching/centromeres-located-autosomal-chromosome/

Cytosine - Adenine, Cytosine, Guanine, and Thymine are the four base nucleotides, or DNA words, that comprise your DNA and are represented in genetic genealogy by the letters A, C, G, and T.

Deletion – A deletion occurs when a segment of DNA is deleted, meaning there is no longer any DNA at that location or those locations. In Y-DNA STRs, this results in a null value, or 0, meaning nothing is there, and in mitochondrial DNA, this results in a "d" appearing after the location as in 8281d.

Derived - Derived means that you have a mutation at a specific location. An ancestral state is the opposite, which means you do not have a mutation and instead match the reference model.

Discover™ Haplogroup Reports - A Y-DNA tool that provides your Haplogroup Story, Country Frequency, Notable Connections, Migration Map, Globetrekker[266], Ancient Connections, Time Tree, Ancestral Path, Suggested Projects, Age Estimates, Scientific Details, and the Haplogroup Compare[267] feature. New features are added regularly.

DNA – Deoxyribonucleic acid is a molecule that coils into a helix and provides genetic instructions for reproducing.[268]

DNA for Native American Genealogy - My book detailing how to use DNA and other sources to find and identify your Native American ancestors. Answers the most common questions and provides a research checklist. Available from Genealogical.com[269] or Amazon.

DNA Pedigree Chart – Incorporating your and your ancestors' Y-DNA and mitochondrial DNA haplogroups into your genealogy research and pedigree chart by finding appropriate people to test, or who have tested.

DNA Sequencing – The process in a genetics laboratory that reads and reports the sequence of nucleotides in your DNA.

DNA Testing – For genealogy, swab or spit tests submitted to testing companies to obtain various types of results, including Y-DNA, mitochondrial DNA, autosomal DNA ethnicity breakdown, and matching information with other testers.

DNA Tests – Genealogical DNA tests are available from four major vendors who provide an autosomal DNA product, including matching. Each vendor provides unique features to their customers. FamilyTreeDNA also provides Y-DNA and mitochondrial DNA testing for genealogy in addition to their Family Finder autosomal product.

DNAeXplain, DNA-Explained - My free website and blog at www.dnaexplain.com where hundreds of articles can be found about how to use genetic genealogy. Keyword searchable.

---

266 https://dna-explained.com/2023/08/04/globetrekker-a-new-feature-for-big-y-customers-from-familytreedna/

267 https://dna-explained.com/2023/10/11/new-discover-tool-compare-haplogroups-more-at-familytreedna/

268 https://en.wikipedia.org/wiki/DNA

269 https://genealogical.com/

DNAPainter – A third-party application created by Jonny Perl that provides a variety of tools, including the ability to associate segments with ancestors and paint those segments on the blank chromosomes of the tester in order to identify matches with common DNA segments, which infers common ancestors.

Double Helix – The familiar shape of both strands of the DNA molecule.

Download DNA - Downloading a file of your raw, sequenced DNA results, often in order to upload it to a different vendor. FamilyTreeDNA accepts uploads from major vendors.

DYS Markers - DYS locations are the names of Y-DNA STR markers, such as DYS393. D stands for DNA, Y stands for the Y chromosome, and S is a unique segment.

Earliest Known Ancestor (EKA) - When referring to Y-DNA and mitochondrial DNA, this means the earliest known ancestor on your direct patrilineal line, meaning your father's father's father's direct paternal line, and for mitochondrial DNA, your direct matrilineal line, your mother's mother's mother's direct maternal line.

EKA – See Earliest Known Ancestor.

Endogamy – The custom of marrying within a community or clan. In genetic terms, the result is that many of the community members share common DNA segments of distant founder ancestors, which increases the number of autosomal matches, sometimes significantly. Endogamy often causes matches to appear to be more closely related than they are.

End-of-branch Haplogroup - The end-of-branch haplogroup or SNP is the most refined possible for a tester with the most high-resolution test possible. Today, for Y-DNA, that's the Big Y-700 test. A man with Private Variants may receive a new haplogroup if another man tests who matches his Private Variants, causing a new haplogroup to be formed. This is contrasted with the end-of-line haplogroup, which is the highest resolution haplogroup at the testing level of the participant - which may or may not be the Big Y.

End-of-line Haplogroup - For Y-DNA and mitochondrial DNA, youngest or closest in time haplogroup at the level that the individual has been tested. If the man has only taken a higher-level test, his end-of-line haplogroup is the haplogroup determined by that test. The end-of-branch haplogroup is the most refined haplogroup possible for an individual, given the best and most high-resolution test, which is currently the Big Y-700.

Ethnicity – Generally speaking, a social group that has a common national or cultural tradition and who identify with each other based on shared attributes. In genetic genealogy, the term ethnicity is used to describe the breakdown of populations and geographies that can be determined (estimated) through the use of population genetics and comparison to reference populations.

Extra Mutations - Mitochondrial DNA mutations in addition to the tester's haplogroup-defining mutations.

False Positive Match - A match that is actually identical by chance (IBC) and not identical by descent (IBD,) meaning it's not a valid match, but without further evaluation, appears to be valid.

Family Finder - FamilyTreeDNA's autosomal DNA test that includes maternal/paternal Family Matching, also known as bucketing, myOrigins, population-based chromosome painting, and ancientOrigins.

Family Matching – Assigning autosomal Family Finder matches maternally, paternally, or both, based on testers linking known relatives to their profile card in the tester's family tree.

Family Tree – See Tree.

FamilyTreeDNA – Pioneering genealogical DNA testing company that offers Y-DNA, mitochondrial DNA, and autosomal DNA testing through their Family Finder product. FamilyTreeDNA's database includes results from people who tested beginning in 2000. FamilyTreeDNA provides the most advanced sequencing and tools for both Y-DNA and mitochondrial DNA. FamilyTreeDNA does not require a subscription for full access if you test with them but has a small unlock fee for advanced tools if you upload your DNA from another vendor.

FASTA File - A special format industry-standard file used for downloading mitochondrial DNA. FASTA files require specialized software to read the nucleotide results.[270]

First Nations – In Canada, groups of indigenous people aren't called tribes, but are referred to as First Nations, Metis, (who are mixed), and Inuit peoples, (who are considered to be circumpolar), arriving at a later date. This terminology is not without discord.[271]

FMS (full mitochondrial sequence, also the mtFull test) - The highest and most refined level mitochondrial DNA test that tests the entire 16,569 locations in the mitochondrial genome, providing the most refined matches and haplogroup. The full mitochondrial sequence includes the HVR1, HVR2, and Coding Regions.

Full Sequence – For mitochondrial DNA, the full sequence refers to testing all 16,569 locations of the mitochondria, as compared to testing smaller portions. Early tests only tested between 500-1000 positions for matching. Today, some autosomal DNA vendors who don't provide mitochondrial DNA tests separately do target-test a few SNP locations in order to provide customers with an estimated high-level haplogroup.

GEDCOM File - GEDCOM is a standard file format for transferring, downloading, and uploading genealogy family trees to and from various genealogy software programs. By exporting your file from a genealogy program in GEDCOM format and uploading it to FamilyTreeDNA, or elsewhere, you don't need to reconstruct your tree at each site.

GEDmatch – A third-party DNA matching database that provides tools independent from any of the testing vendors. GEDmatch does not perform testing.

270 https://en.wikipedia.org/wiki/FASTA_format

271 https://www.rcaanc-cirnac.gc.ca/eng/1100100013785/1529102490303

Genealogical Proof Standard (GPS) – The Genealogy Proof Standard was created as a form of guidance provided to genealogists to ensure thorough, accurate research and reasonable conclusions drawn from as much information as possible. DNA testing, especially Y-DNA and mitochondrial, is an important part of the Genealogy Proof Standard when it's possible to locate testers.[272 273 274]

Genetic Affairs – A company founded by Evert-Jan Blom that provides clustering technology through a variety of tools where customers can view clusters of matches that match each other in addition to the tester. Clusters indicate a common ancestor between cluster members.

Genetic Ancestor - Ancestor whose DNA you carry today, as opposed to an ancestor distant enough in your tree that you did not inherit any of their DNA.

Genetic Distance (GD) - For Y-DNA and mitochondrial DNA, the number of mutations difference between two testers at a specific level of testing. A smaller number means a closer match. A GD of zero (GD 0 or GD0) is an exact match.

Genetic Genealogy – The application of genetic tools to genealogy. Genetic genealogy has the ability to confirm ancestors, reveal ancestors and relationships, and, conversely, refutes both relationships and genealogy, including close relationships. Genetic genealogy results must be interpreted accurately and are sometimes inconclusive.

Genetic Sequence – Some number of adjacent DNA locations that are used for comparison to other testers in genealogy. Identical ranges of specifically selected locations that match are genealogically relevant. Mutations found in genetic sequences are used in both mitochondrial and Y-DNA to determine haplogroups.

Genotype – Your nucleotide results at a specific location or locations, or, more broadly, the genetic make-up of an organism.

Group Projects - Also referred to as Projects, provided by FamilyTreeDNA and formed by volunteer administrators around a surname, a geographic region, a group of people, such as American Indians, or a haplogroup. Testers join projects that are relevant to their genealogical research to collaborate with others. Families can form private Group Projects.

Group Time Tree - Similar to the Discover™ Time Tree, but includes only the results within that project, and includes the Earliest Known Ancestors (EKA) of testers. Individuals are displayed in sub-groups as grouped by project administrators.

Guanine - Adenine, Cytosine, Guanine, and Thymine are the four base nucleotides, or DNA words, that comprise your DNA and are represented in genetic genealogy by the letters A, C, G, and T.

Haplogroup – For Y-DNA and mitochondrial DNA, separately, a group of specific mutations that identify people who share a common genetic clan. Haplogroups, based on a series of mutations, can be traced forward and backward in time. Y-DNA and mitochondrial DNA haplogroup names are not connected or related to each other.

---

272 https://www.familysearch.org/wiki/en/Genealogical_Proof_Standard

273 https://bcgcertification.org/ethics-standards/

274 https://www.familysearch.org/wiki/en/The_Genealogical_Proof_Standard_(National_Institute)

Haplotree & SNPs – A feature provided for FamilyTreeDNA Y-DNA testers showing the entire Y-DNA haplotree in pedigree format, including all tested, untested, and equivalent SNPs. Additionally, this tree can be displayed reflecting geographic locations, surnames, and projects relevant to each haplogroup.

Haplogroup Origins - For Y-DNA and mitochondrial DNA, FamilyTreeDNA compiles the location information provided by your matches about their ancestors, then reports by haplogroup and country, respectively.

Haplogroup Story - In the Discover™ Haplogroup Reports, also known as the Discover™ tool, a summary of countries where your haplogroup is found, its age, parent haplogroup, descendant haplogroups, and a summary pedigree.

Haplotree - For both Y-DNA and mitochondrial DNA, the tree of mankind or womankind that reaches from the tester back to Y-line Adam or Mitochondrial Eve, the earliest male and female to have descendants living today.

Haplotype - Your individual DNA results at specific adjacent locations that are generally inherited together.

Heteroplasmies - Mutations, especially in mitochondrial DNA, where multiple nucleotides are found at the same location at a frequency greater than 20%. Multiple combined nucleotide values above 20% are represented by letters other than A, C, G, and T.

Human Reference Genome - The expected value at a specific genetic location is determined by the value found in the Human Reference Genome (HRG), generally indicated by the word, "reference." The Human Reference genome is updated periodically and referred to as the Genome Reference Consortium (GRC), followed by "h" (for human) plus a number. The current version (in 2023) is GRCh38, also abbreviated as hg38.

HVR1 - Hypervariable region 1 (HVR1) in mitochondrial DNA, extends from location 16,001-16,569. In early DNA testing days, people could purchase just the HVR1 region test.

HVR2 - Hypervariable region 2 (HVR2) in mitochondrial DNA, extends from position 1-574. In early DNA testing days, people could purchase the HVR1+HVR2 tests to receive a total of about 1100 base pairs for matching. Today these tests have been replaced with the full sequence test that tests all 16,569 locations of the entire mitochondria.

Hypervariable Region – See HVR1 and HVR2.

IBC[275] – Identical by Chance (IBC) matches occur when autosomal DNA contributed by the mother and father just happens to align in such a way that a segment of DNA matches another individual. However, the match is not a valid genealogical match because it did not descend from an ancestor of either the mother or the father but was a result of random recombination between the two.

IBD – Identical by Descent (IBD) matches occur when the DNA between two individuals matches because they share a common ancestor, and their DNA descends from that ancestor through the tester's parent.

---

275 https://dna-explained.com/2016/03/10/concepts-identical-bydescent-state-population-and-chance/

IBS – Identical by State (IBS) matches occur when individuals are identical by descent, but the segments are small, generally under the matching thresholds of the vendors, and are a result of being members of a common population. IBS segments are used in population genetics for the assignment of ethnicity by mapping DNA segments to populations.

Identical by Chance – See IBC

Identical by Descent – See IBD

Identical by State - See IBS

Imputation – A scientific methodology designed to statistically estimate the DNA that would logically be found adjacent to known DNA locations, in order to fill in untested regions in situations where DNA raw data files are somewhat incompatible with each other. Incompatibility occurs when test chip versions change, and between different vendors' DNA tests. Imputation at FamilyTreeDNA is quite reliable.

Indigenous – The original inhabitants of a place. The exact definition and how the word is used varies depending on the circumstances. In terms of Native American people, regardless of their tribal or political affiliation, indigenous people are the people originally occupying the Americas prior to European contact or colonization. May also be referred to as aboriginal.

Inheritance – In genetic terms, DNA that people inherit from their parents. Everyone inherits exactly half of each parent's autosomal DNA on Chromosomes 1-22. For females, the X chromosome, number 23, is inherited in exactly the same way as the autosomes, but males only inherit an X chromosome from their mother. Males inherit a Y chromosome from their father, instead of an X,[276] which is what determines their sex. Males and females both inherit mitochondrial DNA from their mothers, but only females pass it on.

Insertion - Insertions happen when a copy error occurs, and multiple copies of a nucleotide(s) are duplicated and inserted between two other locations. In mitochondrial DNA, these are styled as 315.1C where .1 means one copy of a C has been inserted at location 315.

In Common With - Also known as Shared Matching. You select a match and then see which of your other matches they match "in common with" you.

Legitimate Match - A legitimate match, in autosomal DNA, means that the match is identical by descent, meaning that the person matches you because you both received the same segment of DNA from a common ancestor. The opposite of a false positive match.

Markers – Generally referred to in Y-DNA, meaning the STR markers used for genealogical matching. STR markers are tested in panels of 12, 25, 37, 67, and 111 markers and sold as Y-37 and Y-111 tests. The Big Y-700 test provides a minimum of 700 STR markers, including the 111 markers sold in the STR panel tests.

Matches Maps - For Y-DNA and mitochondrial DNA, a map showing the customer-provided locations for their earliest known ancestors (EKA).

276 Rare medical conditions where the X or Y chromosome is duplicated, such as XXY (Klinefelter Syndrome) and XYY (Jacobs Syndrome) exist, but are beyond the scope of this book.

Matching – Vendors compare the DNA of their customers and report matches above a minimum threshold determined by each vendor. It's up to the consumer to interpret the match for genealogical relevance.

Match Matrix – At FamilyTreeDNA, the Matrix tool allows for up to 10 autosomal matches to be selected for comparison to determine which of your matches also match each other.

Match Threshold – Y-DNA and mitochondrial DNA matches are determined by genetic distance (GD), meaning how many single location mutation differences two individuals can have and still be considered a match. An autosomal match threshold is defined by the minimum number of matching centimorgans (cMs) and a minimum number of SNPs. Vendors have different match threshold minimum criteria, and match thresholds change from time to time.

Maternal Side – Your mother's entire side of the tree, which is not to be confused with a direct matrilineal line which is your mother's mother's mother's direct line. Some vendors refer to mitochondrial DNA as your "maternal" DNA. Unfortunately, this leads to confusion about the mitochondrial DNA pathway, misunderstanding which ancestors contributed their mitochondrial DNA to descendants.

Matrilineal – The matrilineal line is your mother's mother's mother's direct line up your tree through only females, which is the lineage of everyone's mitochondrial DNA.

Matrix - Also called the Match Matrix. Autosomal testers can select up to 10 Family Finder matches to create a Matrix to determine if their matches also match each other.

Migration Maps – Y-DNA and mitochondrial DNA each have their own migration maps for each haplogroup showing their path within and outside of Africa.

Mitochondrial DNA (mtDNA) – DNA necessary in humans for the production of energy. However, genealogically speaking, mitochondrial DNA is a valuable tool for understanding our direct matrilineal line, both historically and in terms of genealogical matching.[277]

Mitochondrial Eve - Mitochondrial Eve is the earliest female to have descendants living today. All people worldwide descend from Mitochondrial Eve.

Mitochondrial Public Tree - FamilyTreeDNA's public, free mitochondrial DNA haplotree provides variants and country flags for each SNP confirmed haplogroup along with a Country Report.[278]

Missing Mutations - Especially in mitochondrial DNA, mutations expected to be found in a particular haplogroup, but are missing in a specific tester or group of testers.

MPE - misattributed parental event, see NPE

mtDNA – see Mitochondrial DNA.

mtDNA Journey - A video provided for mitochondrial DNA testers to explain their results. Includes a match to a famous historical figure. This may be replaced by something similar to the Y-DNA Discover™ Haplogroup Reports in the future.

---

277 https://en.wikipedia.org/wiki/Mitochondrial_DNA

278 https://www.familytreedna.com/public/mt-dna-haplotree/L

mtDNA Matches - People who match you at or below the mutation threshold for the level of test you are viewing.

mtFull – Full mitochondrial sequence, see FMS.

Mutation – A change at a DNA location that can (autosomal DNA) or will (Y-DNA and mitochondrial DNA) be passed to future generations.

MyHeritage – A genealogy company that offers both genealogical records for research and MyHeritageDNA autosomal DNA testing. Some features are only available with a premium subscription plan.[279] MyHeritage does accept uploads from other vendors and charges a small unlock fee for access to advanced tools. FamilyTreeDNA accepts uploads from MyHeritage for tests taken after May 2019.

MyOrigins or MyOrigins3 – At FamilyTreeDNA, their ethnicity or population estimate.

MyOrigins Chromosome Painting – At FamilyTreeDNA, their chromosome painting is based on populations and provides a visual representation of where ethnicity segments are located on the tester's chromosomes.

MyOrigins Sharing - At FamilyTreeDNA, the ability to view the ethnicity results, Y-DNA, and mitochondrial DNA Earliest Known Ancestor (EKA) locations of autosomal matches who opt-in to the Origins Sharing feature.

Named Variants - In the Big Y test, a Named Variant is a mutation that has been identified, labeled, and, generally, placed on the Y-DNA haplotree if it passes quality assurance. Unnamed variants are private mutations that have not yet been named because multiple men in this lineage have not yet tested positive for this mutation, or because the reads at that location are not reliable.

NGS Sequencing - NGS, or next-generation sequencing, utilizes parallel scan sequencing technology as compared to the older type of sequencing that reads specific targeted allele locations.[280] [281]

Notable Connections - A fun feature provided by FamilyTreeDNA's Discover™ tool that shows notable connections, both famous and infamous, along with how closely in time you're related.

Novel Variant – See Private Variant.

NPE - Non-parental event, not-parent-expected, non-paternal event - all names for the scenario where, via DNA testing, one or both parents are discovered to not be the biological parent of the tester. This phrase is more commonly applied to the discovery that only one parent is not the parent expected, which is most often the father. Other terms sometimes used for these situations are undocumented adoption and MPE (Misattributed Parental Event).[282]

---

279 https://www.myheritage.com/pricing

280 https://www.illumina.com/science/technology/next-generation-sequencing.html

281 https://www.illumina.com/science/technology/next-generation-sequencing/ngs-vs-sanger-sequencing.html

282 https://dna-explained.com/2019/07/18/concepts-what-are-npes-and-mpes/

Nucleotides – Abbreviated as A, C, G, and T, Adenine, Cytosine, Guanine, and Thymine are the nucleotide building blocks of DNA and are composed of one base plus a sugar molecule and a phosphate molecule. Mutations occur when one nucleotide is substituted for another at a particular genetic location, or a deletion or insertion occurs.

Origins Sharing - The ability to share your myOrigins results with your matches. For Origins Sharing, both people must opt in.

Parental or Trio Phasing – When an autosomal DNA match occurs between two individuals, comparing that match's DNA to both individuals' parents verifies that the DNA descended from one parent and was not randomly combined between both parents to assemble in the child in a way that appears as a match to another human. The process of verifying matches against parents' DNA is known as parental or trio phasing, as compared to statistical or academic phasing that does not utilize the parents' DNA. Parental phasing is the most accurate way to assign specific nucleotides to either the maternal or paternal copy of the chromosome but isn't always possible when both parents aren't available for comparison.

Paternal Side – The entire father's side of the tree, which is not to be confused with a direct patrilineal line. Some vendors refer to Y-DNA as your "paternal" DNA. Unfortunately, this leads to confusion about the Y-DNA pathway, misunderstanding which ancestors contributed their Y-DNA to male-line descendants for testing.

Patrilineal – Your patrilineal line is your father's father's father's direct line on up the tree. In males, the patrilineal line is the source of the Y chromosome, and, in Western cultures, is generally the source of the male's surname as well. Therefore, Y-DNA matching and interpretation are often simplified because the most meaningful matches are generally those with the same surnames.

Phasing – Two types of phasing are used in genetic genealogy, parental or trio phasing and academic/statistical phasing. Phasing occurs when your DNA is assigned to either your maternal or paternal chromosomes, which facilitates phased matching.

Phylotree[283] – A publicly available resource that includes more than 5400 mitochondrial haplogroups, their defining mutations, and links to the NCBI (National Center for Biotechnology Information)[284] data uploads of associated mitochondrial sequences utilized in haplogroup definition. Phylotree is no longer updated.

Population Genetics - A specialized field of genetics that focuses on the composition of populations, their relationships to each other, changes within and interchange between populations, and their distribution around the world.

Population Segments - Segments attributed to various populations, and painted, in myOrigins. Population segments can be correlated with genealogy and attributed to specific ancestors.

Populations – Related inhabitants of a country or region. As pertains to genetic genealogy, testers are interested in information that connects them with their ancestors' historical populations.

283 http://www.phylotree.org/

284 https://www.ncbi.nlm.nih.gov/

Private Variant – Private variants are mutations that have been discovered during Big Y testing, but no one in your lineage yet matches that mutation, so a new haplogroup cannot be named. New haplogroups are "born" when two or more men in the same genetic lineage have matching private variants. I refer to private variants as "haplogroups in waiting."

Projects - Also known as Group Projects, provided by FamilyTreeDNA and formed by volunteer administrators around a surname, a geographic region, a group of people, such as American Indians, or a haplogroup. Testers join projects that are relevant to their genealogical research to collaborate with others.

Public Y-DNA and Mitochondrial Haplogroup Trees – Public, free Y-DNA[285] and mitochondrial DNA[286] haplotrees providing country flags for each SNP-confirmed haplogroup, Country Report, and, for the Y tree, a Surname Report.[287]

rCRS - The rCRS, or revised Cambridge Reference Sequence. The CRS is the mitochondrial DNA reference sequence first published in 1981 using the DNA of a volunteer in Cambridge, England. That sequence was subsequently updated to correct errors in 1999 and is designated as the rCRS. The rCRS haplogroup is H2a2a1.

Random Recombination - Pieces or segments of autosomal DNA passed from parent to child during recombination are selected randomly, meaning that descendants may, or may not, inherit a particular segment from an ancestor.

Recombination – During reproduction, the process where the maternal and paternal copies of each chromosome of each parent divide and recombine into one chromosome, respectively, to be contributed to a child. The child receives half of the autosomal DNA of each parent - one copy of each chromosome that combines with a copy of that chromosome from the other parent.

Reference – The expected value at a specific genetic location is determined by the value found in the human reference genome, generally indicated by the word, "reference," as in reference value.

Reference Populations – Populations against which testers are compared for relevance. Generally, each testing company uses a combination of public sources and its own internal database to define the reference populations against which its customers are compared for ethnicity predictions.

Reverse Mutations - When a value at a specific genetic location mutates to a new value, then mutates back to the old value. Often found in Y-DNA STR markers and sometimes in mitochondrial DNA. Individual reverse mutations are much less important in autosomal DNA since long strings of contiguous DNA nucleotides, more than 500, are compared for matching. Small differences are presumed to be read errors or non-genealogically relevant issues.

RSRS - The Reconstructed Sapiens Reference Sequence (RSRS) published in 2012 updated the mitochondrial DNA rCRS (revised Cambridge Reference Sequence.)

---

285 https://www.familytreedna.com/public/y-dna-haplotree/A

286 https://www.familytreedna.com/public/mt-dna-haplotree/L

287 https://dna-explained.com/2018/09/27/family-tree-dnas-public-y-dna-haplotree/

Segment - A contiguous grouping of DNA nucleotide positions. In autosomal DNA, segments must be of a minimum size to be considered a match.

Shared Matches – Three-way matching, where you and a match both match with a third person.

Shared Origins – At FamilyTreeDNA, the ability to view the ethnicity results, Y-DNA, and mitochondrial DNA ancestor locations of matches who opt in for the Origins Sharing feature.

SNP – A Single Nucleotide Polymorphism is a single mutation at one location.

SNP Pack - For Y-DNA, FamilyTreeDNA bundled logical progressions of SNPs together for specific haplogroups for customers to confirm various SNPs descending down the haplotree. However, with the advent and subsequent price reductions of the Big Y test, and the speed at which the Y haplotree now grows, SNP packs are usually obsolete by the time they can be designed. They no longer make sense, especially since they cannot position you at the tip or end of your branch, and they cannot discover new SNPs to become haplogroups.

Statistical Phasing – Also called academic phasing. Statistical phasing is a technique using probability to statistically assign DNA segments to specific "sides" of a chromosome based on their neighboring DNA when the parents' DNA is not available for parental or trio phasing. Statistical phasing phases or reassembles each chromosome separately, and the parental sides may not be consistently in the same position (top or bottom) on all chromosomes. This type of phasing may occasionally produce switch or strand swap errors within a chromosome.

STR – Short Tandem Repeat markers are markers that measure and report the number of a series of repeats used to compare Y-DNA results for genealogical connections.

Suggested Projects - The Discover™ Haplogroup Reports, also known as the Discover™ tool, suggest Y-DNA projects based on the projects that other men with this haplogroup have joined. A mitochondrial version of Discover™ is expected soon.

Surname Report - For Y-DNA, on the Public Haplotree and on the Haplogroup & SNP page, the Surname Report provides a list of surnames associated with testers within this haplogroup, so long as there are two or more testers and they have opted-in to public display.

Terminal SNP - In Y-DNA, for many years, this was the term used for the SNP furthest down on the tree. meaning the closest in time, for which a man is positive. At that time, many people would purchase individual SNPs or SNP packs, so the terminal SNP could be anything from their predicted haplogroup from STR testing to their Big Y haplogroup, or any place in between. However, sometimes the word "terminal" was interpreted medically as a different kind of "terminal" with a negative connotation, so the term's usage has fallen somewhat out of favor today. When used, it means the haplogroup closest to the present time that has been determined. Terminal SNP has been replaced by the term "end-of-line" haplogroup today.

Thymine - Adenine, Cytosine, Guanine, and Thymine are the four base nucleotides, or DNA words, that comprise your DNA and are represented in genetic genealogy by the letters A, C, G and T.

Time Tree – A haplogroup feature created by FamilyTreeDNA that provides testers with a pedigree type tree that shows time in years between current testers, their most recent common haplogroup ancestor, and ancient and notable connections.

Transition - When a T to C or C to T mutation occurs, or an A to G or G to A mutation occurs. These are more common mutations and more likely to experience reverse mutations. See Transversion.

Transversion - When any mutation other than a T to C, C to T, A to G, or G to A mutation occurs. Transversions are less common mutations and less likely to experience reverse mutations. See Transition.

Tree or Family Tree - A genealogical tree created by you reflecting your direct ancestors. A tree can be created in external software and uploaded to FamilyTreeDNA via a GEDCOM file or created at FamilyTreeDNA. Linking known relatives to their profile in your tree is how FamilyTreeDNA buckets your matches maternally and paternally. Plans exist for FamilyTreeDNA to utilize the MyHeritage trees.

Triangulation – A genetic genealogy technique in which multiple people (at least three) are proven to match each other on the same reasonably-sized segment, confirming that the segment is identical by descent and that the group of matching people share a common ancestor.

Tribes – Within the United States, Native American tribes are legal entities and sovereign nations, governing themselves,

Undocumented Adoption – Adoptions have not always been regulated and documented throughout history, so sometimes, when tests reveal unexpected results regarding parentage, an undocumented adoption has occurred. In other cases, the results are due to an NPE.

Unlock - At FamilyTreeDNA, you can upload an autosomal DNA file from another vendor for free and receive matching, shared matching, family matching, aka bucketing, and other features. However, advanced features like ethnicity, the chromosome browser, chromosome painting, Family Finder haplogroups, and ancientOrigins require the payment of a small unlock fee that is substantially less than the cost of a DNA test.

Unstable Mutations - Mutations of a type or location that are unstable, and, therefore, unreliable. Unstable mutations are found in certain regions of Y-DNA and mitochondrial DNA, are not used for haplogroup definition, and generally not for matching. Mutations near the centromere and sometimes the tips of autosomes, called telomeres, are also not used for matching.

Upload DNA - After downloading a raw DNA sequence file from one vendor, uploading that file to a different vendor instead of purchasing a new DNA test and having your DNA sequenced again.[288]

Variant – Another word for mutation or SNP.

Variant Report - For both Y-DNA and mitochondrial DNA, on the Public Haplotrees, the Variant Report details the variants, or mutations, that define or are equivalent to a specific haplogroup.

---

288 https://dna-explained.com/2019/11/04/dna-file-upload-download-and-transfer-instructions-to-and-from-dna-testing-companies/

X-DNA – The X chromosome has a unique inheritance pattern, eliminating some ancestors as the source, which makes chromosome matches on the X chromosome uniquely useful to genealogists.[289] The X chromosome is tested as part of autosomal testing, but is not reported by some vendors. Of the four major vendors, FamilyTreeDNA and 23andMe both utilize and report X chromosome matching.

Y-DNA – The Y chromosome is only inherited by males and is widely used for matching to other males to determine direct paternal genealogical lineage. STR markers are used in conjunction with SNP data to refine matching to its highest level. The Big Y test provides both types of matching for the best result along with the most granular haplogroup possible.

Y-DNA Chromosome Browser - Big Y testers can view their mutations on a special Y-Chromosome Browsing Tool that displays the results of each forward and reverse scan of the Y chromosome during testing at each location.

Y-DNA Matches - Other testers who match your Y-DNA STR or SNP results equal to or below the matching threshold for the level test you're viewing.

Y-DNA Public Tree - FamilyTreeDNA's public, free Y-DNA haplotree, which provides country flags for each SNP-confirmed haplogroup, a Country Report, and a Surname Report.

Y-DNA Results – The actual values at each location returned by the DNA test for this specific tester. The similarity of results, when compared to other testers, determines matches.

Y-Line Adam - Y-Line Adam is the earliest male to have descendants living today. All males worldwide descend from Y-Line Adam.

289 https://dna-explained.com/2018/02/07/who-tests-the-x-chromosome/

www.ingramcontent.com/pod-product-compliance
Lightning Source LLC
Chambersburg PA
CBHW080916090325
23107CB00025B/319